Saints, Infirmity, and Community in the Late Middle Ages

Saints, Infirmity, and Community in the Late Middle Ages

Jenni Kuuliala

Routledge
Taylor & Francis Group
LONDON AND NEW YORK

First published in 2020 by Amsterdam University Press Ltd.

Published 2025 by Routledge
4 Park Square, Milton Park, Abingdon, Oxon OX14 4RN
605 Third Avenue, New York, NY 10158

Routledge is an imprint of the Taylor & Francis Group, an informa business

ISBN: 9789462983373 (hbk)
ISBN: 9781041185710 (pbk)
ISBN: 9781003703242 (ebk)
NUR 684

Cover illustration: St. Louis IX taking the cross
Source: Paris, Bibliothèque nationale de France, MS Fr. 2829: *Le Livre des faiz monseigneur saint Loys, composé à la requête du cardinal de Bourbon et de la duchesse de Bourbonnois*, fol 17v.

Cover design: Coördesign, Leiden

DOI: 10.5117/9789462983373

For Product Safety Concerns and Information please contact our EU representative:
GPSR@taylorandfrancis.com
Taylor & Francis Verlag GmbH, Kaufingerstraße 24, 80331 München, Germany

Table of Contents

Acknowledgements

While writing this book, I have had the pleasure of working in different research institutions and projects, where the support of many wonderful colleagues has been of crucial importance for finishing the work.

I started the project when working as an EU researcher at the University of Bremen (University of Bremen and the European Union FP7 COFUND under grant agreement n° 600411) as a member of the Creative Unit '*Homo debilis*: Dis/ability in der Vormoderne'. I want to thank especially Cordula Nolte for the support she has shown for my work, as well as all members of the Creative Unit for the many inspiring discussions during my stay.

The book was finished while I was working as an Academy of Finland postdoctoral researcher (project 287483) at Tampere University and the very final edits I made as a University Researcher in the Academy of Finland Centre of Excellence in the History of Experiences, led by Pertti Haapala, at the same university. I extend my gratitude to all my colleagues in the discipline of history at the Faculty of Social Sciences, and especially the members of Trivium – Tampere Centre for Classical, Medieval, and Early Modern Studies there – whose friendship and collegiality always makes work life a pleasure.

During the project I worked several times in Rome. I am grateful to the staff of the Finnish Institute in Rome and especially intendent Simo Örmä for all the help and hospitality during my visits. I also want to thank the staff of the Vatican Library for their services during the archival work needed for this book.

I wish to thank Philip Line for correcting the language, which he has done meticulously and efficiently as usual. All remaining mistakes are my own. Katariina Eskola has been of great assistance in putting together the bibliography for this volume. I am grateful to Amsterdam University Press, and especially the editors of the series *Premodern Health, Disease, and Disability* for accepting this book for it. I also wish to thank the referee whose insightful comments have been very helpful in enabling the book to take its final shape.

Several colleagues have been extremely helpful in discussing the book, its themes, and various different topics with me, always providing their insight and support when needed. My special thanks go to Bianca Frohne, Jussi Hanska, Teemu Immonen, Sari Katajala-Peltomaa, Pia Koivunen, Susanna Niiranen, Rose-Marie Peake, Marika Räsänen, Bernhard Schirg, Raisa Maria Toivo, Lauri Uusitalo, Ville Vuolanto, Reima Välimäki, and

Marita von Weissenberg. I also wish to thank the participants of the conferences 'Disability and Religion', the Tenth Anniversary Annual Meeting on Disease, Disability and Medicine in the Medieval World (held at Swansea University in December 2016) and 'Re-imagining the Christian Body' (held at the University of Turku in November 2017) where I first presented preliminary results of this research. The encouragement and insight of the participants was of great importance for finishing the book.

Tampere, 1 October 2019
Jenni Kuuliala

Abbreviations

AASS	*Acta sanctorum quotquot toto orbe coluntur vel a catholicis scribtoribus celebrantur*, vols. 1-68
BAV	Biblioteca Apostolica Vaticana, Vatican City
BNF	Bibliothèque nationale de France, Paris
PC Bernardino of Siena	*Il processo di canonizzazione di Bernardino da Siena*, ed. Letizia Pellegrini (2009)
PC Birgitta of Sweden	*Acta et processus canonizacionis beate Birgitte*, ed. Isaac Collijn (1924-30)
PC Brynolf of Skara	*Vita s. Brynolphi episc. Scarensis, com processu euis canonizationis*, ed. C. Annerstedt (1876)
PC Catherine of Vadstena	*Processus seu negocium canonizacionis b. Katerine de Vadstenis*, ed. Isaak Collijn (1942-46)
PC Celestine V	*Il processo di canonizzazione di Celestino V*, ed. Alessandra Bartolomei Romagnoli and Alfonso Marini (2015)
PC Charles of Blois	*Monuments du procès de canonisation du bienheureux Charles de Blois*, ed. A. de Sérent (1921)
PC Clare of Assisi	*Santa Chiara di Assisi*, ed. Giovanni Boccali (2002)
PC Clare of Montefalco	*Il processo di canonizzazione di Chiara da Montefalco*, ed. Enrico Menestò (1984)
PC Dauphine of Puimichel	*Enquête pour le procès de canonisation de Dauphine de Puimichel*, ed. Jacques Cambell (1978)
PC Dominic of Caleruega	*Processus canonizationis s. Dominici*, ed. A. Waltz (1935)
PC Dorothea of Montau	*Die Akten des Kanonisationsprozess Dorotheas von Montau*, ed. Richard Stachnik, with Anneliese Triller and Hans Westpfal (1978)
PC Elizabeth of Hungary	*Quellenstudien zur Geschichte der hl. Elisabeth*, ed. Albert Huyskens (1908)
PC Frances of Rome	*I processi inediti per Francesca Bussa dei Ponziani (Santa Francesca Romana)*, ed. Placido Tommaso Lugano (1945)

PC Lawrence Loricatus	Benedict XIV [Prospero Lambertini], *De servorum Dei beatifijicatione et Beatorum canonizatione* (1840)
PC Louis of Toulouse	*Processus canonizationis s. Ludovici ep. Tolosani*, ed. Collegio S. Bonaventura (1951)
PC Margaret of Hungary	*Legenda vetus: acta processus canonizationis et Miracula sanctae Margaritae de Hungaria*, ed. Ildikó Csepregi et al. (2018)
PC Nicholas of Tolentino	*Il processo per la canonizzazione di s. Nicola da Tolentino*, ed. Nicola Occhioni (1984)
PC Thomas Aquinas	*Processus canonizationis s. Thomae, Neapoli*, ed. M.-H. Laurent (1911)
PC Vincent Ferrer	*Procès de la canonisation de saint Vincent Ferrier*, ed. P.-H. Fages (1904)
PC Yves of Tréguier	*Processus de vita et miraculis Sancti Yvonis*, ed. A. de La Borderie et al. (1887)
Vie, Dauphine	*Vie de Ste Dauphine*, ed. Jacques Cambell (1963)
Vie, Elzéar	*Vie de s. Auzias*, ed. Jacques Cambell (1963)

Introduction

Abstract

The starting points for this book are late medieval *imitatio Christi* and the valorization of pain, and their importance for saints' lives. It presents gender and dis/ability as vital concepts for such analysis. Bodily suffering has been seen as a definitive factor for female saint's cults; while this book does not question these conclusions, it stresses the importance of the ambiguity of gender as a historical category and in defining the characteristics of a saint's cult, and approaches dis/ability as a cultural construct incorporating positive connotations of certain bodily variations. The introduction also discusses source-critical aspects that must be taken into account when using medieval canonization processes for the study of saints' lives and the accounts of contemporary witnesses.

Keywords: canonization processes, sainthood, lay piety, infirmity, disability, gender

Approaching Holy Infirmity

Bodily infirmity and sanctity are inseparable in all medieval hagiography. Since late antiquity, saints' miraculous and charitable actions towards their followers were recorded in an endless number of legends and miracle collections, in sermons and *exempla*, in liturgies, in pictorial depictions, and from the thirteenth century onwards, in the protocols of canonization inquests. As a large majority of recorded miracles were healings, hagiographic sources place illness and impairment at the core of lived religion.[1]

1 For lived religion, see Katajala-Peltomaa and Toivo, 'Religion as an Experience'; Arnold, 'Histories and Historiographies of Medieval Christianity'. For lived religion and canonization processes, see Katajala-Peltomaa *Demonic Possession and Lived Religion*. Miracle narratives have been widely used for the study of healing, illness, and disability in the Middle Ages. See e.g. Farmer, *Surviving Poverty*; Farmer, 'Young, Male and Disabled'; Finucane, *Rescue of the Innocents*; Katajala-Peltomaa, 'Demonic Possession as Physical and Mental Disturbance'; Kuuliala, *Childhood*

Kuuliala, Jenni, *Saints, Infirmity, and Community in the Late Middle Ages*.
Taylor & Francis Group 2020
DOI: 10.5117/9789462983373_INTRO

In my earlier research I have mostly focused on miraculous healing, the more famous connection between saints and their devotees. While researching disability and sanctity in late medieval canonization processes,[2] I started to wonder about the other side of the coin. Although much sparser and usually less elaborate than descriptions of miracles healing bodily illness and impairment, the depictions of the sufferings of the saints themselves caught my eye. What meanings did saints' devotees give to the ailments of those they venerated, and how were infirmities used and investigated in canonization proceedings? Some late medieval saints for whom a canonization process was opened, such as St. Louis IX of France (d. 1270) or St. Clare of Montefalco (d. 1308), are known sufferers. What surprised me was that with very few exceptions, in virtually all *inquisitiones in partibus* the topic was approached even when the holy person's death was not in question. At the same time, it soon became evident that despite the established structure of the inquisition into a saintly candidate's *vita*, the reports of their bodily infirmities received very variable nuances and emphases. It were precisely these variations that started to intrigue me. Although there are certain patterns in the ways canonization inquests were conducted and in their development in the course of time, each process is also a unique entity that is influenced by the preferences and practicalities of those conducting it, by the way the witness statements were taken down, and by the local and cultural customs, views, and practices.[3]

The suffering saint is, of course, an age-old and built-in theme in all hagiography. Following in the footsteps of Christ, the very first martyrs were described as facing their gruesome deaths with grace and patience, and infirmity and suffering played a major role in the lives of many of the saints in late antiquity.[4] Similar attitudes and characteristics were attributed to later saints. In the thirteenth century, coinciding with the development of the canonization inquest itself, the idea that a human body could imitate the passion of Christ became prevalent and suffering acquired even more significance among the ideals of holiness.[5] It has even

Disability; Metzler, *Disability in Medieval Europe*, 126-85; Van Mulder, 'Miracles and the Body Social'; Wilson, 'Hagiographical Interpretations of Disability'.

2 For example, Kuuliala, *Childhood Disability*; Kuuliala, 'Disability and Religious Practices'; Kuuliala, 'Heavenly Healing or Failure of Faith?'

3 Already André Vauchez noted in *Sainthood*, 4, that the conformity of witness accounts has been much exaggerated in research.

4 These have been studied in depth in Crislip, *Thorns in the Flesh*.

5 See Cohen, *The Modulated Scream*, 188; Gaposchkin, *The Making of Saint Louis*, 45; Hollywood, 'Inside Out'. In the early thirteenth century the view perhaps received most emphasis

been suggested that bodily suffering became a prerequisite for sainthood in the late Middle Ages, something that conclusively sealed their saintly existence. Suffering thus became valorized and glorified, showing saints as true followers and imitators of Christ. This was emphasized especially in the case of holy women.[6] Suffering appears to have had entirely different connotations for saints than for the ailing *miraculées*. The former faced it with patience and humility, even gratitude, whereas for the later hagiographic texts highlight the unfortunate functional consequences of physical infirmity and sometimes also the physical pain. To emphasize the saint's power, the illnesses and impairments of *miraculées* were placed among the problematic, undesirable aspects of human existence that needed to be remedied.[7] And yet, the two infirmities – those of saints and those of their devotees – belonged to the same cultural sphere of the body, illness, impairment, pain, and healing, and knowing about saints' attitude towards their infirmities could work as a way of coping with one's own experiences.

Sainthood as a concept, as well as the individual saint's sanctity, was always a fluid category negotiated within communities. Sainthood formed as a gradual process, which included conflict and cooperation. It was primarily shaped in everyday interaction between the saints – or people considered to be holy[8] – and their communities and devotees. The agreement that someone was a saint was not fixed, but in many instances continuously

in Franciscan hagiography, as the Franciscans attempted to give the right to imitate Christ's passion solely to their founder; Vauchez, *Sainthood*, 440. Gábor Klaniczay writes that it is precisely the *imitatio Christi* that marked the starting point of the greater awareness of the self and individuality, as well as the importance and knowledge of historical models of life, which he has studied in the context of sanctity. *Imitatio Christi* was already an essential ideal for those attempting to live saintly lives in late antiquity, and gained increasing importance and popularity in eleventh- to twelfth-century religious movements. The old models thus became a prescription for late medieval saints aspiring to a similar lifestyle and similar glory. Klaniczay, *The Uses of Supernatural Power*, 95-110.

6 Cohen, *The Modulated Scream*, 27-28.

7 As will be discussed further in this book, and as shown by recent studies on medieval disability, bodily impairment did not need to be a personal tragedy – this image in hagiographic writings is first and foremost connected to the purpose of the texts and to the need to give sufficient proof for the healing miracle.

8 See Finucane, *Contested Canonizations*, 3-4, and Wetzstein, *Heilige vor Gericht*, 211, on the problems of the term 'saint' with its two meanings: a person considered to be holy, and a canonized saint. To avoid repeating definitions such as 'a putative saint' or 'a person considered to be a saint', I am using the term 'saint' or 'holy person' here to refer to those persons for whom a canonization inquest was opened and who were, therefore, considered to be saints by a group of devotees. As pointed out by Finucane, the problem lies in the Latin word *sanctus/sancta*, which can be either an adjective or a noun. In the witness accounts the word *beatus/beata* is also frequently used.

renegotiated.[9] This naturally pertains also to the views of saints' bodies and infirmities, and their meanings and connotations. In the case of living saints, their community members and devotees saw their symptoms and ailments with their own eyes when interacting with them, either in the public sphere or when visiting them in person. At the same time, we may assume that there were different levels of information spread about saints' suffering from the promoters of the cases. The canonization inquest itself also had an influence on the communal nature of a cult. Although few of the saints under investigation in this book were actually canonized in the medieval period, just the opening of an inquest planted an idea in people's minds that the subject of the inquest had the status of an 'authentic' saint. For this reason this study focuses on what we could label as 'official sainthood', even if a vast majority of saints venerated through the medieval period were never subjects of a canonization inquest.[10]

The purpose of this book is, therefore, to investigate how bodily infirmities of late medieval saints were used to construct sanctity in canonization inquests conducted from the thirteenth to the fifteenth century. I have chosen this particular group of sources because my primary interest lies in the communal views of saints' ailments and in the ways they were negotiated, narrated, and interpreted by the witnesses of canonization inquests. Here the inquests and the testimonies about sainthood are treated as belonging to the sphere of lived religion, in which theological ponderings and institutionalized aspects of belief intermingled with everyday experience and functioned as important background elements. From this viewpoint religion, and consequently the veneration of saints, is viewed as a dynamic process, which 'created a performative space and gave meaning to people's experiences.'[11] In the sources, the issues raised by the conductors of the hearings, the views of the witnesses, and the experiences of the saints under investigation intertwine, creating a fluctuating yet persistent cultural image of 'holy infirmity'.

Because of the way canonization protocols were formed (discussed below), they are the best group of texts to use for analysis of groups of devotees' views and conceptions regarding sanctity. Although there were many saints for whom a canonization inquest was opened and who had a great influence on Christendom at large, some of whom will be discussed in this book, many of their cults were relatively local. In his book *Prophets*

9 Kleinberg, *Prophets*, 4-6.

10 Vauchez, *Sainthood*, 142, 250. See also Kleinberg, 'Canonization without a Canon'.

11 Katajala-Peltomaa and Toivo, 'Religion as an Experience', 2.

in their Own Country: Living Saints and the Making of Sainthood in the Later Middle Ages, Aviad Kleinberg criticizes quantitative analysis of hagiographic texts and rightly points out that it is hard to find a representative saint, because we do not even know exactly what they were supposed to represent, and all saintly people were somehow exceptional. Therefore, one must concentrate on the saint's community instead.[12] Or, as Jacques Dalarun famously put it, saints were exceptions, placing themselves in opposition to the norms,[13] which holds true for their bodies as well. This is also the standpoint of this book. Based on the canonization processes, it is impossible to characterize a 'typical' or 'representative' saintly infirmity, although certain characteristics belonged to the tool kit for reconstructing sanctity. Since saints were exceptional yet human, their infirmities were just that too; they were not immune to the bodily ailments that their communities suffered from. Yet their bodies and minds surpassed those of other people in tolerating pain and discomfort, even surviving extreme asceticism. Although there are certain recurrent characteristics and factors that seemingly have similar connotations in the narrations of saints' physical ailments, each community gave them their own meaning. Furthermore, the canonization inquest itself unavoidably influenced the manner in which witnesses' views and testimonies were written down. Instead of even attempting to draw a synthesis, let alone a quantitative analysis, my intention is to look into the canonization testimonies and the meanings the witnesses as individuals and as groups of devotees gave to a holy person's physical illness, impairment, and suffering.

Although all canonization inquests follow a set of rules, they differed in character.[14] Furthermore, geographical setting, as well as the type of individual saint – both of which have been thoroughly analysed in André Vauchez's seminal study *Sainthood in the Later Middle Ages* (*La sainteté en Occident aux derniers siècles du Moyen Âge*) – had a big influence on the way a saint's body was treated. Vauchez has pointed out that, concerning sainthood at large and not just those saints subject to a canonization process, the Mediterranean region preferred saints who willingly suffered by voluntarily inflicting hardship upon themselves, whereas elsewhere suffering was

12 Kleinberg, *Prophets*, 17. As for the problems of quantitative analysis, Mulder-Bakker 'Invention of Saintliness', 16, reasonably points out that the gender balance in veneration of saints may have been quite different from the balance in quantity of hagiographic material, which is what the modern reader sees; the Virgin Mary, Mary Magdalene, and virgin saints such as Catherine, Barbara, and Agnes were widely venerated, even if male saints were more numerous.

13 Dalarun, *L'Impossibile sainteté*, 237

14 See Vauchez, *Sainthood*, 4-5.

primarily seen as violent death and 'martyrdom'. Of the Mediterranean saints, the vast majority were ascetics and hermits, practising extreme austerity. Mediterranean sainthood was also to some extent defined by the 'emotion experienced by the faithful at the spectacle of an existence renounced'.[15] This phenomenon will also become clear in this book. Although we will see that saints from other regions were reported as having suffered from various infirmities related and unrelated to their ascetic practices, Mediterranean saints appear more corporal as a consequence of the focus on their asceticism, and their infirmities, as witnessed by their devotees, receive more attention in their canonization documents.

The saint's origins and lifestyle obviously had an effect on the way witnesses viewed and constructed his or her possible infirmity. Different aspects of saints' lives were emphasized depending on their position in the society. Generally, the sainthood of hermits and female saints, especially mendicant nuns and anchoresses, was most corporeal by nature, whereas the sainthood of prelates and male members of the secular elite was primarily constructed through their other deeds. During our period of investigation, most saints still came from the nobility or other elite sectors of society, although theological shifts between the mid-twelfth and mid-thirteenth centuries changed the Christian ideal of perfection and brought virtues such as humility, poverty, and asceticism increasingly to the fore. During the late Middle Ages, the number of lay saints began to increase. As a result of the influence of apostolic movements and also heresies, a growing number of laypeople considered it possible to live an 'authentic Christian life' without renouncing the world. In addition, certain royal dynasties promoted their own members as saints, in our period notably the Angevins and the Capetians.[16] Italy, and the Mediterranean as a whole, is a separate region in this sense, since the origins of the saints were significantly more modest than elsewhere. This at least is partly explainable by the strong eremitical tradition.[17]

There are several important conceptual and theoretical viewpoints that will shape the following discussion. One of the most important ones concerning holy suffering is that of gender. Overall, especially saints' *vitae* have been widely used for the study of medieval gender practices, while canonization testimonies about saints' lives have been used for this purpose

15 Vauchez, *Sainthood*, 190-93, 217.

16 Vauchez, *Sainthood*, 175-83, 354-55; see also Goodich, *Vita perfecta*, 127, for friars and clerics; and Vauchez, *Laity in the Middle Ages*, for the importance of lay saints.

17 Vauchez, *Sainthood*, 182-84, 187-89.

only sporadically. Before late 1990s, this research focused primarily on women.[18] In recent years, a more nuanced and balanced view of gender and sanctity – which concerns the handling of male saints as well as female – has gained ground, but there are still relatively few individual studies that compare male and female saints or that focus on male piety.[19] It has been concluded in earlier research that the sources on female saints' lives put far more emphasis on their penitentiary practices, especially fasting, and enduring illness or impairment, than those on men.[20] Among these works, the most influential one has been Caroline Walker Bynum's *Holy Feast and Holy Fast: The Religious Significance of Food to Medieval Women*, in which she studied the religious significance of food for medieval holy women. Although infirmity is not the main topic of her study, it includes a considerable amount of discussion about the significance of suffering for female sanctity, a topic which she also addresses in her collection of essays *Fragmentation and Redemption: Essays on Gender and the Human Body in Medieval Religion*.[21] Many other scholars have taken a similar viewpoint, while a number have also criticized it.[22] Another influential study, useful for my current analysis, is Dyan Elliott's *Proving Woman: Female Spirituality and Inquisitional Culture in*

18 See Lewis, 'Gender and Sanctity in the Middle Ages'. For studies on holy women, see e.g. Bynum, *Holy Feast and Holy Fast*; Dinzelbaher, *Heilige oder Hexen*; Elliott, *The Bride of Christ Goes to Hell*; Elliott, *Proving Woman*; Minnis and Voaden (eds.), *Medieval Holy Women in the Christian Tradition c. 1100-c. 1500*; Goldy and Livingstone (eds.), *Writing Medieval Women's Lives*.

19 See Cullum, 'Feasting Not Fasting', 184-86. For collections focusing on both men and women, see e.g. Riches and Salih (eds.), *Gender and Holiness*; Blumenfeld-Kosinski and Szell (eds.), *Images of Sainthood in Medieval Europe*; for studies focusing on holy men, see Cullum and Lewis (eds.), *Holiness and Masculinity in Medieval Europe*; Weissenberg, 'Generations of Men and Masculinity'; Weissenberg, 'Men, Marriage, and Masculinity'; Cullum and Lewis (eds.), *Religious Men and Masculine Identity in the Middle Ages*. Men as writers of women's sainthood have been analysed in Coakley, *Women, Men, and Spiritual Power*; Mooney (ed.), *Gendered Voices*.

20 This phenomenon is visible elsewhere in medieval religious culture as well. For example, the German *Nonnenbücher* portray illness as a way of *imitatio Christi* and as an equivalent substitute for serving in a monastic *officium*. Garber, *Feminine Figurae*, esp. 20-24, 99, 109. The significance of illness is also highlighted in the lives of beguine saints. Elliott, *The Bride of Christ Goes to Hell*, 181.

21 Fasting and female sanctity is also analysed in Bell's *Holy Anorexia*, in which he contextualizes the fasting of holy women with the modern framework of anorexia nervosa. This view has been criticized by Bynum as anachronistic, a view which I share. The importance of suffering for female saints is also noted in Weinstein and Bell, *Saints and Society*, in which they study certain phenomena related to sanctity by quantitative analysis of saints' *vitae*. This viewpoint, however, omits the communal realities and individual charactersistics of cults; for criticism, see Kleinberg, *Prophets*, 14-16.

22 For this discussion, see e.g. Riches and Salih, 'Introduction', 2-4. Especially the article collections referred to in note 19 have taken a nuanced viewpoint in this discussion.

the Later Middle Ages, in which she brings together the inquisitorial practices of sainthood and heresy and analyses the significance of female religious corporality, suffering and mysticism included, within this framework. Elliott's work is one of the few that systematically uses canonization records for this kind of analysis, although she focuses on a limited number of them. Making the case that corporality was of great importance to female saints need not, of course, imply that it was insignificant for male saints. In her seminal study on pain in later medieval Europe, *The Modulated Scream: Pain in Late Medieval Culture*, Esther Cohen has concluded that female saints had to have a written record of their empathetic pain as evidence of their intimate connection with Christ while men did not, even though there were several male mystics and men were also encouraged to shed tears publicly as sign of empathy.[23]

It is not my intention to compromise the view that medieval culture tended to associate holy women with bodily suffering more readily than holy men. I think, however, that concept of gender and its impact on sainthood should be treated with care, and that to form a comprehensive picture, female and male sanctity should be compared. Studies on (holy) women's religiosity are mostly based on *vitae* written by men, and, as pointed out by Sarah Alison Miller, 'it is a problematic task, then, to determine to what extent such instances of extreme corporeal phenomena [...] bespeak hagiographic enthrallment with the suffering of holy women or the religious praxis of women themselves'.[24] Furthermore, medieval gender categories are not so clear that simply dividing people into 'men' and 'women' suffices for research purposes. Rather, gender was constantly negotiated and fluctuating.[25] Imitating Christ's passion was considered symbolically female, because as women were thought more susceptible to bodily sensations and pleasures, they could more easily share in his suffering. Therefore, despite this discourse being symbolic and ideological, feminine expression of religiosity was not necessarily considered inferior to the masculine.[26] Bynum concluded that

23 Cohen, *The Modulated Scream*, 129.

24 Miller, *Medieval Monstrosity and the Female Body*, 100. See also Elliott, *Proving Woman*, 191, who writes that there was an increasing spiral of physicality that characterized the spirituality of late medieval women, or at least the way in which their spirituality was ultimately represented. See also Hollywood, 'Inside Out', and Scott, 'Mystical Death', for the view that male hagiographers may have been more keen to see suffering as essential for female holy women than the women themselves.

25 Katajala-Peltomaa, 'A Good Wife?', 83.

26 Toivo, 'Gender Performance in Early Modern Religious Life', 172-73; McNamer, *Affective Meditation*, esp. 7, 27.

the gender dichotomy was relatively insignificant for the holy women, 'who saw themselves as human beings – fully spirit and fully flesh', and the whole of humanity as capable of *imitatio Christi*.[27] Damien Boquet and Piroska Nagy have pointed out that the female mystics found authority in their embodied piety, although not without risks.[28] Martha G. Newman has argued, in an article focusing on late twelfth-century Cistercian choir monks and nuns who had saints as their role models, that their corporalities largely depended on their social standing. Of the male monks, the *conversi*, who had a lower social standing, were presented with saints whose holiness was constructed in very corporeal terms as role models. Therefore, in certain times, places, and contexts, social status and hierarchies were more powerful than gender as defining factors of corporality and spirituality.[29] Or, as Sharon Farmer has put it, 'when we fail to incorporate other categories of difference into our analysis of gender constructions, then it is *we*, and not the authors whom we study, who end up constructing simplistic gender categories'.[30]

As the following analysis will show, in the case of canonization inquests, as elsewhere, gender was not the only aspect defining the importance of *imitatio Christi* or suffering in general. The putative saints' other societal roles affected how their corporalities were viewed, and a female saint in whose holiness corporality played a major role could be remembered from her other societal, even 'masculine' deeds. How these mechanisms worked is one of the important questions of this book. As regards the impact of gender, another interesting question would be whether male and female witnesses in canonization inquests interpreted saints' infirmities differently. However, because of the ways the testimonies on the putative saint's *vita* were constructed – a matter discussed further in this chapter – this question can never be resolved conclusively.

Another important framework is that of body, illness, and impairment. During the past decade, medieval dis/ability studies have grown into an independent branch of research, and dis/ability history has also been one of the starting points for this book. In previous research, there has been much discussion of what is meant by 'medieval disability' and if and how modern disability terminology and theory may be applicable

27 Bynum, *Holy Feast and Holy Fast*, 296.

28 Boquet and Nagy, *Medieval Sensibilities*, 204.

29 Newman, 'Crucified by the Virtues'. As pointed out by Sharon Farmer in her introduction to the volume, Newman's article presents a more versatile and nuanced gender categorization than Bynum's *Holy Feast and Holy Fast*. Farmer, 'Introduction', xx-xxi.

30 Farmer, 'Beggar's Body', 171. See also Muravyeva and Toivo, 'Introduction', on gender and societal relations.

to it. Medieval terminology concerning bodily impairments or illnesses is always vague, and there was no consistent umbrella term like 'impairment', let alone 'disability'.[31] Rather, late medieval Latin hagiographic texts label various bodily and mental ailments most often as *infirmitates*, infirmities, which is also the primary term used in this book.[32] As the following analysis will demonstrate, in the hagiographic context, saints' bodily infirmities were rarely specifically diagnosed or defined, and the specific nature of the illnesses or impairments of holy persons did not have a great impact on the way they were used to reconstruct sanctity. To attempt to distinguish 'impairment', 'disability', or 'illness' in the modern, cultural, medical, and political sense of the words would be anachronistic and not very useful.

The fact that saints were extraordinary people whose bodies carried extraordinary messages is of great significance for this study's connection with medieval dis/ability studies.[33] Holiness manifested itself in various ways, of which infirmity was one. Although medieval society valued the soul and depreciated the body,[34] medieval people perceived phenomena that we would interpret as psychological in very physical and material terms.[35] This is in accordance with B. Hughes and K. Paterson's view regarding modern society, that the body itself is a source of knowledge about the world.[36] However, as Sarah Kay and Miri Rubin point out, we can never know other people's bodies, even though we persist in making analogies to our own bodies as a means of knowing others. The body is external and internal, personal and public, life-giving and vulnerable, and it leads to different ways

31 Frohne, *Leben mit 'kranckheit'*, 18-24; Goetz, 'Vorstellungen von menschlicher Gebrechlichkeit'; Kuuliala, *Childhood Disability*, 44-48; Metzler, *Disability in Medieval Europe*, 4-5. On the categorizations of 'illness', 'disability', and 'impairment', see Frohne, 'Moderne Begriffe und Definitionen'.

32 See also Kuuliala et al., 'Introduction'. Especially in earlier centuries, the word *debilitas* was also widely used of various bodily ailments and infirmities. Goetz, 'Vorstellungen von menschlicher Gebrechlichkeit'.

33 Writing about the 'extraordinary bodily quality in women's piety' in later medieval Europe, Caroline Walker Bynum has stated that '[b]ecause preachers, confessors and spiritual directors assumed the person to be a psychosomatic unity, they not only read unusual bodily events as expressions of the soul but also expected the body itself to offer a means of access to the divine'. Bynum, *Fragmentation and Redemption*, 235. Although often emphasized in the case of female pious women and in female saints' *vitae*, this holds true also in the case of many male saints, and the idea can be seen to have penetrated many layers of society, as I hope to show in this book.

34 See e.g. Dinzelbacher, *Körper und Frömmigkeit*, 14-16.

35 Camille, *Gothic Art*, 23.

36 Hughes and Paterson, 'The Social Model of Disability and the Disappearing Body', 334.

of perceiving the human person.[37] Furthermore, the challenge is that the study of the medieval body usually means the study of what was written about the body, and even in that context the focus of the texts was commonly on what the body was supposed to be like, or what it was supposed to do.[38]

Therefore, saints' infirm bodies – and the interpretations given to them in canonization depositions – primarily tell us about the corporality of sainthood. We cannot 'know' saints' bodies or bodily experiences, and neither could their communities, but, at the same time, the sensations of their bodies became public, at least in the later reconstructions of their sanctity. That being said, the veneration of saints had penetrated the whole of medieval society, and the conceptions of saints, and their infirmities, were not born in a vacuum, but from everyday experiences and views of communities. The corporality of saints was not entirely separate from the corporality of other people. However, the 'social model of disability', which sees 'impairment' as a biological state and 'disability' as a consequence of the restrictive practices of a given community does not fit very smoothly with the hagiographic valorization of infirmity, although such a phenomenon has been seen as harmful in modern society, where disability activists have coined the term 'supercrip'.[39] If we want to impose one theoretical model here, saints' infirmities must be viewed in the context of a 'cultural model of disability', in which religion obviously plays a major role.[40] The 'cultural

37 Kay and Rubin, 'Introduction', 7.

38 See Neal, *The Masculine Self*, 127.

39 For example, Rhonda Black and Lori Pretes write that the 'supercrip' representations in the media mean that disabled people or characters are portrayed as someone with great stamina and courage, who overcome their physical limitations because of their determination and therefore motivate non-disabled people; Black and Pretes, 'Victims and Victors'. If we want to play with this idea, some saints can, in their religio-cultural context, be seen as 'supercrips' of their period, where they were able to endure excessive pain and discomfort gratefully and without complaint, performing their other duties (such as those of a bishop or an abbess) with perfection. However, it is reasonable to ask if this view of them had much effect on the way society viewed infirmity in general. Furthermore, the negative consequences of the 'supercrip' figure cannot be transferred as such to the later Middle Ages, where the whole cultural concept of 'disability' was significantly different from ours.

40 Another model that could be used when analysing saints' infirmities is the so-called 'religious model of disability', first proposed by Edward Wheatley in his discussion of blindness. However, Wheatley's supposition is that the medieval 'religious model' is a similar paradigm to the 'medical model' of modern society, which sees disability as a personal tragedy that needs to be cured, and that the medieval church would, through its views and institutionalization, have diminished disabled people's agency. Wheatley, 'Blindness, Discipline, and Reward', 197; Wheatley, *Stumbling Blocks before the Blind*, 12. For criticism of this model, see Eyler, 'Introduction', 7-8, who points out its 'top-down approach'. Saints' infirmities certainly were formulated according to a 'religious model', but in a completely different way than Wheatley's classification suggests.

model' is especially suitable for the study of premodern dis/ability history, because it sees the concept of 'impairment' as fluid and culturally defined, and dis/ability as a cultural construct. Furthermore, the model allows an analysis of the body in both its material and symbolic dimensions.[41] The current study therefore offers a window onto one of the many ways, often overlapping and occasionally contradictory, in which physical infirmity was viewed and explained in late medieval culture. It connects infirmity with one crucial aspect of lived religion, the veneration of saints. Whereas studies of miracle narrations have revealed mainly negative attitudes to infirmities, in the lives of saints infirmities were primarily seen in a positive light. However, as the following analysis will show, this was not always the view, as even the desirability of holy infirmities was subject to varying views and negotiations.

Furthermore, although emotions are not the primary object of this study, canonization records show that they had an important role in reconstructing holy infirmity, which brings together the 'cultural model of dis/ability' and the history of emotions. Groups of saints' devotees can be defined in the framework of 'emotional communities', as established by Barbara H. Rosenwein. An 'emotional community' denotes a group of people that adhere to the same emotional experiences and also value and devalue the same emotions.[42] These communities were not static, but the veneration of saints was nevertheless a deeply emotional practice, and especially in miracle accounts, emotions follow each other in a certain order, from despair and affliction to hope and joy.[43] Veneration of saints meant experiencing and witnessing emotional events, which in turn confirmed and created communities and strengthened the sense of belonging.[44]

Saints' infirmities can also be viewed in terms of 'emotional practices'. Monique Scheer has defined them as actions, which are learned and transferred between people intergenerationally and/or through a socialization process between adults. Emotions-as-practices are conscious and subconscious bodily acts of experience and expression, which allow people to 'communicate to themselves who they are.' Furthermore, they include rituals and habits, which assist in attaining a certain emotional state. Scheer presents Christian penitential acts as an example of a practice that helped

41 Frohne, 'The Cultural Model of Dis/ability'. See also Eyler, 'Introduction'.

42 Rosenwein, *Emotional Communities*, 2.

43 See Devaney, 'Everyday Miracles in Seventeenth-Century Spain', 193-94; Katajala-Peltomaa, *Demonic Possession and Lived Religion*.

44 See Boquet and Nagy, *Medieval Sensibilities*, 217.

in achieving an emotional goal, a corporeal experience of regret.[45] The same framework would help to interpret saints' ways of representing the pain they felt and its connection to *imitatio Christi*, as well as the community members' participation in it by observing and interpreting the holy people's practices and expressions that generated emotions in them. Medieval lived religion and emotional practices are inherently interlinked with infirmity. A saint's infirmity was, at the same time, a lived practice, and a tool used for inquisitorial needs as well as a tool used by the community to achieve certain emotional states.

The discussion of saints' infirmities and how they were used to construct holiness is divided into four chapters. The first one will highlight the way infirmity functioned in conversion narratives. The idea that a holy figure's often sudden illness or impairment stimulated conversion that secured a saintly lifestyle and a later *fama* can be read as a hagiographic *topos*. The most famous saint of our period whose dramatic conversion was prompted by infirmity was St. Francis of Assisi. According to the earliest *Life*, written by Tommaso di Celano, his conversion was partly triggered by a long bout of infirmity.[46] As Jacques le Goff explained, we do not know much about Francis's illness during this time, but it established his physical and spiritual personality as a sick man, even if it was not the sole reason behind his change of lifestyle.[47] We may expect this to have been an important example for the hagiographers of the thirteenth and fourteenth centuries, especially in Franciscan circles.[48] At the same time, each (future) saint's situation at the time of the conversion, or 'turnaround', to use André Vauchez's term,[49] was different, and so are the means by which the information about such an event was transferred. Therefore, even if physical infirmity or suffering had a role in this process, its emphases and characteristics varied. Among the saints whose canonization protocols we have, such a dramatic infirmity-conversion chain of events is very rare, but it is somewhat more common for infirmity to play some role at the 'outset' of their journey to sainthood. Therefore, the chapter will focus mostly on the other significant roles infirmity played at the outset of these figures' saintly careers.

In the established pattern of a saintly lifestyle, two aspects that were tightly interlinked with their corporality were patience, *patientia*, and

45 Scheer, 'Are Emotions a Kind of Practice?', esp. 202.

46 Tommaso di Celano, *Vita prima*, 20. Other *vitae* of Francis also give evidence that he suffered from bouts of ill health even in his early life. See Trembinski, 'An Infirm Man', 273.

47 Le Goff, *Saint Francis of Assisi*, 25-26. See also Vauchez, *Francis of Assisi*, 117.

48 See also Goodich, *Vita perfecta*, 120.

49 Vauchez, *Francis of Assisi*, 117.

penitence, including *abstinentia* and the corporeal forms of devotional practices. *Patientia* and *penitentia* were most tightly interlinked with imitating Christ's passion as well as purifying one's soul, and therefore suffering in one way or another is integral to these concepts. The second chapter of this book will address the question of *patientia* and how infirmity was, or was not, used to reconstruct it in canonization depositions. Raptures and ecstasies are included in this analysis. In this chapter the question of (un)diagnosing 'holy infirmity' will also be addressed, asking which aspects of it were essential to record in the hearings of different saints. At the end of this chapter the discussion will move on to the ways a family member's infirmity, especially in the lives of married saints, was used in the construction of their patience. In the third chapter, the discussion will turn to abstinence and penitentiary and devotional practices. Abstinence was one of the key features of late medieval saints' lives, and was therefore also investigated intensely in canonization inquests. For the topic of this book, the most essential element of abstinence and penitence is the way a holy person's community reportedly attempted to delineate austerity and devotional practices when they had corporeal forms. My main interest lies in non-self-inflicted infirmities, but austerity was often delineated precisely on grounds of its causing or aggravating infirmity. My viewpoint will therefore be centred on infirmity as a factor defining austerity and the role various community members played in this process.

The final chapter of the book will move away from the framework of delineators of sainthood and focus on saints' infirmities and their cultural and communal meanings on a more general level. We will first turn our attention to the ways community members interacted with a living saint and the roles infirmity played in this. How was a saint's infirmity presented in the depositions concerning such encounters? In this chapter the question of saint as medical practitioner will also be addressed, especially from the viewpoint of charity and the medical pluralism of the period,[50] asking if and how the saint's own bodily suffering influenced these activities. In the end, the question of the benefits of infirmity will be addressed. As mentioned above, late medieval society valorized pain and suffering, and the concept of 'holy infirmity', as depicted in canonization protocols, is a part of this discourse. How, then, did saints manifest the beneficial side of infirmity, especially when there were attempts to treat their ailing bodies,

50 The concept of 'medical pluralism' means that people sought the help of educated medical practitioners, various types of folk healers, and religious healing methods side by side. See Gentilcore, *Healers and Healing*, for this concept.

and is their attitude to their bodily suffering comparable to the attitudes to it within their communities?

In this analysis, saints and other well-known persons will be referenced by the established English versions of their names. The names of people testifying in the canonization inquests will appear in the Latin (or occasionally Italian or French) form, as recorded in the original document. All translations and transcripts from manuscript sources are my own, unless stated otherwise.

Canonization Processes as Sources for Holy Infirmity

This study uses the testimonies of canonization inquests conducted between the early thirteenth and the mid-fifteenth century as the main source material, which determines the saints who will be its focus. There are some important holy figures of this period strongly associated with corporality or suffering, the most obvious examples being St. Francis of Assisi[51] (1181/1182-1226) and St. Catherine of Siena[52] (1347-1380), who were canonized but not subjects of official canonization inquests and who therefore appear

51 St. Francis is perhaps the saint most closely associated with suffering, although, as noted by Donna Trembinski in her studies on his physical illness and disability, this aspect of his life has been largely ignored in research and subdued in most of his *vitae*. Trembinski, 'An Infirm Man', 269-70. Trembinski analyses Francis's disabilities thoroughly in her forthcoming monograph *Illness and Authority: Disability in the Life and Lives of St. Francis of Assisi*. As portrayed in his *vitae*, in Francis's later life, he began to suffer pain in his eyes and his vision gradually worsened, he suffered from fevers, and evidently received the painful *stigmata*. During the last years of his life, when he was in his forties, he was almost blind and often so weak he could not get up from bed on his own. Modern scholars have attempted to diagnose Francis's ailments – the conditions suggested are, for example, glaucoma, iritis, trachoma, corneal ulcers, leprosy, malaria, or dropsy. As Trembinski has convincingly shown, there is no evidence that Francis's infirmities were considered to be caused by leprosy, but they were regarded as having separate causes. See Trembinski, 'Illness and Authority', 114-17. For criticism of the leprosy diagnosis, see also Klaniczay, 'Illness, Self-inflicted Body Pain and Supernatural Stigmata'; for Francis's suffering, see also Wells, 'Exemplary Blindness of Francis of Assisi'.

52 Beside St. Birgitta of Sweden, Catherine is one of the most controversial yet influential fourteenth-century religious women. Her visions and mystical marriage to Christ, excessive penitence and fasting, political role in attempting to get the pope to return to Rome, and her *stigmata* are recorded in various writings, the most influential of them being Raymund of Capua's *Legenda major*. Nocentini, 'The *Legenda maior* of Catherine of Siena'. Especially the claims of her having been stigmatized like St. Francis made her canonization a problematic issue, and, despite the widespread veneration of Catherine as a saint during her life and after her death, Stefano Manconi and Tommaso da Siena (or Tommaso Caffarini) only succeeded in organizing a diocesan hearing, known as the Processo Castellano. Catherine was finally canonized in 1461

only as comparative cases. The characteristics of the hearings addressed below will influence the analysis, as those saints whose inquests tackled the question of infirmity most profoundly will receive the most attention. Each saint and her or his hearing will be introduced when first discussed in the course of the analysis.

Papal canonization is usually considered to have started in the early thirteenth century, although there were some earlier saints whose cases occasioned a process.[53] Their inquests, however, were conducted in a rather summarized form, with a short biography followed by some miracles,[54] so the image of infirmity in these early canonization protocols is not very detailed. From 1230 on, there had to be a wider recognition of sanctity for a canonization process to be opened,[55] and an established local cult was a prerequisite for this. The case was then brought to the knowledge of the Holy See by its promoters.[56] If the pope found there was enough reason (usually politics played an important part here), he sent a commission to investigate the life, deeds, and merits of the putative saint. During the hearings dozens or even hundreds of people testified about the miracles they had witnessed or experienced and related what they knew about the saint's life. The inquests were conducted according to a number of principles. The basic rules were set by canon law, but there were only a few of them. The major rulings concerning the implementation of the processes were issued during the early thirteenth century,[57] but each process put these principalities into practice in a different way. Nevertheless, the protocols can be compared with other legal documents of the period.[58]

The witness statements given in canonization inquests have been widely used as source material in the recent decades, especially for questions

by the Sienese pope Pius II. On Catherine's process and canonization, see Klaniczay, 'The Power of the Saints', 131-32. See also p. 85 n. 194 below.

53 The earliest processes used in this study are those of St. Dominic (1233) and St. Elizabeth of Hungary (1235). Dominic's hearing is the first one in which *articuli interrogatorii* was specifically referred to. Vauchez, *Sainthood*, 506. Elizabeth's inquest is important for the development of the canonization procedure because the famous *testes legitimos* was first included in it; it provides the standard set of question for the commissioners to use so as to determine the cogency of the witness statements. Klaniczay, 'Proving Sanctity', 123-24; Wetzstein, *Heilige vor Gericht*, 538-39.

54 See Vauchez, *Sainthood*, 324.

55 Vauchez, *Sainthood*, 327.

56 For the different parties of the canonization process, see Katajala-Peltomaa and Krötzl, 'Approaching Twelfth-Fifteenth-Century Miracles', 21-23.

57 These include *audivimus, venerabilii*, and *testes legitimos* (*interrogatorium*). Katajala-Peltomaa and Krötzl, 'Approaching Twelfth-Fifteenth-Century Miracles', 17-21.

58 On the legal development of the canonization process, see Paciocco, *Canonizzazioni e culto dei santi nella Christianitas*; Wetzstein, *Heilige vor Gericht*.

related to lay piety, lived religion, family, gender practices, and the social history of medicine. In these analyses it is precisely those depositions that concern miracles which have gained most attention, although the testimonies on saints' lives have been analysed as well.[59] In their discussion of miracles, Laura Ackerman Smoller and Michael Goodich have pointed out that although the language of the documents belongs to the notaries who recorded the depositions for other civil servants, the messages in them belong to the witnesses.[60] There is no need to assume that this was not also true of testimonies concerning saints' lives, although there the preferences and practicalities for those conducting the inquests may have been even more pronounced. After all, there had to be a public cult for a canonization inquest to be opened. This, in turn, had to be welcomed and accepted by an ecclesiastical institution, and therefore collaboration between clergy and laity, the elements of the lay religious life or 'popular' religion and ecclesiastical influence are intertwined.[61]

Both miracles and an exemplary life were of crucial importance in constructing and examining the authenticity of sainthood. There are some indications that while miracles were the most visible and crucial aspect of sanctity for the larger public, many theologians emphasized the beneficial side of saints' lives. Thomas Aquinas, for example, stressed the virtue of saints as an example for others, implying that sacrifice and sanctity were intertwined.[62] Exactly how much weight was given to a saint's life in the inquest varied. André Vauchez states that the processes increasingly emphasized the saint's life instead of their thaumaturgic powers in the course of the thirteenth and fourteenth centuries. For example, in the early thirteenth century there were still inquests into saints who had died recently, such as Ambrose of Massa in 1240-41, that focused on their miracles, whereas the process of Brynolf of Skara (d. 1317) in 1417 includes a much higher

59 For studies analysing testimonies to *vitae*, see e.g. Archambeau, 'Remembering Countess Delphine's Books'; Elliott, *Proving Woman*; Kleinberg, *Prophets*; Smoller, 'Northern and Southern Sanctity'; Vauchez, *Sainthood*. For a recent historiography of canonization processes, see Katajala-Peltomaa, 'Recent Trends in the Study of Medieval Canonizations'. For the historiography of miracles, see Katajala-Peltomaa and Krötzl, 'Approaching Twelfth-Fifteenth-Century Miracles', 9-15.

60 Smoller, 'Miracle, Memory, and Meaning', 430-31. See also Goodich, '*Mirabilis Deus in sanctis suis*', 143-44. One of the principal rules of the hearings was to faithfully record the witnesses' statements and read them back to them, and the failure to do this could result in the failure of the case. Wetzstein, *Heilige vor Gericht*, 45.

61 Katajala-Peltomaa and Krötzl, 'Approaching Twelfth-Fifteenth-Century Miracles'; Vauchez, *Sainthood*, 142, 250.

62 Goodich, *Miracles and Wonders*, 19.

proportion of depositions on his life.[63] However, in the fifteenth-century hearings used in this study there appears to be a balance. The processes of St. Frances of Rome (1440, 1443, 1451) and St. Bernardino of Siena (1448-49) were indeed carefully built around sets of articles on their *vitae*, but the number of healing miracles investigated was substantial. At the same time, the 1457 process of St. Rose of Viterbo, who lived in the thirteenth century, focuses almost entirely on miracles undoubtedly also because of the long time span between the saints' death and the inquest.

In the testimonies on saints' lives, their corporality and infirmity included, the framework of a holy life, constructed around virtues, played a crucial role. Ideally, the inquests were conducted based on *articuli*, a list of propositions related to the saintly candidate's life and miracles. In most cases, the *articuli* were collected beforehand by the procurator of the hearing, and in them the pattern of sainthood intermingled with the details of the saint's life. The articles demonstrate the 'profile' that the promoters of the cause hoped to get recognition for, and therefore they guided, channelled, and restricted the future witness accounts and the focuses of the hearings.[64] The conductors of canonization inquests were mostly preoccupied with ascetic and moral virtues, with chastity emphasized in all hearings. However, although some educated, clerical witnesses could emphasize theological virtues in their testimonies or otherwise use the classification of virtues by established authors, the *articuli* include a more traditional model of sanctity, inspired by hagiographic literature.[65] As already mentioned, among the *articuli* touching on the topic of *infirmitas*, the most important are those related to *patientia* and *penitentia*.[66] However, there is great variation in the length, detail, and level of organization in the articles between various processes, and in some cases they were crafted only after the interrogations or are lacking altogether.[67] Even if the inquest in question was not conducted based on *articuli*, these concepts were investigated, albeit with some variation.

63 Vauchez, *Sainthood*, 499-505.

64 See e.g. Menestò, 'The Apostolic Canonization Proceedings of Clare of Montefalco', 109. The articles record certain concepts, but at the same time the details of saints' lives are often left quite vague. Vauchez, *Sainthood*, 302 has emphasized this notion regarding St. Thomas Cantilupe's humility, but the same holds true for many other hearings and concepts as well.

65 Vauchez, *Sainthood*, 518-19.

66 Especially *abstinentia*, and within it fasting, was one of the most important ways of acquiring spiritual perfection. This is why the conductors of canonization proceedings invested so much time and effort in exploring this particular subject. Vauchez, *Sainthood*, 191; see also pp. 111-12 below.

67 Wetzstein, *Heilige vor Gericht*, 505-6; Smoller, 'Northern and Southern Sanctity', 292-93; Katajala-Peltomaa and Krötzl, 'Approaching Twelfth-Fifteenth-Century Miracles', 23-24. See also note pp. 67-68 below.

Despite the variations in the *articuli*, the importance of sanctity for medieval culture was such that witnesses are likely to have known which aspects of the saint's life were essential, especially those specifically called to testify about the matter. These witnesses were a specific set of people, which is of great importance for any analysis based on canonization protocols.[68] Although a large variety of people benefitted from saints' powers in receiving miraculous assistance when they had difficulties, and although saints were venerated at all levels of society, only a very particular group of people were given the chance to present their views about their lives. Clerics and men from the secular elite were valued most as witnesses, especially when a saint's *vita* was investigated; in the case of miracles, women are more common as witnesses.[69] Additionally, servants and companions were interrogated in some inquests. The commissioners valued the word of those who had known the saint personally or even lived with them; this is the case especially with monks and cloistered nuns, many of whom came from elite families.[70] As for laity, women were only summoned to testify about a saint's *vita* if they were of 'good reputation', usually meaning *matronae* known to be pious and to have a religious lifestyle, but even they were rare among the witnesses unless they personally knew the putative saint. Their voice is most often heard in the processes of Dauphine of Puimichel (1363) and St. Frances of Rome, whose companions and spiritual daughters frequently testified.[71] Therefore, although sainthood was communally formed, the picture of a *vita* we get from canonization protocols was constructed largely by the saints' innermost circle, and the view we get is also often quite masculine.[72] Some

68 See e.g. Lett, 'La parole des humbles', 233-34.

69 On gender, wealth, and the selection of witnesses, see Farmer, *Surviving Poverty*, 50-55; Katajala-Peltomaa, *Gender, Miracles, and Daily Life*, 32-42; Lett, *Un procès de canonisation*. See also Esch, 'I processi medioevali', 42; Golinelli, 'Social Aspects in Some Italian Canonization Trials', 170-71; Goodich, 'Politics of Canonisation', 177, for women as witnesses. For women's significance in giving testimony on children's miracles, see Lett, *L'Enfant des miracles*, 32.

70 See also Park, 'Relics of a Fertile Heart, 120. In the case of St. Margaret of Hungary, for example, the majority of the nuns in her monastery had been royal princesses or widows or daughters of higher aristocracy. Klaniczay, *The Uses of Supernatural Power*, 102. Concerning the sanctity of King (St.) Louis IX of France (1214-1270), one of the 'ailing saints' also discussed in this book, M. Cecilia Gaposchkin has concluded that even among the miracle beneficiaries, the elite had some kind of personal tie or knowledge of him, so that his miraculous powers were a more personal matter for them, while the poor travelled to his shrine and created the culture of the miraculous at Saint-Denis. Gaposchkin, 'Place, Status, and Experience', 249-66.

71 In Frances's case, this is particularly striking, as virtually all the men testifying about her life were clerics. Esposito, 'St. Francesca and the Female Religious Communities', 198.

72 As an example, in Louis IX's canonization inquest there were only three female witnesses out of thirty-nine to his *vita*. Of the thirty-six men, two were Louis's family (his son and brother),

information was disseminated to the general public in everyday discussions, sermons, and *vitae*, but in many cases the view of the holy person's life was presumably somewhat vague outside their inner circle.[73]

Despite the similar principles behind all canonization inquests, the amount of information we get about the saintly candidates' lives, and their infirmities, varies greatly. The length of the depositions varies from process to process; while some of them record the witness statements in detail, others are much more summarized, presumably after a series of rewritings and edits.[74] As mentioned earlier, there is also a change over time in that the witness statements in the earliest inquests are less structured or sketchier than those in later ones. Furthermore, from the turn of the fourteenth century onwards, there was a growing need to investigate (especially female) saints' mystic experiences more thoroughly and in medical terms,[75] which influences the level of detail in these processes. This need coincides with a growing tendency to highlight and investigate the legendary aspects of a holy life.[76] Letizia Pellegrini has recently pointed out that because there was a significant gap in the canonization inquests following the Western Schism, the tradition of conducting them was to some extent lost. Therefore, the commissioners of the mid-fifteenth-century inquests could 'start anew' and form a new set of preferences.[77] In all processes under investigation here, some witness depositions were also recorded in more detail because of their value. Therefore, although all inquests are similar to a certain degree because of their common method and purpose, the differences between the protocols and testimonies must be taken into account when making any comparisons, especially when researching a specific topic such as *infirmitas*.

one was the son of the king of Jerusalem (Jean of Acre, 1258-1296), eleven were clerics of various ranks and titles, eight were titled *monseigneur* and/or *chevalier* (one of them was also Louis's chamberlain), six other witnesses also belonged to Louis's staff, as mentioned above one was his surgeon, and the rest were other distinguished laymen. Many of the witnesses had accompanied him on his crusades. Guillaume de Saint-Pathus, *Vie de saint Louis*, 7-10; O'Tool, 'Caring for the Blind', 92-93.

73 See Gaposchkin, 'Louis IX and the Liturgical Memory'; Gaposchkin, 'Place, Status, and Experience', esp. 252, on this matter in the context of Louis IX's sanctity.

74 Katajala-Peltomaa and Krötzl, 'Approaching Twelfth-Fifteenth-Century Miracles', 20.

75 Elliott, 'The Physiology of Rapture and Female Spirituality', 157, 161-64.

76 Vauchez, *Sainthood*, 527-34.

77 Pellegrini, 'Testifying to Miracles'.

Infirmitas Leading to Saintly Life

Abstract
This chapter discusses the importance of infirmity for the narrations of the beginning of a saintly candidate's path to holiness. While traditional conversion narratives waned in popularity and are next to non-existent in the canonization processes, infirmity could be underlined in the narratives regarding other important aspects of the early stages of a saint's life. It could mark a moment when the (future) saint made an important decision that defined his or her saintly life, or influence the holy person's lifestyle and choices. In the case of lay female saints, it could be seen and used as a factor that justified their marital relations or helped to achieve a celibate marriage.

Keywords: hagiography, sainthood, conversion, marriage, lay sainthood, celibacy

A person living in medieval society had to choose a social persona from those that were on offer,[1] and their community had to interpret and accept it. The narratives about saints' childhood in canonization testimonies usually repeat the topos of *puer senex/puella senex*, in which holiness manifests itself already in their early years. Sometimes the formation of a persona as a saint was, however, portrayed as a dramatic transformation. The saints either made a complete conversion, or their saintly path faced obstacles or included moments of crisis that defined their future holiness.[2] These moments are among the most dramatic ways infirmity could be used to reconstruct or even create sanctity. There is the trope of a saint converting to a religious life as a result of physical ailment, or being prompted by illness or impairment to change his or her habits and lifestyle. This motif is common in the

1 Rubin, 'The Body, Whole and Vulnerable', 21.

2 See Bejczy, 'The *Sacra infantia* in Medieval Hagiography', for these two models of a saint's childhood and youth. See also Kieckhefer, 'Holiness and the Culture of Devotion', 296-97.

Kuuliala, Jenni, *Saints, Infirmity, and Community in the Late Middle Ages.*
Taylor & Francis Group 2020
DOI: 10.5117/9789462983373_INFIR

numerous *vitae* of saints,[3] but not so commonly depicted in the canonization processes. One reason for this apparent void is that redemption narratives become less popular in the late thirteenth century, at least when it comes to official sanctity.[4] The few examples we have of infirmity leading to the path of sainthood are, nevertheless, worth discussing before moving on to the more common ways infirmities were used in constructing sainthood.

Infirmity, Conversion, and the Path to Sainthood

How big a role an alleged conversion as an aftermath of ill health played in a saint's *fama* varies greatly. Among the saints that had an official canonization process, John Buoni (1168-1249) is perhaps the one for whose later reputation such a conversion is recorded as having most significance. What is known for certain is that after his conversion at the age of about 40, John became a hermit at Bertinoro, near Cesena. During the following forty years, a great number of men followed him, forming a group called the Giambonites, or 'Zamboniti'. People in Cesena and Mantua started to venerate him. There is one nearly contemporary source, a Fiorentine *codice* Cod. Plut. 90, sup. 48, datable to between 1236 and 1342, which records that John's conversion was prompted by an illness. Later versions, like Agostino da Crema's *vita* from 1484 records that during an illness John Buoni made a vow that he would abandon his riches and was immediately cured of this illness.[5] Later *vitae* specify that John spent a considerable time as an entertainer and juggler in several towns and courts before the illness.[6]

3 Le Goff, *Saint Francis of Assisi*, 26; for examples, see Goodich, *Vita perfecta*, 119-21; Weinstein and Bell, *Saints and Society*, 156. As mentioned in the introduction, the best-known and most influential late medieval conversion narrative where illness plays a role is that of St. Francis of Assisi. See pp. 25-26.

4 Vauchez, *Sainthood*, 514.

5 Mattei, 'Introduzione', 27. See also 25-26 for the early life of John Buoni and the improbability that he actually had a wealthy background. A case that has some similarity to John Buoni's is that of the hermit Franco Lippi of Grotti (1211-1291). He was a bandit or a highwayman for a long time, until he suddenly became blind at the age of 50, and this prompted his conversion. He confessed his sins and made a pilgrimage to Santiago de Compostela, where he received a miraculous cure. He heard a sermon given by Ambrose Sansedoni, converted, and became a Carmelite recluse. See Goodich, *Vita perfecta*, 120. Augustine Novello, on the other hand, was reportedly wounded in the Battle of Benevento in 1266 and promised to adopt a religious vocation if he were cured of the illness. This happened, and he joined the Augustinian hermits. 'Vita b. Augustini Novelli ord. erem.', *AASS*, Maii IV, 618.

6 'Processus apostolici, de b. Joanne Buono', *AASS*, Oct. IX, 698-701, 746. The author of a fifteenth-century *vita*, Ambrosio Calepino (1440-1510), defined this illness as *languor*; 'Vita, Auctore Ambrosio Calepino, ordinis eremitarum S. Augustini', *AASS*, Oct. IX, 748.

The idea that John's path to sainthood was initiated by a dramatic, instant conversion thus lived on. But when we think about those testifying about his life in the canonization inquest of 1251-54, the situation appears to be different. The other Giambonites were those giving depositions about his life, and they did not mention any infirmity leading to conversion – in fact, they did not even talk about the conversion itself. They had known John Buoni during the latter half of his life, and this is what constructed his sanctity for them.[7] It is impossible to know if already at that time there was some common *fama* about his conversion, but for the other brothers his ascetic lifestyle and his miracle-working abilities were the signs of his holiness. Most likely this was also the case for those conducting the inquest, as no questions regarding the conversion are recorded in the document.

Physical infirmity could also be represented as an event formulating the future saint's life path in a different way, prompting a seemingly more minor change that would later become a key element of the person's sanctity. This kind of narrative is more common in canonization records. The best-known saint in whose life illness was, at least in retrospect, interpreted in such terms is St. Louis IX of France (1214-1270), the only canonized French king (by Boniface VIII in 1297). Louis, who became a king at the age of 12, expressed his piety in many different ways: he lived an exemplary personal life, favoured the mendicant orders, purchased the Crown of Thorns from Baldwin II, helped to enact religious reforms in France, and funded many religious institutions.[8] All these were essential in the creation of his sanctity, but, above all, Louis was a crusader king – and infirmity played a crucial role in his becoming one.

The source situation concerning Louis is tricky when studying canonization inquests. The majority of the records of Louis's hearing, held at Saint-Denis in 1282-83, have been lost. Only the testimonies of three miracles and a fragment of the testimony of his brother Charles of Anjou (1227-1285), king of Sicily (1266-85), have survived.[9] However, the material concerning

7 See also Mattei, 'Introduzione', 25.

8 Until his majority, Louis's mother Blanche of Castile (d. 1252) acted as a competent and powerful regent. She is also considered to have been the main influence in Louis's life, establishing her own devout beliefs and religious values in her son. Louis married Margaret of Provence in 1234. The matrimony was arranged by his mother on political grounds, as Margaret was the eldest daughter of the count of Provence. For a concise biography of Louis, see Gaposchkin and Field, 'Introduction', 1-13. The definitive biographical study of Louis is Le Goff, *Saint Louis*. For Louis's cult and canonization, see Gaposchkin, *The Making of Saint Louis*.

9 The miracle testimonies have been edited in *Fragments de l'enquête faite à Saint-Denis en 1282 en vue de la canonisation de Saint Louis*, ed. Delaborde, and Charles's deposition in *Déposition*

Louis's life, his miracles, and his sanctity in general is extensive. As for the canonization inquest, Guillaume de Saint-Pathus, a Franciscan friar who was the confessor of Louis's widow Margaret, compiled his *Vie et miracles* based on the canonization records in around 1303. It is generally accepted that the miracle accounts especially are very faithful towards Guillaume's source. As for Louis's life, Guillaume used the original depositions but rearranged the material on various aspects of Louis's sanctity according to saintly virtues, in which respect he followed Bonaventure's *Legenda major* of St. Francis and Franciscan ideals.[10] Although this work cannot be treated as if it were canonization protocols, it is an invaluable source for our current topic.

Louis's *Vie* by Guillaume de Saint-Pathus, as well as several other texts concerning his sainthood, portray the events in the abbey of Pontoise in 1244. Louis, then 30 years old, had already succumbed to dysentery two years earlier, during a military campaign against the English and their allies in Poitou, but the illness had not fully healed and he had a relapse expected to be fatal. Guillaume de Saint-Pathus describes Louis's illness and recovery as an event that led to his becoming a crusader and, consequently, a saint. He tells us of this occasion in the part of his work dealing with the strength of Louis's faith ('de sa ferme creance').[11] The connection between the cure and Louis's future saintly path is made explicit when Guillaume states that as the illness worsened and everybody believed Louis to be dying, 'Our Lord lengthened his life by a miracle', so that Louis could follow his good intentions and serve God, thus providing an example to others.[12] Guillaume is referring to the whole of Louis's life, but undoubtedly to his future status as the crusader saint in particular,[13] as it was during this illness that Louis

de Charles d'Anjou pour la canonisation de saint Louis, ed. Le comte Riad. An English translation of the latter is included in Jackson, *The Seventh Crusade*, 115-20.

10 On the documents, see Gaposchkin, *The Making of Saint Louis*, 37-39; Farmer, *Surviving Poverty*, 7-9. On Louis IX's canonization, see Gaposchkin, *The Making of Saint Louis*, 19-65; Goodich, *Vita perfecta*, 186-91. The section concerning miracles has been edited by Percival B. Fay as Guillaume de Saint-Pathus, *Les miracles de saint Louis*, and the part concerning his life by H.-F. Delaborde as Guillaume de Saint-Pathus, *Vie de saint Louis*.

11 Guillaume, for instance, relates that Louis 'delivered a great and profitable sermon and arranged in his malady all his things and did what a good Christian should do', thus formulating the narrative according to what was expected of a holy person and a ruler who was dying. Guillaume de Saint-Pathus, *Vie de saint Louis*, 21. See also O'Tool, 'Caring for the Blind', 78-79. For the 'requirements' of a holy person's death, see Goodich, 'Death of a Saint'.

12 Guillaume de Saint-Pathus, *Vie de saint Louis*, 21: 'et croit l'en que Nostre Sires li aloigna sa vie par miracle'.

13 For the importance of crusading for Louis's sanctity, see esp. Gaposchkin, 'The Captivity of Louis IX', 90; Gaposchkin, 'The Place of the Crusades in the Sanctification of Louis IX'. The matter and its connection with Louis's infirmities will be further discussed later in this book.

took the cross. After he was cured, Louis assembled the prelates and barons of his kingdom, and after some time and preaching, his 'brothers and many prelates' followed his example and took the cross.[14]

As usual, Guillaume does not tell us how many witnesses of the canonization hearing actually mentioned this incident, how much emphasis it received in the original testimonies, or the nature of them. Although he does so elsewhere in his work, here he does not even mention any witnesses by name. The incident was, however, an established part of Louis's *fama*.[15] The famous chronicler and the author of *Histoire de saint Louis*, Jean de Joinville (1224-1317) recounts the same incident precisely as Louis making a vow to lead a crusade if he was cured. Joinville's work as well as other sources say that some objected to his decision, especially Louis's mother Blanche, who even made him renounce the vow on the grounds that he had been ill at the time – this merely resulted in Louis taking the cross again in sound health.[16] The renunciation under pressure from Blanche and remaking of the vow is unusual when compared with miraculous cures in general. After all, in narrations of cures a vow was often made precisely at the time of illness, and there was a tendency for it to be made at the most desperate time.[17] William Chester Jordan points out that many chroniclers and hagiographers, like Guillaume de Saint-Pathus, do not place emphasis on the voices of doubt concerning Louis's decision, although there are other texts, for example by Matthew Paris, which show that after decades of crusading and the Capetians' strong involvement in the campaigns, there was criticism of Louis's decision.[18] These dissimilarities in the narrations may demonstrate not just Guillaume's personal preferences but also those of the parties of the canonization inquest in creating a certain kind of a narrative about the infirmity and its immediate consequences. That being said, it is worth pointing out that Jean de Joinville was himself among the witnesses to the inquiry. Whether or not he reported Blanche's reluctance to see her son campaign on the grounds of her son's faltering health is a matter for conjecture.

Louis most likely saw crusading as his destiny – after all, his three immediate predecessors, Louis VII, Philip Augustus, and Louis's father Louis VIII, had all been crusaders. Moreover, the vow has been interpreted as Louis's final and successful attempt to free himself from his mother's power. Gaposchkin and Field, 'Introduction', 6; Jordan, *Louis IX and the Challenge of the Crusade*, 8.

14 Guillaume de Saint-Pathus, *Vie de saint Louis*, 21-22.

15 For a later example, see the late fifteenth-century version of Louis's *vita*, *Le Livre des faiz monseigneur saint Loys, composé à la requête du cardinal de Bourbon et de la duchesse de Bourbonnois*, BNF, MS Fr. 2829, fol. 19v.

16 Jean de Joinville, *Histoire de saint Louis*, 39.

17 See Smoller, 'Defining the Boundaries of the Natural', 345.

18 Jordan, *Louis IX and the Challenge of the Crusade*, 1-8.

As Louis's case shows, physical illness could be seen as significant for a holy person's saintly path without signifying a complete change in their lifestyle of the type recorded in the *vitae* of St. Francis of Assisi or John Buoni. Already in Louis's own family, his sister Isabelle of France (1224-1270)[19] had fallen severely ill in childhood, an experience that reportedly had a big impact on her later refusal to marry and ultimately her decision to choose a religious vocation and found the convent of Longchamp. She died with an air of sanctity and miracles reportedly occurred at her grave. Her *vita* was written by the convent's prioress Agnes d'Harcourt.[20] To take another example, St. Vincent Ferrer (1350-1419), a Dominican preacher venerated especially in Brittany, wrote a letter to (anti)pope Benedict XIII in 1412, informing him of events in the late 1390s, during the Western Schism. Vincent recounted how he was seriously infirm, and in his sleep had a vision of St. Dominic and St. Francis of Assisi praying at the feet of Christ. The vision continued with Christ coming to Vincent and touching his face, giving him the task of preaching penitence and preparing his listeners for the arrival of the antichrist. This healed Vincent and, having received a licence from Benedict, he began his preaching mission, which largely formulated the last twenty years of his life as well as his reputation as a saint.[21] However, the significance of the letter for Vincent's subsequent sanctity was not so much his recovery from illness but the licence to preach obtained from Christ himself.[22] His illness had the potential to be of similar importance in defining his sanctity to the illness of St. Louis IX, but it never became the defining factor.

Puer senex is a common trope in medieval hagiography, and only occasionally is infirmity a part of the narrative, as in the case of Isabelle of

19 For Isabelle, see Field, *Isabelle of France*, and also Jordan, *Louis IX and the Challenge of the Crusade*, 9; Klaniczay, *Holy Rulers and Blessed Princesses*, 237.

20 *The Writings of Agnes of Harcourt*, 58; 'Vita gallice scripta per Agnetem de Harcourt', *AASS*, Aug. VI, 792-808; Field, *Isabelle of France*, 13-36. Isabelle was beatified only in 1521, apparently because the papacy was reluctant to further strengthen the power of the Capetian dynasty in the thirteenth century, although her brother Charles of Anjou made a plea for her sainthood when giving a witness account in Louis IX's canonization inquiry; Klaniczay, *Holy Rulers and Blessed Princesses*, 237.

21 This incident is reported in Pietro Ranzano's *vita*; 'Vita s. Vincenti Ferrerii', *AASS*, Apr. I, 491. During the Schism, Vincent remained a supporter of the Avignon pope. On the letter and its significance, see Smoller, *The Saint and the Chopped-Up Baby*, 133-34. For Vincent's cult and canonization, see Smoller, 'Defining the Boundaries of the Natural'; Smoller, 'Miracle, Memory, and Meaning'; Smoller, 'Northern and Southern Sanctity'; Smoller, *Saint and the Chopped-Up Baby*. For his life, see Daileader, *Saint Vincent Ferrer, his World and Life*.

22 Smoller, *The Saint and the Chopped-Up Baby*, 6.

France. The one example of this among the saints of our period for whom we have the canonization protocols is St. Dorothea of Montau (1347-1394), an anchoress and mystic, whose cult flourished in Prussia and especially in the areas around Gdansk.[23] Her process is one of those where the informative and detailed testimonies to her life are given by a very specific set of people, mainly clerics who had been influential in her life. The most influential of them was her confessor Johannes Marienwerder, who gave a sermon after her death, wrote a vernacular *Life*, the so-called *Vita Lindana* and a Latin *vita*, and acted as the procurator of the canonization inquest held in 1404. His influence on the *fama* of Dorothea's sainthood was crucial,[24] and his own truncated clerical career inspired him in these enterprises. Johannes also gave a long witness account in the hearing, whose documents include *Libellus de vita, virtutibus et miraculis* of Dorothea by him.[25] In all sources, Dorothea's sanctity is constructed in very corporeal terms, her fervent asceticism and self-chastisement intermingled with her mystic experiences. The texts also record that already at the age of 7, God wounded her.[26] Johannes Mönch, bishop of Marienwerder, testified that he had heard from Dorothea herself that her mother's servant had accidentally poured boiling water over her

23 Dorothea was born in Groß Montau as the daughter of a wealthy Dutch farmer. At the age of 16, she was married to a sword-smith called Adalbrecht of Gdansk, with whom she had nine children, eight of whom died of the plague. The sources portray him as a stern and even cruel husband. After Adalbrecht's death in 1390, Dorothea moved to Marienwerder, and was hugely influenced by Johannes Marienwerder. She became an anchoress of the local cathedral, and lived as a recluse for the last four years of her life. For an overview of Dorothea's life, see e.g. Stargardt, 'Dorothy of Montau'; Kieckhefer, *Unquiet Souls*, 22-24. Dorothea, her mystic experiences, and her relationship with her confessor have been profoundly studied, with special attention being given to the two *vitae* Johannes of Marienwerder wrote. See e.g. Classen, 'Wounding the Body and Freeing the Spirit'; Elliott, 'Authorizing a Life'; Heβ, *Heilige machen*, 245-331; Signori, 'Anchorites in German-Speaking Regions', 56-58; Suerbaum, 'Urban Housewife as a Saint'.

24 There are sporadic exceptions to this. For example, Margaretha Creuczeburgische testified to the article about the matter and stated that she believed it to be true, having heard about it from Dorothea's mother. *Die Akten des Kanonisationsprozess Dorotheas von Montau*, ed. Stachnik (PC Dorothea of Montau), 100.

25 Elliott, 'Authorizing a Life', 168-69; Elliott, *Proving Woman*, 130-31. For the canonization process, see Heβ, *Heilige machen*, 264-70. Both Johannes Marienwerder and Johannes Reyman gave such a *libellus* to the commissaries before giving their statements, to secure their deposition in case they died before the investigation. Johannes Reyman withdrew his *libellus* but Johannes Marienwerder read it aloud, and it is included in the protocols edited by Stachnik. See PC Dorothea of Montau, 297 and Heβ, *Heilige machen*, 271. The text is in PC Dorothea of Montau, 300-19, and it is referred to often in the depositions of Johannes Marienwerder and Johannes Reyman.

26 The third set of articles records that at the age of 7 she had boiling water poured over her and that the Almighty saved her and freed her of all injuries. PC Dorothea of Montau, 25.

so that she had lesions from her head to the soles of her feet. Dorothea had told the bishop that she thought she heard God's voice saying: 'I will make you a new human'. From then on, God had often wounded her. Dorothea had also explained that she had been very infirm because of the accident, so that she had to be carried in a linen cloth.[27] In his witness statement, Johannes Marienwerder was rather laconic about the matter. He simply specified that since the age of 7, God had inflicted wounds upon Dorothea, which she deliberately accepted.[28]

In the two clerics' depositions, Dorothea's wounds create an important spiritual imagery throughout the texts, carrying with them specific symbolism, in which the most notorious characteristic is of course Christ's passion. At the same time, deliberately receiving wounds, which could be fatal, was not generally accepted because it could denote suicide.[29] Therefore, the type of the wounds she suffered had to be defined. One of the methods was to specify their starting point, placed in her childhood and therefore set in the framework of the narrations about her as *puella senex*.[30] At the same time, even the clerics do not seem to have given very much emphasis to the early childhood injuries – childhood events were usually not among the most important ways of constructing the life of a saint.[31] All in all, these testimonies are the ones in Dorothea's hearing that most probably leave a modern reader wondering if Dorothea could indeed have acquired a 'genuine' physical infirmity in her childhood, which was interpreted as a gift from God, perhaps inspired by her religious mother,[32] and which the clerical witnesses later used to reconstruct her sanctity.[33] This is the

27 PC Dorothea of Montau, 411-12.

28 PC Dorothea of Montau, 261, 280; see also 303; 'Vita b. Dorotheae Lindana', *AASS*, Oct. XIII, 506-7; Suerbaum, 'An Urban Housewife as a Saint', 181.

29 Classen, 'Wounding the Body and Freeing the Spirit', esp. 419-21. The portrayal of the wounds, and in general the tendency to portray Dorothea as a martyr saint, is in accordance with the ideals of the Teutonic Order, who strongly promoted her cult. For the Order, fighting wars on the frontiers of western Christendom, martyrdom was important imagery. Hartmann, 'Bridal Mysticism', 111.

30 For the portrayals of Dorothea's childhood in the *vitae*, see e.g. Heß, *Heilige machen*, 256-57; Suerbaum, 'An Urban Housewife as a Saint', 181-83.

31 See Vauchez, *Sainthood*, 507-8.

32 See also Hartmann, 'Bridal Mysticism', 105. Dorothea's mother Agatha was considered a saint by many. She too developed an extremely close relationship with her confessor in her widowhood – to the point that the two decided to die at the same hour, which they almost did. They were even buried in the same tomb. Elliott, *Spiritual Marriage*, 213. See also Vauchez, *Sainthood*, 508, for praising the religious vocation of saints' parents.

33 I share Caroline Walker Bynum's views on the dangers of trying to retrospectively diagnose or define such physical marks of sainthood. See Bynum, *Holy Feast and Holy Fast*, 206-7, 391, n. 82, for this discussion, also concerning Dorothea and *stigmata*. Richard Kieckhefer is one

case especially with the deposition of Johannes Tiefensee, the custodian of the Marienwerder church. He testified to having heard from Dorothea's confessors that from her ninth until her seventeenth year she had a wound in her spine, which was thought by her parents to have protuberances or a hump. Later she had more wounds in her body. Johannes appears to have made a rare distinction between these wounds and those of a more spiritual kind, since he also stated that only God truly understood the wounds of the heart.[34] It is unclear how important the wounds were for Dorothea's common *fama* at the time. The information about the childhood wounds was, however, widely disseminated by Johannes Marienwerder's vernacular *vita*, and it is probably no coincidence that her canonization process includes a high number of miracles in which a child is saved from an accident involving boiling water or fire.[35]

What sets the testimonies about Dorothea's childhood accident and the resulting wounds apart from other 'conversion' infirmities in the canonization testimonies is the lack of any straightforward cure narrative. Admittedly, the *vitae* describe her as being healed through Christ's intervention,[36] but, at the same time, some of the testimonies give the impression that she continued to receive wounds. An uncured infirmity as a catalyst to a holy life is also a feature of the *fama* of St. Margaret of Castello (1287-1320), a Dominican saint. According to the two *vitae*, written later in the fourteenth century but apparently based on contemporary documents,[37] she was born 'blind, small, and deformed' ('cecam, parvulam ac diformen'). In her childhood, Margaret was taken on a pilgrimage to the grave of James of Castello to be cured of her blindness, but after that failed, her parents left her in the town. She was eventually taken to a local convent where she continued her saintly

of those who has attempted to diagnose Dorothea, proposing that her wounds may have been caused by a 'pemphigoid condition'; Kieckhefer, *Unquiet Souls*, 27. By contrast, Raymond Van Dam describes attempts to diagnose beneficiaries of miracle cures in modern terms as deprecating of medieval people's experiences, portraying them as unable to cope with their own lives. Van Dam, *Saints and their Miracles in Late Antique Gaul*, 84. The same applies to saints' ailments. Attempting to 'diagnose' their conditions in such terms undermines the medieval experience and understanding of their infirmities. See also Yarrow, *Saints and their Communities*, 10-11.

34 PC Dorothea of Montau, 472. These wounds were reported in the *Lives* as well. 'Vita b. Dorotheae Lindana', *AASS*, Oct. XIII, 494; Stargardt, 'Dorothy of Montau', 477.

35 See e.g. PC Dorothea of Montau, 62-63, 124, 334, 396-97, 443. For children's accidents in miracle accounts, see Finucane, *The Rescue of the Innocents*, 101-49.

36 Stargardt, 'Dorothy of Montau', 476. However, a cure narrative is also missing from the Latin *vita*; 'Vita b. Dorotheae Lindana', *AASS*, Oct. XIII, 506-7.

37 Goodich, *Vita perfecta*, 50.

life. The *vitae* use her blindness, or rather her 'inner vision', to construct her sanctity, but ignore her other impairments.[38] As a rare example, in the case of these two women, infirmity played a decisive role in initiating their saintly careers, but only because it was *not* fully cured.

Ailing Health and Chastity in Marriage

Although infirmity as the impetus for a religious or saintly life is very rarely investigated in a later medieval canonization hearing, there is one group of saints in whose case it appears frequently either as a concept, a parallel, or as a specific topic: the married lay saints, whose number greatly increased in the late Middle Ages, and whose marital life could be defined or validated by an infirmity. Especially in the case of female lay saints, chastity in marriage was often presented as a profound element of their holy lives. At the same time, for those female saints who did marry – or to those promoting their sanctity – this issue could bring about some kind of a controversy or inner conflict.[39] The principal hagiographic role models for the aspiring saints who had to marry were St. Cecilia, forced to marry a nobleman against her wishes, and St. Alexis, who disguised himself as a beggar in order to avoid marriage and follow his religious calling.[40]

A young woman forced to enter marriage against her vows, or at least against her inner devotion, and acquiring some kind of infirmity as a reaction was a narrative trope, and it was sufficiently common for the saints, their devotees, and the petitioners and commissioners of a canonization process to know how to reconstruct a holy life that fitted the pattern.[41] This was the case also with the marriage of Dauphine Puimichel and St. Elzéar of

38 *Vita Margaritae de Città de Castello*, ed. Laurent, esp. 120-22; *Vita beatae Margaritae virginis*, ed. Poncelet, esp. 23-25. The description in the *vitae* of her parents' feelings of disgust towards their disabled daughter are very rare in late medieval hagiographic texts, and cannot be considered representative of parental emotions towards children with physical impairments. Miracle accounts do occasionally include parents who prayed for relief for themselves and from their worry and weariness, however. See Kuuliala, *Childhood Disability*, esp. 206-30, 145-48.

39 Among the saintly couples choosing to live together in chastity, in the majority of cases the initiative was the woman's, while men appear to have been more inclined to abandon the relationship and/or enter a religious order. Elliott, *Spiritual Marriage*, 5, 208-9. For the 'lost virginity' of St. Birgitta of Sweden, see Salmesvuori, *Power and Sainthood*, 41-61.

40 On the legends of these saints as a model for other medieval saints' *vitae*, see Golinelli, '*Velut alter Alexius*'.

41 See Elliot, *Spiritual Marriage*, 208-11, 222-23. See also Goodich, *Vita perfecta*, 177, for examples of similar lifestyles among saints.

Sabran, whose chaste marriage is one of the best known and most heavily researched among such marriages in the later Middle Ages.[42] Dauphine (1283-1358) was born to a noble family in Provence. She was orphaned at the age of 7, and was in the custody of her two uncles. The sources tell us that she made a vow of chastity as a child, which is also a trope in medieval hagiography.[43] Dauphine's decision to live in chastity was important for her 'official' sainthood, and it was investigated in her canonization inquiry, conducted in 1363 in Apt and Avignon (she was never officially canonized).[44] According to the articles, she wished her estates would be burnt and said she would rather die than consummate a marriage.[45] Her Occitan *Life* adds that she wished to become blind or acquire a severe deformity to be despicable in the eyes of the world and thus be able to give herself completely to God,[46] a trope also recorded in the earlier canonization inquests of St. Elizabeth of Hungary (1207-1231)[47] and her niece St. Margaret of Hungary (1242-1271),[48] which mention the two women threatening to cut off their noses if forced to

42 See esp. Vauchez, *Laity in the Middle Ages*, 194-97, who points out the problematic nature of their marriage for sanctity, and how the Franciscan François de Meyronnes referred to these models when petitioning the pope for Elzéar's canonization.

43 See *Enquête pour le procès de canonisation de Dauphine de Puimichel*, ed. Cambell (PC Dauphine of Puimichel), 33, 209-11, 313-14. According to the witnesses, the information about this aspect of the saint's life usually had come from herself or from her sister Alasacia. See also Sigal, 'Les témoins et les témoignages', 464-65. For Dauphine's childhood, see Elliott, *Spiritual Marriage*, 283-85.

44 On the process and Dauphine's cult, see Archambeau, 'Healing Options during the Plague'; Archambeau, 'Tempted to Kill', 51-54; Sigal, 'Les témoins et les témoignages'.

45 PC Dauphine of Puimichel, 33-35.

46 Dauphine's *Vie de Ste Dauphine*, 136-37. Dauphine's and Elzéar's Occitan double *Lives* have been published as *Vies occitanes de saint Auzias e de sainte Dauphine*, ed. Cambell. Elzéar's *Life* titled *Vie de s. Auzias* (*Vie, Elzéar*) is on 41-127, and Dauphine's *Vie de Ste Dauphine* (*Vie, Dauphine*) on 129-246.

47 *Quellenstudien zur Geschichte der hl. Elisabeth*, ed. Huyskens (PC Elizabeth of Hungary), 124. St. Elizabeth was the daughter of Andrew II of Hungary and Gertrude of Meran. As a child she was engaged to Louis, the heir apparent of the landgrave of Thuringia. She spent her youth at their court and married Louis, who had already succeeded his father, in 1218. The couple had three children together. Louis IV died in 1227, after which she lived a religious life. She did not enter a monastic order, but spent her remaining years at a Franciscan hospital. Elizabeth was canonized only four years after her death, after a campaign by her confessor Conrad of Marburg, Emperor Frederick II, and the Ludowing dynasty, among others. The Arpad dynasty also invested in her cult. Klaniczay, *Holy Rulers and Blessed Princesses*, 202-3, 201-18.

48 Several witnesses testified that when Margaret's father King Bela IV (r. 1235-70) wanted to marry her to the king of Bohemia, the girl threatened to cut off her nose and lips. *Legenda vetus: acta processus canonizationis et Miracula sanctae Margaritae de Hungaria*, ed. Csepregi et al. (PC Margaret of Hungary), 156-57, 214-15, 208-9, 240-41.

marry.[49] Yet, at the age of 15 Dauphine's uncles married her to Count Elzéar of Sabran and Ariano (b. 1285, can. 1371). After Elzéar's death in 1323, she renounced hear earthly wealth and position.[50]

Although not mentioned in the canonization process, the account of Dauphine's wish for deformity was likely widely known, as the Occitan double *Lives* of Dauphine and Elzéar were presumably intended for a lay audience.[51] However, infirmity appears more important in the context of the events *after* their marriage. In these narrations, physical illness is portrayed as a tool in Dauphine's aspirations in a rather singular light. The tenth article states that after Dauphine had agreed to marry Elzéar, she told him that she wished to guard her virginity and follow the example of St. Cecilia, St. Valerian, and St. Alexis. However, Elzéar, then only 13 years old, put pressure on his bride to consummate their marriage. It then happened that Dauphine became ill with a grave fever. She had her husband brought to her and told him that unless he agreed to stop harassing her to engage in carnal relations, she would not rise from her bed alive, as she would much rather die than consent to his advances. She continued that she wished that if Elzéar consented to her will, God would cure her and they would both live 'to the glory and honour of God'.[52] The texts continues by stating that Elzéar, who 'tenderly loved' his wife, made the promise of chastity to her. The couple lived their lives as Tertiary Franciscans.[53]

Many witnesses in Dauphine's hearing attested that her *fama sanctitatis* began at the time of Elzéar's death, when she gave up her earthly possessions and status, but especially those who had been close to her also recounted earlier events. Usually Dauphine herself was their informant.[54] Their testimonies about the tenth article provide inconsistent information

49 Cutting off a nose was a reference to a mutilation used as a punishment for adulterous women, and it was also the most visible of the medieval corporal punishments. Wolf, ed. and trans., *Life and Afterlife of St. Elizabeth*, 204, n. 36; Metzler, *Social History of Disability*, 24.

50 On Dauphine's life, see e.g. Elliot, *Spiritual Marriage*, 216-20; Vauchez, *Laity in the Middle Ages*, 73-82.

51 See Weissenberg, 'What man are you?', 121, n. 40, who writes that the vernacular *Life*'s audience was presumably lay whereas the Latin *vita* was directed to a clerical audience, most likely within the Franciscan communities to whom the saint's cult is attached.

52 PC Dauphine of Puimichel, 35-37: '"Scias, Elziari, quod, nisi michi consenseris quod de carnali copula me ulterius non inquietabis, nunquam ab hoc lecto viva resurgam, cum scias me velle pocius mori quam copule carnali consentire. Si vero tibi placuerit michi in hoc consentire, spero quod Deus michi graciam faciat; et ab hac infirmitate evadam, et vivemus ambo simul amplius ad Dei gloriam et honorem."'

53 PC Dauphine of Puimichel, 37.

54 See Vauchez, *Laity in the Middle Ages*, 191-92.

about the origins of Dauphine's illness.[55] Bertrandus Iusberti, the guardian of the Franciscan convent in Apt, who had been Dauphine's *familiaris* and confessor, testified that he had heard from Dauphine that when she told Elzéar she would die if he did not consent to her virginity, he started to cry for fear of losing her, because he loved her dearly. Concerning the severity of Dauphine's fever, Bertrandus further reported that contrary to the statements in the article, Dauphine was *not* so gravely infirm that she could not get up from her bed, but she told Elzéar that to make him agree to live in chastity.[56] Durandus Andree, who was Dauphine's confessor and physician,[57] reported that Dauphine had one confidant, a noble widow living a holy life, Garsenda Alphante de Ansoysio, who knew about her secret promise. After talking over the matter with Garsenda, Dauphine started to pretend to be gravely infirm, and, staying in bed and accepting the 'diet of the infirm' ('dietam tenuit infirmorum'). Shortly afterwards a real fever or squincy ('squinancia') struck her, to the point that the physicians were indeed despairing of her life. She said to Elzéar that she did not believe she would be cured unless he promised her a chaste marriage.[58]

Here Durandus's background as a physician played a role. Medical professionals frequently testified in the hearings, in which their task was to provide scientific evidence for miracles and saints' physical conditions.[59] Diet was an important element in the six non-naturals regulating health, and in the interaction between a physician and a patient; following the administered diet was one of the patient's responsibilities.[60] All this gave

55 Catherina de Podio, a noblewoman who had lived with Dauphine, did not give a specific testimony to the article. She however reported having heard from Dauphine's sister and women living with her that she had had many 'turbaciones' at the time of her marriage. PC Dauphine of Puimichel, 385.

56 PC Dauphine of Puimichel, 212-13.

57 It was common, especially in the early and high Middle Ages, for physicians to be clerics. In the later medieval period these two functions started to move apart, but as the case of Durandus Andree shows, it was still not uncommon for a household or court physician to be a cleric. According to Danielle Jacquart's calculations, in the fourteenth century around 14 per cent of French physicians were clerics. Jacquart, *Milieu médical*, 363, 383. For the corresponding figures in Aragon, see McVaugh, *Medicine before the Plague*, 72-73. Most often the pattern among 'physician-theologians' was to first study medicine and then theology. See Courtenay, 'Curers of Body and Soul'.

58 PC Dauphine of Puimichel, 242-43.

59 Ziegler, 'Practitioners and Saints'. The role of physicians in canonization inquests increased in the early modern period; for this development, see Bouley, *Pious Postmortems*, and Duffin, *Medical Miracles*. See pp. 127-28 below for further discussion.

60 See e.g. Pomata, *Contracting a Cure*, 26-28; Siraisi, *Medieval and Early Renaissance Medicine*, 42, 120, 137.

weight to Durandus's testimony, although he had not been treating Dauphine at the time. He did not know if the contents of the article were publicly known, as he had heard about the matter in private. When he had talked about it with Dauphine, nobody else had been present, and when with the household members, other household members had been present.[61] Bertranda Bartholomea, Dauphine's *socia* for forty-seven years, did not add anything to the tenth article, but according to her, within the kingdom of Naples the matter was known in Naples, Caserta, and Ariano, and in Provence in Apt, Cabrières-d'Avignon, Ansouis, La Motte d'Aigues, and the *castrum* of Puimichel.[62] How big a role the infirmity played in this *fama* remains unclear, but as Dauphine's illness was recorded in her Occitan *Vie*, it undoubtedly held some significance for a larger group of devotees later on. The text does not refer to any pretence of illness but records that she really was ill and doctors feared for her life.[63] The canonization inquest of 1363 was held before the composition of Dauphine's *Lives*,[64] so the author omitted the varying tones of the narrative, which obviously would not have served his purpose.

The article and the testimonies portray Dauphine's infirmity as the catalyst for the sanctity of both spouses, implying that it was God-sent. The gift promised to God to obtain the cure in the manner of miracle narratives was from Elzéar when he renounced his rights as the husband; only later on was his heart enlightened to truly value this decision.[65] Unfortunately, Elzéar's canonization hearing survives only as a summary, and we do not know if this matter was brought up by the witnesses – Dauphine being among them.[66] Although Elzéar's Latin *vita* describes at length his conversion to

61 PC Dauphine of Puimichel, 249.

62 PC Dauphine of Puimichel, 303-4.

63 *Vie, Dauphine*, 154-55.

64 For the dating of Dauphine's *Lives*, see the introduction to *Vie, Dauphine*, on p. 18.

65 See Kelly, *Performing Virginity*; Lewis, 'Male Saints and Devotional Masculinity in Late Medieval England', 119-20, for the fluidity and importance of male virginity and celibacy; for laymen and sanctity in general, see the articles in the compilation, Cullum and Lewis (eds.), *Religious Men and Masculine Identity in the Middle Ages*, and for St. Elzéar specifically, Weissenberg, 'What man are you?' For Elzéar's sanctity, his virginity and 'monklike' lifestyle were crucial. Although he was a secular leader, his leadership appears subdued in representations of his sanctity. André Vauchez writes of him that one cannot even talk 'of the penitential ideal, since the goal he set himself was not the expiation of his faults at the cost of some renunciations but the preservation of his impeccability'. Vauchez, *Sainthood*, 363.

66 See 'Le sommaire de l'enquete pour la canonisation de s. Elzear de Sabran, TOF (d. 1323)', ed. Cambell, 445. Dauphine played an active role in the canonization process of Elzéar. One of the witnesses in her hearing reported her intelligence and capability when she was in Rome promoting the case. PC Dauphine of Puimichel, 539.

chastity and how he came to terms with the decision, Dauphine's infirmity is not mentioned,[67] and his Occitan *Vie* does not record the illness after the wedding. As discussed by Dyan Elliott, virginity appears to have held less importance for Elzéar than for Dauphine, mostly marking the beginning of his saintly and mystic path. At the same time, the balance of their spirituality is noteworthy.[68]

The other famous late medieval female lay saint in whose *fama* a wish for chastity and infirmity interlink was St. Frances of Rome (1384-1440), originally Francesca Bussa di Ponziani. She was born to a noble family of Paolo Bussa and Iacobella Roffredeschi. At the age of 12 she was married to Lorenzo Ponziani, the son of a wealthy family from Trastevere in Rome and commander of the papal troops. Later on, Frances became an important pious figure among the Roman upper class, especially among residents of Trastevere and Campitelli; she practised charity and founded the monastery of Tor de' Specchi, the home of the Oblates of St. Frances, where she moved after Lorenzo's death in 1436.[69]

The first process to establish Frances's sanctity is dated 8 August 1440, only five months after her death, which meant that there were many people who had known her and who could testify about her virtues – this being specifically mentioned in the documents. The first hearing, conducted between 21 September and 18 November, was based on 140 articles. The second hearing was conducted in 1443 based on 75 articles, and the third one, between 5 and 19 April in 1451, based on 151 articles. In addition, a few testimonies from 1453 are included in the dossiers.[70] Frances was eventually canonized in 1608 by Pope Paul V. Despite the short time frame of the three inquests, there is little continuity in them. In the first hearing, the articles and testimonies were somewhat vague in their formulation. Many times the testimonies

67 'Vita s. Elzearii de Sabrano, conf.', *AASS*, Sept. VII, 540-41.

68 In addition to initiating the chastity, Dauphine taught her husband to read, which was not exceptional among lay nobility, and also taught him the Hours of the Virgin and the Divine Office. Elliott, *Spiritual Marriage*, 289-90. Furthermore, Bertrandus Iusberti testified that before his death Elzéar had said that he himself was a bad man saved by a good woman. PC Dauphine of Puimichel, 205.

69 For a biography of Frances, see Esch, 'Francesca Bussa, santa', in *Dizionario Biografico degli Italiani*, XLIX (1997), www.treccani.it/enciclopedia/santa-francesca-bussa_%28Dizionario-Biografico%29/ (accessed 20 May 2018). For the wealth of the Ponziani family, see e.g. Esch, 'Die Zeugenaussagen', 120-23.

70 Esch, 'I processi medioevali', 40-41. On Frances's canonization and cult, see Bartolomei Romagnoli and Picasso (eds.), *La canonizzazione di santa Francesca Romana*; Bartolomei Romagnoli (ed.), *Francesca Romana: la santa, il monastero e la città alla fine del Medioevo* Esch, 'Die Zeugenaussagen'.

were grouped, and new questions were sometimes added during the course of the interrogations. The hearings of 1443 and 1451 were better organized and also present Frances more as a conventional saint.[71] In his analysis of the witnesses in the canonization proceedings, Arnold Esch has shown that both the witnesses and the miracle beneficiaries in the hearing come from a politically specific group of people; most of them were members of the pro-Colonna nobility who participated in governing the last free commune of Rome (1395-98), or from families who had belonged to the popular party who lived in Trastevere and Campitelli, where most of the miracles investigated had occurred. As already mentioned in the Introduction, the majority of the witnesses to Frances's life were oblates of Tor de' Specchi.[72]

The second article in Frances's first two hearings is about her adolescence. As in the case of Dauphine, she is reported to have decided to live as a virgin, but her father decided she should marry. After moving to her husband's house, she was seized by a severe infirmity, so that she could neither take in food nor move herself, and it was eventually believed she would die. At some point a *malefica* came in, wanting to treat her with sorcery, which she refused. In the end, she had, quite appropriately, a vision of St. Alexis, who asked if she wanted to be cured. To this Frances replied yes, if it pleases the Lord. She woke up fully healed.[73] The couple had three children, Battista, Evangelista, and Agnese, and started to abstain from sex only twelve years before Lorenzo's death.[74] Several witnesses were mentioned as having given testimony to the article, most of them intimate with the saint, but as usual in this source, they do not add new information to the article. Nevertheless, the number of witnesses who had known Frances personally, as well as the remarks of some of them who had heard about the matter from elsewhere, show that this dramatic beginning to Frances and Lorenzo's marital life was a known aspect of Frances's *fama sanctitatis* in their circle, if not among the larger public. Frances's infirmity had an important role in explaining and justifying her controversial sanctity as a married, societally active laywoman

71 Esch, 'I processi medioevali', 41-43, 47-48; according to Esch, this is even more pronounced in the frescoes of Tor de' Specchi, in which Frances's role as a noble citizen of Rome was erased.

72 Esch, 'Die Zeugenaussagen', esp. 96-97, 107-8; see also Esposito, 'St. Francesca and the Female Religious Communities', 197-99.

73 *I processi inediti per Francesca Bussa dei Ponziani* (*santa Francesca Romana*), ed. Lugano (PC Frances of Rome), 10. See Elliott, *Spiritual Marriage*, 223, on the redemptive element of the vision of St. Alexis, and also Golinelli, '*Velut alter Alexius*', 146.

74 PC Frances of Rome, 10-11. Although the process of 1451 investigated her decision to remain a virgin and her reluctance to marry, her illness is not mentioned in the article or testimonies. PC Frances of Rome, 226.

who had children, especially as God decided to heal her through the merits of St. Alexis so that she could go on living in this way. This was the case for the witnesses but possibly also for Frances herself, as here again she had been the one to inform the witnesses about the matter. In Dauphine's case, on the other hand, the infirmity was equally important in highlighting the divine will that she and Elzéar would remain virgins.

Frances's illness also had further connotations. The *vita* written by Frances's confessor Johannes Matteotti connects her own infirmity at the beginning of her marriage to her charitable actions towards other infirm people, for which she was famous, as he writes that 'after she was restored to good health, she started to administer care to other infirm people'.[75] While a similar direct connection is missing from the canonization processes, they investigated her charity at length.[76] As will be discussed further in this book, she was a known benefactor and medical practitioner among the sick of her circle, as her spiritual daughters, daughter-in-law, and other people testified. Some of these accounts connect her own later infirmity with her charitable actions.[77] Therefore it appears that for her followers and devotees, her own infirmities indeed had a role in her charity, which in turn largely marked her sainthood.

Although there are no examples in the canonization processes, it was not rare for a male saint to marry or enter into a carnal relationship reluctantly, and infirmity could also help them to fulfil their wishes. One earlier saint in whose *vita* this idea is pronounced is St. Alfred (d. 899). According to his legend, as a young man he realized that he was unable to resist the temptations of the flesh, and he therefore prayed to God that He would bring some illness upon him which would make this possible but which would allow him to continue in his duties. As a result, he was struck by a painful condition during his wedding feast. Alfred's recorded experience resonated with many men in subsequent centuries, and his case was strongly promoted by King Henry VI of England (r. 1422-61), presumably, as suggested by Katherine J. Lewis, because of his own ill health.[78] The ability to resist the temptations of the flesh was one of the key elements of male saints' sanctity,[79] and infirmity could be used to achieve this goal as well.

75 'Acta Francisca Romana vidua', *AASS*, Mar. II, 92: 'Postquam autem pristine sanitati reddita est, aliorum infirmorum copeit curam genere.'

76 PC Frances of Rome, 33-36, 234-37.

77 See pp. 162-64 below.

78 Lewis, 'Imitate, too, this king in virtue', 142.

79 For example, Alison More points out that in the accounts of the physical aspect of conversion, the physicality of men was commonly depicted as resisting sexual temptation, whereas for women

The married female saints and their hagiographers, but most likely also those venerating them, had to find a way to negotiate their corporality, marriage, and sainthood. In their case, infirmity could act as a convincing proof of their unwillingness to consummate a marriage when they were unable to decide for themselves. It was portrayed as an agent that helped to determine their path to holiness. Similarly, healing, which occurred at God's wish, served a purpose in making the path to sainthood explicit. I will address the theme of living saints and attempts to heal their bodily ailments later in this book, but already in the cases discussed above a clear pattern is visible. A healing was portrayed not as being initiated by a wish to remove bodily discomfort or incapacity, but as a process justified by and leading to the saintly path. In a way these healings are comparable with the miraculous cures of saints' devotees. Their healed state was often defined precisely by their ability to fulfil their social roles,[80] which was the primary definition of health in premodern society.[81] For saints, the corresponding social role was their holiness.

accounts of illness were not uncommon. More, 'Convergence, Conversion, and Transformation', 37. Although it is clear that the depictions of male saint's tribulations with their sexuality were fairly common, in my opinion the various accounts of male saints' physical infirmities to some extent diminish the bodily differences between male and female saints in conversion narratives. See also Weissenberg, 'What man are you?', 121.

80 See e.g. Kuuliala, 'Heavenly Healing or a Failure of Faith?'

81 Gentilcore, *Healers and Healing*, 185-86.

Patientia and the Borders of Holy Infirmity

Abstract

Saintly patience towards earthly tribulations is one of the key characteristics of saints' lives, and it was frequently investigated in canonization inquests. The tribulations could include, for example, deaths of loved ones or troubles with earthly rulers. In most canonization inquests the topic of bodily infirmity, especially the saintly candidate's patient attitude towards it, was also investigated. However, the way such patience comes up in the process varies greatly: it could be used and investigated to highlight aspects of a saint's life that the witnesses and the conductors of the hearing considered important, such as preaching, spiritual raptures, or earthly duties. Here the saint's gender and status in society and the geographic origins of their cult all played major roles.

Keywords: hagiography, sainthood, patience, suffering, mysticism

Of the characteristics attributed to saints, the one which is most closely connected to their non-self-inflicted bodily suffering is *patientia*, patience. It means the saint's acceptance of various earthly tribulations and is closely linked to their *imitatio Christi*, often also to their raptures and other spiritual experiences. *Patientia* is among the key features in the *articuli* of the canonization hearings. Depending on the process in question, the aspects of the saints' patience that were accentuated and the importance physical suffering had in them varied.[1] It is often quite difficult to deduce the origin of the dissimilarities between various processes or between individual witness accounts, that is, whether they were the choice of the procurators or commissioners or a result of the communal negotiations regarding their

1 On patience and sanctity, see Bynum, *Holy Feast and Holy Fast*, 102-4. On patience at large, see Waugh, *Genre of Medieval Patience Literature*.

Kuuliala, Jenni, *Saints, Infirmity, and Community in the Late Middle Ages*.
Taylor & Francis Group 2020
DOI: 10.5117/9789462983373_PATIE

holiness and therefore inherent in the saint's *fama*. Since the two factors constantly interacted, both had an influence on how much weight was given to the saint's infirmity and how it was reconstructed in the hearing. As will be shown in the discussion below, it is evident, however, that the saint's social status, the events of their life, their gender, and their geographic origin all played an important role in the emphases the commissioners and the witnesses gave to bodily infirmity.

(Un)diagnosing Holy Illness and Impairment

Although there was a common tendency to highlight the suffering of female saints, for individual communities of devotees, as well as those promoting a candidate's sainthood, the matter was not straightforward. Suffering could either be highlighted or play a side role, regardless of the holy person's gender. As an example of 'non-suffering' male saints, the patience of St. Thomas Aquinas (process held in Naples and Fossanova, 1319/21)[2] and St. Yves of Tréguier (1253-1303)[3] was proven by their attitude to other types of hardships; in their case tolerating ill health was only essential at the time of their final illnesses. Thomas Aquinas's sainthood was occasionally constructed through his corporality, largely through his big size and beauty, and his devotion to the crucified Christ was constructed through his vision and understanding of it, but not through his own suffering.[4] As for St. Yves, for saintly secular priests corporality was not an essential factor in their sanctity, although it is possible that geography plays a role as Yves could be labelled a northern saint.[5] As will be shown below, infirmity was not always as minor a factor for male saints as it was for Aquinas and St. Yves, and it could be emphasized.

It is perhaps more surprising that there are some female saints whose canonization records are also relatively silent about bodily suffering. St.

2 *Processus canonizationis s. Thomae, Neapoli*, ed. Laurent (PC Thomas Aquinas), 287, 332, 378-79. For Thomas, his canonization and later veneration, see e.g. Gigon, 'Histoire de la canonisation de s. Thomas d'Aquin'; Räsänen, 'Making a Saint for the Monastery of Fossanova'; Räsänen, *Thomas Aquinas's Relics*.

3 See e.g. *Processus de vita et miraculis sancti Yvonis*, ed. De La Borderie and others (PC Yves of Tréguier), 17, 25, 50, 57, 62, 66-67, and pp. 151-52 below for further discussion. Yves was of noble origin, born to the family of Helori, lord of Kermartin. He studied civil law at the University of Paris and canon law at the University of Orleans. He became the *officialis* of Rennes and later of the bishop of Tréguier. The canonization inquest was conducted in Tréguier, and he was canonized in 1347 by Clement VI. See also Cassard, *Saint Yves de Tréguier*.

4 Räsänen, *Thomas Aquinas's Relics*, 42-44, 238-39.

5 Vauchez, *Sainthood*, 260, 313-14.

Margaret of Hungary was a mendicant saint known for austerity and extreme devotional practices. However, her canonization records show very little sign of interest in somatic ailments, even though they record that she was ill for a long time before her death.[6] The matter seems to have held some importance for the nuns testifying in the inquest, but the view of those conducting the hearing appears otherwise, as they did not further investigate the infirmity the nuns referred to.[7] Overall, the process is exceptional in its relatively little focus on *patientia*; Margaret's devotion, humility, and asceticism were examined much more carefully. Another example is St. Birgitta of Sweden (1303-73). Her canonization inquest (Sweden, Spoleto, Naples, and Rome, 1376-80)[8] focuses on her revelations, charity, attempts to promote the moral reform of the church, and the numerous miracles. Although there are hints here and there that she had some infirmities, they are never the focus, and even the *articuli* are concerned with the deaths of her loved ones and some earthly tribulations. Only when recording her patience at the time of her final illness and death do they touch on the issue of infirmity.[9]

An individual hearing may thus have paid very little attention to a holy figure's bodily infirmities, even if it records that they occurred. At the same time, in some saints' cases the infirmity manifesting *patientia* was delineated by corporeal and spiritual characteristics. One of the saints in whose canonization inquest bodily infirmity is clearly articulated is St. Nicholas of Tolentino (1245-1305). As an Italian eremitical saint, corporality was an important part of his *fama*. Nicholas was a priest and a member of

6 PC Margaret of Hungary, 184-85.

7 The witnesses to Margaret's life were primarily nuns of her convent at the Rabbit island on the Danube, nowadays known as Margit island. Margaret had been given up to the Dominican monastery as a young child. It has been estimated that the establishment could have housed seventy nuns and servants; thirty-nine of them testified. Although the convent was supposed to enable a world of renunciation, there was a constant royal presence on the island. Klaniczay, *Holy Rulers and Blessed Princesses*, 261. For further discussion of her devotion and humility in taking care of other sisters, see pp. 158-59 below.

8 The most comprehensive study on the process is Nyberg, 'Canonization Process of St. Birgitta of Sweden'.

9 *Acta et processus canonizacionis beate Birgitte*, ed. Collijn (PC Birgitta of Sweden), 17-18, 20-21. As one of the most famous saints of our period, St. Birgitta, her cult, miracles, canonization, and revelations have been the subject of numerous studies. See e.g. J. Adams, *Revelations of St. Birgitta*; Fanous, 'Becoming the Theotokos'; Fröjmark, *Mirakler och helgonkult*; Katajala-Peltomaa, 'Bishops Fighting with Demons in Swedish Canonization Processes'; Heβ, *Heilige machen*, 99-204; Katajala-Peltomaa, 'Fatherhood, Masculinity and Lived Religion in Late Medieval Sweden'; Krötzl, *Pilger, Mirakel und Alltag*; Morris, *St. Birgitta of Sweden*; Nieuwland, 'Motherhood and Sanctity in the Life of Saint Birgitta of Sweden'; Nyberg, 'Canonization Process of St. Birgitta of Sweden'; Sahlin, *Birgitta of Sweden and the Voice of Prophecy*; Salmesvuori, *Power and Sainthood*.

the Hermits of St. Augustine, ordained in 1270. He was a popular miracle-worker and enjoyed a wide reputation as a living saint in Tolentino and the surrounding areas of Marche, where, although living apart from other monks of the monastery of Tolentino, he 'lived [his] religious experience in a communal context'.[10] His canonization process was conducted in 1325, but he was officially canonized by a fellow Augustinian, Pope Eugene IV, only in 1446.[11]

The protocols of Nicholas's hearing provide a fine example of how those conducting the inquest and the community of the devotees could differ in their construction of the corporeal elements of a person's sainthood. The dossiers concerning Nicholas's *vita* are structured around twenty-two articles. Article 16 states that he was 'patient and of calm spirit' in his bodily infirmities, not hindered by the 'many diabolic temptations and impediments'.[12] Although attacks of demons were an important aspect of the lives of heroic desert fathers, providing a model for later ascetics and monastics,[13] connecting bodily infirmity and diabolic temptation in such a manner is exceptional in the canonization processes of the era.[14] The topic of physical wounds caused by demons or the devil was expanded on in the twentieth article, which records the saint's battles with demons at length. It records that once the devil entered his house, found him praying, and attacked him with blows so numerous that scars were seen on his body for several days.[15]

Wounds received at the hands of demons or the devil have a multilayered hagiographic meaning, since enduring them and battling malign spirits and the devil were both ways of following Christ.[16] In the sources of this study, the process of St. Frances of Rome is the most elaborate in examining this side of

10 Vauchez, *Sainthood*, 332, 335.

11 On Nicholas and his process, see Katajala-Peltomaa, *Gender, Miracles, and Daily Life*; Lett, *Un procès de canonisation*. For the canonization, see Krafft, *Papsturkunde und Heiligsprechung*, 947-54.

12 *Il processo per la canonizzazione di s. Nicola da Tolentino*, ed. Occhioni (PC Nicholas of Tolentino), 19: 'Item quod in infirmitatibus sui corporis patiens erat et benignus non obstantibus multis temptationibus et impedimentis diabolicis.'

13 Lewis, 'Male Saints and Devotional Masculinity in Late Medieval England', 113-14.

14 For Nicholas's battles with demons, see Lett, *Un procès de canonisation*, 103-5, 136. Saints were the primary, or only, true followers of Christ in these battles, and for them battling against demons was one aspect of their *imitatio Christi*. For an overview of this topic, see Dinzelbacher, 'Der Kampf der Heiligen mit den Dämonen'.

15 PC Nicholas of Tolentino, 20: 'Tertio: quod per ostium domus loci, in qua dictus Nicolaus habitabat, diabolus cum furia et terrore intrans et ad dictum orantem accessit ipsumque verberibus sic afflixit, quod per multos dies vulnerum cicatrices in toto suo corpore apparebant.'

16 Although not very common, being literally wounded by a demon or the devil had its precursors in earlier hagiographic literature. See Dinzelbacher, 'Der Kampf der Heiligen mit den Dämonen', 662-66.

sainthood, as her battles with demons were an important aspect of her *fama*, recorded by her confessor Johannes Matteotti and depicted in the frescoes of Tor de' Specchi.[17] The processes of 1440 and 1443 examine an incident where demons attacked her while she was reading 'scripturas divinas' in the secret chamber in her family's house. The witnesses to this assault were Johannes, Frances's spiritual daughters Rita Covelli and Jacobella de Brunomonte, and *frater* Ypolitus. The demons threw ashes on her and struck her face so that she looked like a 'monster'; Rita Covelli testified that her face was so 'bruised and beaten' that she hardly recognized her.[18] However, unlike in Nicholas of Tolentino's inquest, the numerous attacks of demons were not otherwise connected with Frances's infirmities and even this attack was not reported as causing any long-term scars or symptoms.

The witness accounts given in Nicholas's inquest give a picture of his deteriorating health towards the end of his life, either through old problems worsening or new ones multiplying.[19] Usually the witnesses mentioned his difficulties in walking, or his need to walk with a stick.[20] Unlike in most other processes analysed in this book, in Nicholas's hearing quite a large array of laypeople, both men and women, gave a short testimony about his *fama sanctitatis*. Most of these witnesses belonged to the Guelph elite of the area, so again, they are from a restricted group of people.[21] Their views about a saint's *fama* were largely formatted into a pattern by the notaries, while the mass of devotees was excluded from enunciating Nicholas's *fama* and its characteristics, even if they shared the witnesses' view of it.[22]

In the articles of the hearing, Nicholas's infirmity was divided into two separate sections to prove two aspects of his sanctity, but his devotees did not necessarily make such a distinction. Regardless of whether they were

17 The frescoes have recently been analysed in Scanlan, *Divine and Demonic Imagery at Tor de'Specchi*. Unfortunately I did not get her work in time to use it in the present study.

18 PC Frances of Rome, 55-56; Rita's testimony states: 'facies vero beate adeo erat infecta et percussa quod ipsa testis vix eam cognoscebat; apparebat eius faceis cuiusdam monstri et eius vestimenta non muliebria sed quoddam ludibrium apparebant'.

19 An Augustinian friar called Thomas de Mathelica testified that he had known Nicholas for only six months before his death, but he specified that the holy man had had 'infirmities especially in his tibias'; PC Nicholas of Tolentino, 546. A *frater* named Guillermus, for his part, testified to the sixteenth article, stating that he too had seen Nicholas infirm *pluries et pluries*. PC Nicholas of Tolentino, 463.

20 Although this can be read as an indication of his final, fatal illness, hagiographic texts frequently indicate a condition severely affecting the person's mobility or bodily strength by referring to the need for an aid of some kind. See e.g. Kuuliala, *Childhood Disability*, 48-50.

21 For the selection of witnesses, see Lett, *Un procès de canonisation*.

22 Lett, 'La parole des humbles', 238.

testifying to article 16 or to article 20, most witnesses referring to Nicholas's infirmity did not mention its origins or specific diagnosis at all.[23] An exception was an 80-year-old man, Mancinus Fortis de Castro Sancti Angeli.[24] Mancinus was born around 1245 and was therefore of similar age to the saint himself. He had known of Nicholas for seventy years and more. In his testimony to the sixteenth article, Mancinus reported that he saw Nicholas in a state of infirmity 'dozens of times'.[25] In this part of his testimony, Mancinus stated that he had been acquainted with Nicholas for thirty years and had never seen him disturbed by or lamenting any impairment that he had. Instead of referring to demons, Mancinus specified *gutta salza* as the infirmity Nicholas suffered from, reporting that he had a great wound in his shin, and that the saint himself had said that God gave him this wound. He gave testimony to article 20 as well, but only confirmed its contents based on what he had heard.[26] The other witnesses who mentioned the onset of Nicholas's infirmity or wounds referred to the demonic battles. Only one of them mentioned any long-term effects of these incidents. *Frater* Iohannucius de Tholentino, who had been Nicholas's infirmarian for two years, testified that Nicholas had asked for his help because he was so badly beaten by the devil. The commissioners asked if Iohannucius had seen the wounds, and he described black swellings, particularly in his upper body. In answer to the next question, he said that Nicholas had lain burdened ('gravatus') by them for twenty days.[27]

23 For the vagueness of testimonies to article 20, see Lett, *Un procès de canonisation*, 104; see also Boureau, *Satan the Heretic*, 136.

24 For Mancinus, see Lett, *Un procès de canonisation*, 347, 367. His deposition is in PC Nicholas of Tolentino, 250-61. On witnesses of such advanced ages, see Krötzl, '*Sexaginta vel circa*'.

25 PC Nicholas of Tolentino, 256: 'vidit eum pluries et pluries in infirmitatibus suis ut supra dixit'.

26 PC Nicholas of Tolentino, 256-57. *Gutta salza* [sic], 'salty gout', is a very rare condition in canonization records, and the only other reference I have come across concerns a miraculous healing of a skin condition. In the hearing of Lawrence of Subiaco, a boy was cured of a condition which some thought to be *gutta salsa*, some *phlegma salsa* ('salty phlegm'), and some *vero lepra* ('true leprosy'). The inquest survives in the Archivio Apostolico Vaticano MS Archivum Arcis, Arm. 1, XVIIII, 3328 and has been (partly) edited in Benedict XIV (Prospero Lambertini), *De servorum Dei beatificatione et Beatorum canonizatione* (PC Lawrence Loricatus), 676-77. See pp. 117-18 below. Furthermore, in the *vita* of pope Celestine V (Peter of Morrone), a boy was cured of *gutta salsa*, which caused ulcers to appear all over his body, 'as if he was leprosus' (*Die ältesten Viten Papst Cölestins V. (Peters vom Morrone)*, ed. Herde, 177) and the thirteenth-century *vita* of Blessed Umiliana of Cerchi by Vito of Cortona describes the cure of a boy and explains that his illness was called *papici* in the vernacular language, or *ignis volatilis*, and otherwise *gutta salsa*. 'Vita, Aemiliana seu Humiliana', *AASS*, Maii IV, 396. This is also the only reference to *gutta salsa* given in Du Cange et al., *Glossarium mediae et infimae latinitatis*, IV, col. 142c.

27 PC Nicholas of Tolentino, 482-83. *Frater* Augustinus also testified to having seen wounds all over Nicholas's body. PC Nicholas of Tolentino, 565.

Spreading information about Nicholas's wounds and the battles with the devil are intriguing from the point of view of spreading his saintly *fama*. The information of those witnesses who mentioned this aspect of his life originated among the members of the saint's order,[28] but lay members of the community could be active as well. According to Iohannucius, as well as Ventura de Tholentino (also from Nicholas's order), the holy man wanted to keep the battles with the devil a secret, but it turns out that the order was willing to distribute information about them.[29] How widely this idea had spread in the local community, or how often Nicholas's general infirmity was interpreted as being of diabolic origin, is hard to know, as the information comes from clerical or, in rare cases, lay elite witnesses. The testimony of the notary Berardus Appillaterre, whose family members were some of the most faithful, if not *the* most faithful, devotees of the saint and significant distributors of his *fama*,[30] further illustrates the order's actions. Berardus testified that he had seen the scars made by the devil. The commissioners wanted to know how this was possible, and Berardus explained how four years before Nicholas's death, one brother of the order, who had come to ask Berardus's wife Margarita for some bread, had told him about them. Berardus had followed the brother to visit Nicholas, and there they, with the help of the prior, had persuaded the reluctant saint to show them the scars.[31] This is a telling, albeit somewhat rare, example of a saint's lay devotee (who was not a servant) actively searching for information about the corporeal side of sainthood as well as interpreting and distributing it. As will be demonstrated below, most often this kind of information came from people who had been residing with the saint and had somehow taken part in their daily, corporeal experience.

28 For instance, Nucius Rogerii de Sancto Angelo reported that he had got his information about the wounds' diabolic origin from Nicholas's associates; PC Nicholas of Tolentino, 550.

29 PC Nicholas of Tolentino, 403-4, 482-83.

30 Berardus Appillaterre was a notary who had been an official in many other Italian cities. Berardus and his wife Margarita were well acquainted with Nicholas, although the testimonies often emphasize Margarita's role, and he performed miracles on several of their children, both *in vita* and after his death. The family and their relationship with the saint have been extensively analysed in Katajala-Peltomaa, *Gender, Miracles, and Daily Life*, 124-28, 256-62, and in Lett, *Un procès de canonisation*, 392-97. The testimonies of Berardus and his daughters Berardescha and Ceccha Appillaterre are in PC Nicholas of Tolentino, 116-30, 235-47. For example, Iohannucius de Tholentino, the *infirmarius* of Nicholas, reported that he had heard about the saint's *fama* precisely from Berardus Appillaterre and his daughters. Another witness, Dina Angeli, reported that her source of information about Nicholas's *fama* was Margarita, as did even one of the friars, Augustinus de Tholentino. PC Nicholas of Tolentino, 270, 478, 562.

31 PC Nicholas of Tolentino, 121-22.

It seems that the idea of diabolic wounds and the stress on battles with the devil and demons primarily originated from the requirements of the inquiry.[32] In spreading the information about the wounds and the battles as a part of Nicholas's holy life, his order was first and foremost responding to the concerns of the church. The church questioned and investigated the meaning of the battle between the hermit and the devil to determine whether its violence was caused by authentic sanctity or sinful nature,[33] and this seems to have been the case in Nicholas's inquiry. The deposition of the infirmarian Iohannucius de Tholentino is one proof of the commissioners' requirements. Although Nicholas was known to have been infirm for a long time, and although the topic comes up often in the testimonies, the infirmarian was interrogated more intensely about the physical aftermath of the diabolic battle than about article 16, whose contents were less controversial.[34]

Especially for the 'ordinary' devotees who venerated Nicholas as a saint and beneficiaries or witnesses to his thaumaturgic abilities, his infirmity was crucial as a widely known sign of his patience. At the same time, its origins held little significance for them. Presumably the commissioners did not even interrogate them about the details of the holy man's infirmity, because of their status as witnesses, and because witnesses were asked only the questions they were thought to know the answers to.[35] Furthermore, lack of interest in aetiology is typical in all medieval hagiographic material,[36] and this was even more so in the case of saints themselves. It has been argued that as the use of medical language and expertise in medical and non-medical contexts increased in late medieval society, there was 'a rise of medicalization'. However, this medieval 'medicalization' differed from that in the modern world, which pathologizes human variation. As Julia Singer writes, 'the use of medical language does not necessarily imply a concession of authority to the medical domain'.[37] The testimonies to St. Nicholas's infirmity are a fine example of the twofold nature of this medicalization process. As will be discussed later in this chapter, visions and raptures were increasingly investigated and differentiated from somatic conditions in medical terms, and physicians were often present at testimonies about saints'

32 See Lett, *Un procès de canonisation*, 105.

33 Vauchez, *Sainthood*, 331.

34 His testimony to article 16 is in PC Nicholas of Tolentino, 481.

35 See Katajala-Peltomaa, *Gender, Miracles, and Daily Life*, 39.

36 On this aspect in earlier hagiography, see Sigal, *L'Homme et le miracle*, 228, and for later medieval canonization processes, Kuuliala, *Childhood Disability*, 44-48.

37 McVaugh, *Medicine before the Plague*, 190; Singer, *Blindness and Therapy*, 7-8.

ascetic habits and final illnesses.[38] At the communal level, similar precision or medicalization was rarely of importance in the case of other types of infirmities manifesting sainthood, and whether or not the medical domain received any authority varied greatly. In Nicholas's hearing, Mancinus Fortis was the only one giving an exact diagnosis, and he appears to have reported it on his own initiative. Furthermore, as Nicholas's infirmarian as well as the brother of the *medicus* of his monastery were not asked about the matter,[39] it seems evident that the commissioners did not consider the precise nature of his condition important either. However, when the case was brought to the papal curia, the exact nature of the infirmity which Nicholas endured with *patientia* was considered important. In the *relatio* of the process, drawn by Cardinal Guillermo Godin, his testimony is quoted at length and his statement about the name of the infirmity and the wounds is repeated verbatim.[40]

As corporality was important for Italian eremitical sainthood, it is no surprise that the other male saint whose infirmity was a very important aspect of his sanctity to his devotees was John Buoni. Nevertheless, the records of his inquest show that even in the case of eremitical saints the meanings given to bodily infirmity varied. The brothers testifying in his inquest gave uniform reports about his infirmity during the last years of his life, which manifested itself in *fluxum sanguinis*. As a sign of its severity, many of them specifically mentioned the cloth he wore under his habit to prevent the blood from ruining it.[41] The Bollandists define John Buoni's illness as haemorrhoids, which was a serious threat in medieval medicine and, perhaps consequently, a condition that got lot of attention in medical treatises and other types of writings. Then again, the symptoms could also denote dysentery.[42] The diagnosis was, in the end, left vague, as the brothers simply testified that John showed *patientia* at the time of his tribulations. Probably they counted his infirmity as one of these tribulations, but they specified its type and symptoms when talking about his clothes and his asceticism, including his refusal to use medical help (discussed later in this

38 See pp. 152-53 below. Making a distinction between a spiritual and a somatic ailment also became important in the case of demonic possession. See Katajala-Peltomaa, *Demonic Possession and Lived Religion*.

39 See PC Nicholas of Tolentino, 221, 478-82.

40 Vatican City, Biblioteca Apostolica Vaticana (BAV), MS Vat. lat. 4027, fol. 8r.

41 'Processus apostolici, de b. Joanne Buono', *AASS*, Oct. IX, 816, 822, 823, 831, 842.

42 'Processus apostolici, de b. Joanne Buono', *AASS*, Oct. IX, 839; for haemorrhoids and dysentery, see DeMaitre, *Medieval Medicine*, 260-65, 270-75; Siraisi, *Medieval and Early Renaissance Medicine*, 183.

book).[43] Their statements are rather similar in form, which undoubtedly derives partly from the notarial process of writing them down. It is also likely that the community of brothers, who had lived with the holy man for years or even decades and who actively promoted his canonization,[44] had formed a collective memory of the meanings given to his infirmity.

Again, it is impossible to ascertain how much of the emphasis given precisely to the connection of asceticism and infirmity stems from the communal memory and how much derives from the way the canonization inquest, which was an early one, was conducted. The articles do not record any details about John Buoni's life, and as the Bollandists point out in their introduction to the process, in the first inquiry there was much more interest in his miracles *post mortem* than in his life.[45] Nevertheless, comparisons between all the processes referred to above show that the weight of saints' infirmities investigated under *patientia* did not lie in their definitions or diagnoses, but in the varying religious, cultural, and legal meanings given to them.

Perhaps the most influential type of sainthood from the point of view of infirmity and suffering is mendicant sainthood. In the cults of saints associated with Franciscans and Dominicans suffering was often emphasized, especially in the case of female saints, although St. Francis and St. Dominic did not promote the search for suffering for its own sake.[46] Emphasizing physical suffering in the case of these female saints was not automatic or without exception, however. St. Elizabeth of Hungary has been called one of the first members of the Third Order of St. Francis, founded in 1221, but this has been strongly questioned.[47] Nevertheless, canonized in 1235, she became one of the most famous saints associated with the Franciscans, with charity towards the sick and poor being the most celebrated element of her sainthood. She was a 'role model' for many other royal women of the time, as well as for future aspiring female saints.[48] As she was not a nun, she was able to 'best [realize] the ideal of St. Francis in this sphere'.[49] Elizabeth was only 24 at

43 'Processus apostolici, de b. Joanne Buono', *AASS*, Oct. IX, 822, 823, 831, 840.

44 See pp. 135-36 below.

45 'Proemium ad processus in causa canonizationis b. Joannis Boni confectos', *AASS*, Oct. IX, 769.

46 Vauchez, *Sainthood*, 350.

47 See e.g. Wolf, ed. and trans., *The Life and Afterlife of St. Elizabeth of Hungary*, 69, n. 133.

48 On Elizabeth and her importance, see Bartlett, *Why Can the Dead Do Such Great Things?*, 71-76; Wolf, ed. and trans., *The Life and Afterlife of St. Elizabeth*; Elliott, *Proving Woman*, 85-116; Klaniczay, *Holy Rulers and Blessed Princesses*; Klaniczay, 'Saint Elizabeth: A European Saint'; Klaniczay, 'Sainte Élisabeth comme modèle'.

49 Vauchez, *Sainthood*, 375. In the late medieval Italian hagiographies, both her and St. Margaret of Hungary's royal background were emphasized, even though this was precisely what they had tried to avoid. Klaniczay, *Holy Rulers and Blessed Princesses*, 385-86.

the time of her death, and so it is perhaps not surprising that the testimonies to her life given by her handmaids in 1235, the *Dicta quatuor ancillarum*, include little information about any long-term infirmities.[50] Admittedly, there are occasional references to the bodily aspects of Elizabeth's sanctity, in particular the punishments she endured at the hands of her infamous confessor Conrad of Marburg.[51] Despite his enthusiastic chastising of her, Conrad of Marburg did not highlight Elizabeth's infirmity in his *Summa vitae*, sent to the curia to promote her canonization, beyond the discomfort her extreme charity caused her.[52] Only one of the handmaids, Irmingard, testified that often when Elizabeth was *infirmata*, she would spin wool, and if the handmaid tried to take the spindle from her hands to spare her, she would begin to pull and card the wool with bare hands in order not to appear lazy.[53] She thus used this unspecified infirmity to highlight her diligence; having been a part of her daily activities, such incidents undoubtedly held specific meaning to the servants, although they were not used in the official construction of her sanctity.

Chronologically, the next canonization process conducted for a female mendicant saint is that of St. Clare of Assisi (1194-1253). Her case shows more clearly how the aspects of sainthood emphasized in *vitae* and in later *fama* in general may appear somewhat different from the image given by the witnesses of the inquest. Born into a noble family as Chiara Offreduccio, Clare famously left her father's house after hearing St. Francis of Assisi's preaching and became a nun against her parents' wishes.[54] Eventually Clare became the abbess and leader of her religious order, the 'Poor Clares', under the guidance of St. Francis.[55] Because of this, the majority of witnesses to Clare's life in her 1253 canonization inquest were nuns of her order.[56] Their

50 Furthermore, the relatively lengthy testimonies of Elizabeth's handmaids on her death have little to say about any details of her final illness. See PC Elizabeth of Hungary, 138-39. *Summa vitae*, 94 (also PC Elizabeth of Hungary, 159-60), records that she was ill for twelve days before her death.

51 See p. 122 below for this incident.

52 PC Elizabeth of Hungary, 155-60; English translation in Conrad of Marburg, *Summa vitae*, ed. and trans. Wolf.

53 PC Elizabeth of Hungary, 129; for English translation, see *Dicta quatuor ancillarum*, ed. and trans. Wolf, 208.

54 The scholarship on Clare's sanctity is too vast to cite here in full. See e.g. Debby, *The Cult of St. Clare*; Knox, *Creating Clare of Assisi*; Mooney, '*Imitatio Christi* or *Imitatio Mariae*?'

55 Clare's rule itself was a combination of Francis's Later Rule and the Rule of St. Benedict, and evangelical poverty was the core of it. Knox, *Creating Clare of Assisi*, 3-4, 40-41.

56 Clare's canonization was in the interest of the church. Pope Innocent IV mentioned his belief in her sanctity already when giving her funeral mass, thus indicating a similar attitude to her as to St. Francis, in whose case no canonization inquest was even considered necessary. Cardinal Rainaldo, the protector of the Poor Clares, however intervened and persuaded the pope to take

testimony to Clare's infirmity was mostly about its connection with her death,[57] but reading between the lines reveals that the nuns remembered her suffering from ill health for quite a long time. One of them, Pacifica de Gelfutio, testified to Clare's curing five sisters of their illnesses. When the commissioners asked when this happened, she responded that it occurred before the lady herself became infirm. They then inquired exactly when St. Clare acquired this long infirmity, to which Pacifica responded that it occurred twenty-nine years earlier, which would mean 1224.[58]

Those conducting Clare's process did not use her apparently long-time infirmity in constructing her *patientia*. Instead, the process demonstrates how the witnesses could use it to highlight an aspect of sainthood that was important for their community. Based on Pacifica's testimony, Clare would have acquired some kind of infirmity at the age of 30. There are only two other references to this in the hearing. Sister Benvenuta de Peroscia reported an incident of 1240, where Saracen mercenaries of Fredrick II attacked her convent and were repelled by the brilliance of a crucifix when seeing Clare holding a monstrance. According to Benvenuta, at that time Clare was 'seriously infirm' ('gravemente inferma').[59] This aspect of the story was also recorded in Tommaso da Celano's *Vita prima beati Francisci*,[60] which helped to underscore the heroism of Clare's act. In another case, Sister Francesca de messere Capitaneo reported that once Clare was unable to get up from her bed due to her infirmity and asked for a napkin. A kitten living in the monastery brought it to her. Clare said to the animal that it would not be able to take care of such a task without letting the napkin touch the floor, but after the kitten had heard her words, it carefully carried the napkin.[61]

his view that a proper canonization inquest was useful, both to follow legal regulations and because of the possibility that there would be protests from friars about a swift canonization of a woman with a strict interpretation of Francis's rule. Knox, *Creating Clare of Assisi*, 47.

57 On Clare's death and its importance for the local community, see Knox, *Creating Clare of Assisi*, 44-45.

58 *Santa Chiara di Assisi*, ed. Boccali (PC Clare of Assisi), 446: 'Adomandata in que tempo fu che le predecte Sore fuorono liberate, disse: prima che epsa madonna se infermasse. Adomandata de che tempo incominciò ad sancta Chiara quella longha infirmità, respose che se credeva fussero vinti nove anni.'

59 PC Clare of Assisi, 452. See Debby, 'St. Clare Expelling the Saracens from Assisi', and Debby, *The Cult of St. Clare*, 24-27, for this incident, which is also a frequent theme in the iconography of Clare. Debby proposes that it can be interpreted as 'compensation' for Clare's failed attempt at martyrdom; instead, it provides another way of triumphing over the infidels. Furthermore, Fredrick II was widely hated in Franciscan circles, which explains why the story was so popular among them.

60 Debby, 'St. Clare Expelling the Saracens from Assisi', 645.

61 PC Clare of Assisi, 473.

This seemingly random instance is perhaps best interpreted in parallel with St. Francis's known affection for animals and thus a connection to Franciscan ideals, which were in turn linked to earlier hagiography and hermits' close bond with nature.[62]

As will be discussed further in this book, usually somatic and self-inflicted injuries were treated separately in the hearings, although this was not always the case. Clare's process is among the early, less thorough ones, which at least partly explains the lack of further questions regarding her infirmity. At the same time, for the nuns who had just lived with her, her infirmity – which was by no means an extraordinary matter – as well as the incidents connected to it, were still fresh in their memory. However, especially other hagiographic texts regarding her life suggest that she inflicted the injuries that made her infirm upon herself. Tommaso di Celano's *vita* mentions that long periods of excessive asceticism made Clare a subject to infirmities and caused her to lose her bodily strength,[63] and a *vita* written at the time of her canonization states that '[s]he tormented her body with different afflictions' so that '[h]er body begins to grow weak, her body is consumed/ with a long-lasting ailment'.[64] Although mendicant women differed considerably from their male counterparts in their search for tormenting their own flesh,[65] the descriptions of Clare's suffering are reminiscent of those of her spiritual father St. Francis.[66] The prominent role of infirmity in Clare's hagiography other than the canonization documents may be explained by developing Franciscan ideals and the general tendency to emphasize female saints' corporality and excessive penitence.

Regarding the corporality of sanctity, the early date of the processes of Saints Elizabeth and Clare makes them difficult to compare with the later inquests under scrutiny here. Especially in Elizabeth's process, the inquiry into her life and merits was still recorded without fully following the procedure that became established later.[67] It is nevertheless interesting from the viewpoint of gender that in neither of these inquests is the

62 See e.g. Sorrell, *St. Francis of Assisi and Nature*, 48-50.

63 Cited in Bynum, *Holy Feast and Holy Fast*, 100. Francis also tried to rein in Clare's excessive asceticism. See pp. 122-23 below for further discussion.

64 Armstrong, ed. and trans., *The Lady: Clare of Assisi; Early Documents*, 241-42. See pp. 113-14 below for this idea in the canonization testimonies.

65 Vauchez, *Sainthood*, 350.

66 See Trembinski, 'Illness and Authority', 119.

67 See Klaniczay, *Holy Rulers and Blessed Princesses*, 421, who points out that the first legend of Elizabeth after her canonization, written by Caesarius von Heisterbach, organizes the elements of her life portrayed in earlier testimonies according to the more traditional adjustments of the genre.

corporality of female mendicant saints emphasized, although it is clearly present. As pointed out by Dyan Elliott, the usage of inquisitorial procedure in the late Middle Ages resulted in the need for tangible proofs of sanctity. She writes, regarding the corporality of female spirituality, that '[a]lthough these requirements may have been more the concern of a holy woman's clerical supporters than of the woman herself, they would nevertheless make inroads into an individual woman's spirituality – if only through models of female piety already in circulation'.[68] This viewpoint is valid for the topic of the corporality of sanctity at large, male saints included, and the question should be extended to the communities of devotees. In canonization inquests there were requirements for tangible proofs of all aspects of sanctity, and the process itself educated the witnesses as well as influencing circulating models of sainthood in their communities.[69] The requirement of details regarding corporality and suffering made its way into the procedure gradually and in varying degrees.

The role of suffering in mendicant ideals is clearly visible in the cult of St. Louis IX of France, who was a great supporter of the two orders.[70] Among the male saints for whom a canonization process was opened, he is perhaps the one most closely associated with suffering, despite the obvious importance of his kingship and the ideal of the *rex justus* for his cult and canonization.[71] We have already seen how his path to becoming a saint was reportedly initiated by infirmity, and his hagiographers and those testifying about his life in the canonization inquest constructed his holy suffering through detailed depictions of a series of events that were painful for both his body and soul during and after the Seventh Crusade (1248-54). They linked the essential aspect of lay (male) sanctity, the propagation and protection of the Christian faith, to his physical hardships.[72] This makes his suffering special in the sense that it was so profoundly rooted in actual historical events. The crusade was a military fiasco and famously resulted in Louis being captured by the Muslims in 1250, freed on payment of a huge ransom and the return of Damietta.[73] Although Louis IX was the leader of the failed

68 Elliott, 'Flesh and Spirit', 33-34.

69 Smoller, in 'Defining the Boundaries of the Natural', has convincingly demonstrated how canonization inquests educated the witnesses about a proper miracle narrative, and the same is undoubtedly relevant for the ways of remembering a saint's life.

70 See Gaposchkin, 'Louis IX and Liturgical Memory'.

71 Gaposchkin, 'Boniface VIII, Philip the Fair, and the Sanctity of Louis IX'. See also Boquet and Nagy, *Medieval Sensibilities*, 166-69; Vauchez, *Sainthood*, 359-60.

72 Vauchez, *Sainthood*, 359-61.

73 Gaposchkin, 'The Captivity of Louis IX'.

crusade, the disaster enhanced his reputation.[74] The two campaigns (the seventh and eighth crusades, during which he died) are generally seen to have been the primary reasons for his coming to be considered a saint.[75]

In his surviving testimony, Charles of Anjou recounted the events of Louis's captivity and ransom, but he also gave insight into his brother's illness during this time. He described its outbreak among the army as well as its symptoms, such as suffering in teeth and gums, 'fluxum ventris', and dark spots on the tibiae or shins.[76] This illness, also recorded by Jean de Joinville in his early fourteenth-century *vita* and reported by the saint himself in a letter he wrote to his subjects,[77] has been interpreted as scurvy or dysentery, but possible diagnoses may also have included malaria, typhoid, and diphtheria.[78] In any case, its impact on the Christian army was devastating,[79] and Louis himself also fell ill with the malady. Charles gave an explicit description of its effects, stating that in 'informal moments he [Louis] showed [his] brothers extensive dark patches on one of his legs'.[80] Later on, he had to dismount from his horse several times due to the *fluxum ventris*, which he had with the other previously mentioned infirmities.[81] Shortly after this, Louis as well as his men were taken into captivity.[82] The rest of Charles's fragmentary testimony largely concerns the ransom

74 This, however, is not to say that there were no critical voices towards Louis and the whole campaign. Matthew Paris, for example, thought Louis's rapaciousness was a reason for the catastrophe, and Jean de Joinville himself expressed some criticism of Louis's actions and tactics in Damietta. Gaposchkin, 'The Captivity of Louis IX', 107.

75 Gaposchkin, 'The Place of the Crusades in the Sanctification of Louis IX', 195-96. See also Vauchez, *Sainthood*, 360.

76 *Déposition de Charles d'Anjou pour la canonisation de saint Louis*, ed. Le comte Riant, 170: 'Patiebantur autem in dentibus et gigivis, et fluxum ventris, et habebant infirmi in tibiis vel cruribus aliquam plateam nigram.'

77 Edited and translated in Jackson, *The Seventh Crusade*, 40.

78 Jackson, *The Seventh Crusade*, 115, n. 189. See also O'Tool, 'Caring for the Blind', 80.

79 Together with other problems, it forced the army to retreat. The situation rapidly deteriorated, especially after the Battle of Fāraskūr, in which the Muslim historian Sa'd al-Din Ibn Hamawiya claimed that 30,000 Franks were killed. Gaposchkin, 'The Captivity of Louis IX', 92-94.

80 For an English translation Jackson, *The Seventh Crusade*, 115; the original Latin text is in *Déposition de Charles d'Anjou pour la canonisation de saint Louis*, ed. Le comte Riant, 170: 'rex cepit illo morbo quoad omnia laborare, et plateam latam et nigram in uno crure suo fratribus familiariter ostendit'.

81 *Déposition de Charles d'Anjou pour la canonisation de saint Louis*, ed. Le comte Riant, 171: 'Et ipsa noctequa Macorra recesserunt, rex fuit multum gravatus, et oportuit eum pluries de equo descendere propter fluxum ventris quem habebat cum aliis infirmitatibus supradictis.' For an English translation, see Jackson, *The Seventh Crusade*, 115.

82 Gaposchkin, 'The Captivity of Louis IX', 94-95.

negotiations and the immediate aftermath of Louis's captivity.[83] Guillaume de Saint-Pathus's *vita* also records the impact the illness had on the king, carefully specifying its type. According to his narrative, in which he refers to the testimony of Louis's servant Ysembarz,[84] Louis's teeth were rickety, his skin was blotched and pale, he had severe flux, and he was so thin that his spine appeared to stick out. Furthermore, Yzembarz had to carry the king 'to his necessities'.[85] A perhaps even more graphic description of the severity of his dysentery was later given by Jean de Joinville, who wrote that because the king had to use the latrine so often, it became necessary to cut away the lower part of his drawers.[86]

Because of the source situation, it is not known under which article or articles his suffering at the crusade was investigated. Guillaume de Saint-Pathus, who reorganized his material under certain topics essential for constructing sainthood,[87] placed information on the king's infirmity during the crusade under the eighth chapter on devotion, stating that during the time he never failed to say his prayers,[88] and the thirteenth chapter on patience.[89] It is quite likely that this connection was made in the original hearing as well. In the latter case Guillaume's narration about the illness is more detailed and drawn largely from the testimony of Ysembarz. This part of the text also refers to Louis's emotional suffering caused by the failure of the crusade.[90]

83 Other sources, however, narrate that Louis's ill health continued during his captivity, but the Sultan Tūrān Shāh's physicians treated him and he gradually got better. Louis was treated well by his captors, being provided some comforts. This kind of treatment was not, however, extended to other Frankish prisoners. See Gaposchkin, 'The Captivity of Louis IX', 95-96.

84 Guillaume de Saint-Pathus, *Vie de saint Louis*, 112-13. Ysembarz (or Ysembart) is listed as a witness on 10, as 'Yzembart, le queu de benoiet saint Loys, homme de meur aage et riche, né de Paris, de lv ans ou environ'.

85 Guillaume de Saint-Pathus, *Vie de saint Louis*, 56: 'il fu si malades que les denz li [lochoient] et sa char estoit teinte et pale et avoit flus de ventre mout grief et estoit si megres que [ses os] de l'eschine du dos sembloient touz aguz.'

86 Jean de Joinville, *Histoire de saint Louis*, ch. 41, p. 101. Louis's confessor Geoffrey de Beaulieu, who started to write his *vita* a couple of years after the king's death, did not choose to depict the symptoms or the type of Louis's illness during his captivity, although he mentioned it and stated that Louis was in mortal danger. Geoffrey de Beaulieu, *Vita*, ch. 25. For the English translation, see 'Geoffrey of Beaulieu's *Life and Saintly Comportment of Louis, Former King of Franks, of Pious Memory*', 102-3; for Geoffrey and his work, see Gaposchkin and Field, 'Introduction', 18-38.

87 Gaposchkin, *The Making of Saint Louis*, 39-40.

88 Guillaume de Saint-Pathus, *Vie de saint Louis*, 56.

89 The chapter on *devotement* is on Guillaume de Saint-Pathus, *Vie de saint Louis*, 54-58, and the one on *pacience* on 112-19.

90 See Gaposchkin, 'The Captivity of Louis IX', 97, 107. As pointed out by Gaposchkin, Louis's emotional state appears to have been known in Europe, as, for example, Matthew Paris wrote

The elaborateness of the descriptions of Louis's illness illustrate well how the saintly king's body and its functions were no taboo in medieval society, either for those witnessing it or for those reporting it. Rather, although the texts do not directly say so, it is easy to imagine that the events during the crusade, including the king's severe illness, were a strong and emotional memory for Charles, Ysembarz, and other members of the campaign who had been close to Louis. Narrating them served the purpose of highlighting his suffering and, consequently, his sanctity.[91] Without psychologizing the witnesses' sentiments too much, possibly the narration process also provided a means for the witnesses to come to terms with a traumatic event.[92] How big a part all this played in the mind of an occasional layperson is more difficult to ascertain, as for the laity miracles were usually the most evident sign of sanctity. However, as analysed by M. Cecilia Gaposchkin, especially the Franciscan liturgy of Louis emphasized precisely his suffering during the crusades, comparing it with Francis's *stigmata* and the *compassio* of Christ. As the liturgies largely constructed his sanctity for the wider public – especially those who had not witnessed or experienced a miracle – Louis's suffering must have been an important aspect of his image among the laity.[93]

While Louis's suffering during the crusade was a widely known element of his *fama sanctitatis*, for his inner circle another instance of infirmity also had great significance. Guillaume de Saint-Pathus's *vita*, and therefore also the canonization protocols, describe an infirmity on the basis of the testimony of the knight Pierre de Laon and possibly others. The text records that Louis had a malady that seized him a few times every year. During these bouts, the king 'could neither eat nor sleep and he complained and wailed'

about the events of 1250 that there was a fear among the Saracens that 'the king should die of sorrow; for, indeed, he would not eat or drink anything for two days after his capture, and wished for death'. *Matthew Paris's English History*, II, ed. and trans. Giles, 378; see also Boquet and Nagy, *Medieval Sensibilities*, 166, on Louis's sadness. Interestingly, the chronicler did not consider Louis's grave illness essential for this description, which further highlights its importance *precisely* for the hagiography of Louis. Louis's sense of responsibility was also reported by his brother, as he testified that Louis offered to remain in captivity so that his men could be released. Gaposchkin, 'The Captivity of Louis IX', 102. Louis's experiences during the crusade changed his personality and his later reign. This has been extensively analysed in Jordan, 'Anti-corruption Campaigns', and *Men at the Center*. See also Gaposchkin, 'Louis IX, Crusade and the Promise of the Joshua'. O'Tool, 'Caring for the Blind', discusses Louis's experience of ill health as a reason for his charity towards the Parisian blind.

91 See also O'Tool, 'Caring for the Blind', 83.

92 Testifying about miracles has been interpreted as a way for people to make sense of their losses and traumatic experiences; see Klaniczay, 'Speaking about Miracles', at 369. For this idea in the case of children's deaths, see Smoller, 'Miracle, Memory, and Meaning', 433.

93 Gaposchkin, 'Louis IX and Liturgical Memory'.

and 'could not get up from his bed by himself'. When he began to recover, his right foot became red and swollen.[94] This account uses infirmity in a rather atypical way to construct saintly patience. The way Guillaume describes the king's symptoms has similarities with the conditions of many of the *miraculées* cured by his intercession. The inability to eat and sleep, and especially the inability to get up from bed without assistance, are recurring themes specifying conditions causing mobility impairments in St. Louis's *miracula*, as well as in the hagiographic genre in general.[95] The point of this narrative becomes clear when the text describes an incident where an old servant called Jehan la Guete, who had been in the service of Louis's grandfather Philip II, let a burning droplet fall on the king's ailing leg, making him stretch on his bed and cry out in pain. Still, the king did not 'hold anything against' the servant.[96]

The instance was certainly witnessed by several people, as according to the text, many *chevaliers* and one or two chamberlains slept in Louis's room. The narrative uses the severe symptoms as a way of highlighting his kindness towards his household staff, which is a frequent theme in medieval hagiography.[97] That Louis was visibly in pain, made worse by Jehan's lapse, added to his righteousness. Guillaume de Saint-Pathus does not give a clear time frame for this malady, although he mentions it after reporting Louis's experiences in captivity. In any case, it is noteworthy that it lasted for years, and even if it did come and go, it nevertheless troubled Louis regularly. One may only speculate whether this other infirmity would have received more attention without Louis's captivity and his suffering during the crusade, or what the balance between these two infirmities was in the original witness accounts.

94 Guillaume de Saint-Pathus, *Vie de saint Louis*, 116: 'La quele maladie estoit tele que, quant ele prenoit le benoiet roy, il n'entendoit pas bien ne n'ooit endementieres que la dite maladie le tenoit, et ne pooit mengier ne dormer et se compleignoit en gemissant. Et einsi la dite maladie le tenoit iij jours, aucune foiz plus aucune foiz moins, si que il ne pooit issir par soi du lit.'

95 See Guillaume de Saint-Pathus, *Les miracles de saint Louis*, 39, 46, 58, 126, 131, 144, 159, 171. For further discussion, see Kuuliala, *Childhood Disability*, 52-53.

96 Guillaume de Saint-Pathus, *Vie de saint Louis*, 117: 'mon seigneur Pierres de Loon [*sic*] dit par son serement que onques a nul tens il n'aperçut que il fust pour ce de riens meu contre le dit Jehan'.

97 The text also contrasts Louis's behaviour with that of his grandfather. It states that Louis also said to Jehan that his grandfather had dismissed him from his living quarters for a lesser reason. According to Pierre de Laon's testimony, Jehan then told him and the other chevaliers present that when serving Philip II, Jehan had been thrown out of his lodgings because he had placed a bundle of twigs on the fire, which had increased its strength and apparently caused some kind of danger. Guillaume de Saint-Pathus, *Vie de saint Louis*, 117. Charles of Blois was also frequently reported as a good master. See also Cassard, 'Les coulisses de la sainteté?', 4. For saints and their household staff, see Boanas and Roper, 'Feminine Piety in Fifteenth-Century Rome', 181-82, and Bell, *Holy Anorexia*, 138, on similar remarks concerning St. Frances of Rome.

St. Louis IX is, of course, a very special saint because of his status as a king, and therefore the meanings given to his infirmities are also unusual. Among the saints whose canonization protocols we have, the other military leader is Charles of Blois (1319-1364),[98] who inherited the title of the count of Blois from his father and the duchy of Brittany through his wife, Joan of Penthièvre, also known as Jeanne Boiteuse (*c.*1319-1384). The couple were involved with the Breton War of Succession, fought between those supporting Joan and Charles (who was a nephew of Philip VI of France) and those supporting John of Montfort. The war soon became entangled with the Hundred Years' War (1337-1454), and Charles became the official French candidate for the duchy, while John of Montford formed an alliance with Edward III of England. In time things became bad for Charles and his army, and eventually, at the Battle of La Roche-Derrien in 1347, he was taken prisoner and sent to the Tower of London for five years. A treaty was signed in 1353, and Charles was appointed the duke. The war, however, resumed in 1363. Charles's troops had some initial success, until the Battle of Auray in 1364 ended the conflict with his death. The peace of 1365 appointed John IV of Montford as duke of Brittany.[99]

The political situation remained tense after Charles's death. His family, with the help of Breton Franciscans, undertook to obtain an official recognition of his sanctity,[100] while John IV attempted to prevent the inquest.[101] Charles's canonization inquiry was held in the Franciscan church of Angers in 1371. The inquest was conducted without a ready-made questionnaire;

98 The most complete copy of the inquest is preserved in the Vatican Library manuscript Vat. lat. 4025; there is also a copy in the French National Library manuscript Fr. 5381. The process has been edited as *Monuments du procès de canonisation du bienheureux Charles de Blois*, ed. De Sérent (PC Charles of Blois).

99 See e.g. Allmand, *The Hundred Years War*, 14-21, for details.

100 Héry, 'Le culte de Charles de Blois'; Smoller, *Saint and the Chopped-Up Baby*, 26-30. There is a fascinating miracle account in Charles's hearing that reflects the continuing political tensions. There was a fresco of Charles in the Franciscan church of Dinan, which John IV ordered to be whitewashed 'by the suggestion of Englishmen'. However, after insulting words by the English, the hidden image started to bleed, and several witnesses testified that it was indeed real blood and not a fabrication. MS Vat. lat. 4025, fols. 121v-123v, 125v, 175v, 176v; PC Charles of Blois, 283-84, 286-87, 291-92, 406-7. This was to become 'an important episode in the agitation in favour of Charles' canonization'; Goodich, *Miracles and Wonders*, 60. See also Smoller, *The Saint and the Chopped-Up Baby*, 28. See Vauchez, 'Canonisation et politique au XIVe siècle', and Vauchez, *Sainthood*, 229-31, for the birth of Charles's cult and its political character. According to Vauchez, the whole canonization process originated in the political will of Louis of Anjou.

101 Vauchez, 'Canonisation et politique au XIVe siècle', 385.

instead, it was constructed afterwards by the proctor Raoul de Kerguiniou.[102] Nevertheless, the testimonies to Charles's *vita* show that the witnesses were not allowed to relate their memories freely, being posed questions relevant to the ideals of sanctity in an organized way. The most prominent feature of his life in the inquest was his piety. This is typical of the processes and cults of male saints, especially if they were rulers, because their lives fitted the pattern of holiness very poorly. By being very pious, they excelled in their secular roles.[103] Thus, Charles's frequent gifts to the mendicant orders, the scorn his lifestyle received from his peers, as well as his penitence and devotion, play a big role in the testimonies.[104] In this respect Charles's *fama* resembles that of St. Elzéar of Sabran, whose life was constructed in terms spiritual masculinity.[105]

As for Charles's military campaigns, the losses he suffered during them were mentioned by virtually all witnesses to his life when they testified about his *patientia* and also *humilitas*.[106] The details of his campaigns and imprisonment were, however, mostly downplayed – undoubtedly because Charles's campaigns were conducted for entirely secular reasons, whereas Louis IX was a crusader.[107] Most likely this tendency also reflects the current political tensions and the cult promoters' need to highlight his piety. Yet,

102 Vauchez, 'Canonisation et politique au XIVe siècle', 388, writes that this was one of the arguments raised by the cardinals against the case.

103 Weissenberg, 'What man are you?', 112-13.

104 See Cassard, 'Les coulisses de la sainteté?', 2-3; Vauchez, *Sainthood*, 229, 363-67. Although Joan of Penthièvre was not called to testify in the hearing, there are several hints letting the reader assume that the marriage was a happy one. Joan did not share all of Charles's devotional and penitentiary practices, but they had at least six children together; Joan lived as a widow for twenty years, although her remarriage was considered; and at the time of her death, she possessed several of Charles's relics. Jones, 'Politics, Sanctity and the Breton State', 220. See pp. 118, 129 below for Charles's penitentiary practices.

105 Weissenberg, 'What man are you?', 121-25.

106 For example BAV, MS Vat. lat. 4025, fols. 11v, 13v, 16r, 23v, 33v, 37r; PC Charles of Blois, 27-28, 32, 38-39, 56, 81-82, 90. There are differences in which aspects of these the witnesses narrated. The most detailed information about Charles's *patientia* at the time of friends' deaths was given by Colinus Audigerii, who was Charles's *familiaris*. BAV, MS Vat. lat. 4025, fol. 33v; PC Charles of Blois, 81. A curious example of this is, for instance, the deposition of a 30-year-old *miles* Guillelmus de Carrimel, who had been to war with Charles for eight years before his death. Yet his testimony gives a very brief and general statement about Charles's *patientia* in the face of adversities. The commissioners asked for details of these adversities, but Guillelmus responded he did not remember any, although he remembered well what Charles's attitude had been. BAV, MS Vat. lat. 4025, fols. 24v-25r; PC Charles of Blois, 60-61.

107 Charles's sanctity differed from that of Louis IX in his relationships with and attitudes towards the clergy. While Louis, albeit always supporting the church, could also stand up to the bishops and even the pope when they made excessive demands to royalty or trespassed on

there were some witnesses in the inquest who had been close to Charles and for whom the memory of his life, including the military campaigns and Charles's infirmities during them, held specific importance.[108] Yvo Crenan, Charles's servant of twenty-five years, narrated that before the Battle of Auray, Charles was so infirm for seven weeks that he could not stay on his feet. Although the servants reprehended him for wanting to go to a battle in a state of such 'debility', the duke responded that he would go to defend his people.[109] Presbyter Alanus Radulphi and presbyter Guillermus Berengarii also mentioned that he had been severely ill before the fateful battle when testifying to Charles's patience and devotion.[110]

Undoubtedly some, especially the devotees of Charles who knew about his illness before his final battle, saw him as a political martyr.[111] In medieval literature, the knight typically faces death magnificently and heroically, maintaining all his proper values such as honour, glory, and piety.[112] Especially Yvo's testimony connects deliberate martyrdom and the willingness to die for one's subjects with this idea. But there are also testimonies in the inquest which report that Charles suffered from infirmity during the earlier remarkable battle, that of La Roche-Derrien. Alanus Radulphi mentioned it as well when testifying regarding Charles's *patientia*. Furthermore, Charles's *medicus* Georgius Lesnen, the canon of Nantes, gave specific details about this.[113] In his testimony about Charles's *patientia*, Georgius asserted that he was severely wounded before being captured by the English in 1347, adding that he suffered seventeen wounds which the witness saw, and was lying on a bed with a feather mattress. A knight named Thomas Dagorne had the

their prerogatives, Charles defended the clergy in all the disagreements it had with his own officers. Vauchez, *Sainthood*, 361, 366.

108 Charles's process has an exceptionally high number of *milites* and *armigeri* testifying about their miraculous cures of war wounds. These miracles are, generally, *post mortem*, but one knight also recounted a cure of an old wound he had acquired during the Battle of La Roche-Derrien. MS Vat. lat. 4025, fol. 132r-v; PC Charles of Blois, 307-8. For this miracle, see Frohne and Kuuliala, 'The Trauma of Pain'.

109 BAV, MS Vat. lat. 4025, fol. 38r; PC Charles of Blois, 93: 'et dum per istum et alios cubicularios suos reprehendebatur pro eo quod ac conflictum ire volebat in tali debilitate, ipse dicebat: "Ego ibo defendere populum meum, placeret modo Deo quod contencio esse solum inter me et adversarium meum, absque eo quod alii propter hoc morerentur."' For the term *debilitas* in medieval hagiography, see Goetz, 'Vorstellungen von menschlicher Gebrechlichkeit'.

110 BAV, MS Vat. lat. 4025, fols. 23v, 35r; PC Charles of Blois, 57, 85.

111 See also Goodich, *Miracles and Wonders*, 60.

112 Heng, *Empire of Magic*, 170. For crusaders' deaths and wounds as *imitatio Christi*, see Tamminen, 'The Crusaders' *Stigmata*'.

113 On Gerogius de Lesnen's importance as a witness, see Ziegler, 'Practitioners and Saints', 216.

mattress taken from under Charles to cause him indignity, so that Charles was left lying on straw, for which he thanked God.[114]

The details of the capture and the wounds are generally known and recorded elsewhere as well, but it is surprising how little attention they received in the hearing. Thomas Dagorne was Sir Thomas Dagworth (d. 1352), leading the army which took Charles's troops completely by surprise at the battle, and two of his men, Nicholas Lovayn and John of Isplyngrode, captured the duke and took him to England.[115] *Les grandes chroniques de France* states that Charles was wounded in seven locations, more than one of the wounds sufficient to be fatal,[116] and the wounds were also recorded in Richard Lescot's chronicle.[117] Georgius de Lesnen remained in Charles's company throughout his captivity, which explains its significance to his memories. But although his description of the wounds multiplies their number compared with the chronicle, even he focused on the other hardships Charles faced during his long captivity.[118] Furthermore, the *armiger* Iohannes de Fourneto, who testified to Charles's usage of a hair shirt, mentioned that the duke had an injury to his shoulder, which had been penetrated by a javelin.[119] His testimony concerns the event after the capture, and it is likely that it refers to the wounds caused at La Roche-Derrien, but he did not give more importance to them either.

The wounds would have provided intertextual possibilities for constructing the sanctity of a duke who suffered from political injustice in addition to having a saintly character.[120] The few references to the matter indeed strongly resemble the way Guillaume de Saint-Pathus used *infirmitas* in proving the devoutness and patience of St. Louis IX. This is hardly a surprise, given that in many respects Louis IX can be considered the model for Charles's saintly activities;[121]

114 BAV, MS Vat. lat. 4025, fol. 11v; PC Charles of Blois, 27-28.

115 See e.g DeVries, *Infantry Warfare*, 189-90; C. Rogers, 'Sir Thomas Dagworth in Brittany'.

116 *Les grandes chroniques de France*, IX, ed. Viard, 304: 'si li demanderet qu'il se rendist, ausquiex il respondi que ja à Anglois il ne se rendroit, et qu'il avoit plus chier à souffrir mort, ja soit ce qu'il fust navré de VII plaies.' C. Rogers, 'Sir Thomas Dagworth in Brittany', 150, n. 95, has shown that there are several errors in the chronicle account of the battle, especially regarding Charles's attitude towards his captors. The detail about Charles being wounded, however, seems to be true.

117 *Chronique de Richard Lescot*, ed. Lemoine, 79.

118 BAV, MS Vat. lat. 4025, fols. 11v-12r; PC Charles of Blois, 28. *Les grandes chroniques de France*, IX, ed. Viard, 305, reports that it took over a year before Charles was transported to England, because he had to be cured of the wounds before undertaking such a long journey.

119 BAV, MS Vat. lat. 4025, fol. 26r; PC Charles of Blois, 66.

120 In medieval literature, wounds are often portrayed in the context of Christ's passion, and as objects of meditation and *imitatio Christi*. See e.g. Kirkham and Warr, 'Introduction'; Rubin, *Corpus Christi*, 302-6.

121 See Cassard, 'Les coulisses de la sainteté?', 6.

and it demonstrates that even when infirmity was not an established factor in a saint's *fama*, those reporting it modelled their narratives according to previous examples. But, although they held personal importance for some witnesses, the wounds were not crucial for Charles's *fama sanctitatis*. In addition to the need to highlight other aspects of his sanctity than his role as a secular military leader, the established forms of warfare narrative in medieval culture must have had an influence on this, as canonization hearings or hagiographic literature have their roots deep in the narrative culture of the time. In romances and epics, when an individual in battle is referred to only two outcomes are portrayed: the knight either dies or survives uninjured. A knight's wounds that were not fatal were not usually included.[122]

The case of our two military leaders is, of course, distinct in terms of sanctity and gender where the ideals of traditional warriors, crusaders, and clerical masculine ideas intermingle. The idealized masculinity of clerics, and the role of infirmity in it, is much better documented in the two preserved full canonization processes of a saintly bishop: Philip of Bourges or Philip Berruyer (d. 1261, inquest conducted in 1265/66), and St. Thomas Cantilupe (1218-1282, inquest conducted in 1307). Philip was first a canon at Saint-Martin and the cathedral of Tours, then the archdeacon at Beaugency, and then archdeacon at Tours. He was elected archbishop of Tours but he rejected the chapter's appeals, while accepting the see of Orleans in 1234 and later Bourges in 1236.[123] Thomas Cantilupe, on the other hand, was first the chancellor of the University of Oxford, and was appointed the bishop of Hereford in 1275.[124] Philip's and Thomas's sainthoods were largely constructed through their actions as ideal bishops. In Philip's process his performance of liturgical functions, the building of churches, and his

122 Bouchard, *Strong of Body*, 117; Metzler, *A Social History of Disability*, 41. This has most likely also influenced the types of miracle nobility and members of the elite reported, for although they witness in canonization hearings often, their long-term disabling conditions are rare among miracle accounts. See Koopmans, *Wonderful to Relate*, 42; Kuuliala, 'Nobility, Community and Physical Impairment'.

123 For an overview of Philip's canonization process, see Vauchez, *Sainthood*, 63, n. 6. The process has been used as a source in e.g. Goodich, *Miracles and Wonders*; Goodich, *Violence and Miracle*; Kuuliala, *Childhood Disability*.

124 On the Cantilupe process, see Bartlett, *The Hanged Man*, 11-21; Finucane, *Miracles and Pilgrims*, 173-90; Katajala-Peltomaa, *Gender, Miracles, and Daily Life*; Krötzl, 'Prokuratoren, Notare und Dolmetscher', 126-28; Vauchez, *Sainthood*, 487-94. It has been extensively used as a source for medieval social history, for example in Bartlett, *The Hanged Man*; Finucane, *The Rescue of the Innocents*; Finucane, *Miracles and Pilgrims*; Hanska, 'The Hanging of William Cragh'; Katajala-Peltomaa, *Gender, Miracles, and Daily Life*; Kuuliala, *Childhood Disability*. See also Finucane, *Miracles and Pilgrims*, 177, and Vauchez, *Sainthood*, 219-24, on the life cycle of the cult.

pastoral visits were in focus. The witnesses also referred to him suppressing revolts.[125] Thomas Cantilupe's devotees put great emphasis on the image of him as an idealized bishop and a learned man, focusing on his career and the ways he took care of his office and the people in his diocese. In all this, their sainthood was constructed following the model of St. Martin of Tours, who was a model for all medieval holy bishops.[126]

The witnesses in the hearings of the two bishops gave elaborate testimonies about their *patientia*, in which infirmity played a role that appears both subdued and important at the same time. As is common, those witnesses who mentioned this aspect were the bishops' servants or others close to them. In Philip of Bourges' inquest such references mostly pertain to his final illness.[127] A few depositions, however, give a more wavering timeline of the matter. Philip's servant of sixteen years called Gaufridus de Amaireio stated that in bodily adversities Philip thanked the Lord, and that as long as he was with him, he saw the bishop entering the bed clothed in a tunic or close-fitting body garment ('corsetus'), and he believed that this was done because of an infirmity.[128] Similarly, Johannes, a deacon and presbyter from Bourges, as well as *curatus* Johannes, testified that they saw Philip 'several times' when he was infirm, being patient and thanking Christ for whipping him. They also heard the archbishop saying 'Hic ure, hic seca' ('here burn, here plague'), mostly during his last infirmity.[129] *Hic*

125 Vauchez, *Sainthood*, 299-300; he also writes that Thomas Cantilupe and the holy Swedish bishops Brynolf of Skara (d. 1317) and Nicholas of Linköping (d. 1391) had in no manner experienced the lives of the priests they were supposed to rule.

126 On the *Vita Martini* by Sulpicius Severus as a model for all medieval bishop saints, see Vauchez, *Sainthood*, 288, 290-91. The importance of characteristics typically attributed to a bishop saint is highlighted in an interesting way in the connection of Philip of Bourges and Louis IX of France. Philip had, for example, taken the crusader's vow in 1245, which he was later permitted to renounce with the king's approval. All this, however, is completely absent from the canonization testimonies and the *vita*, despite the importance of the crusade for Louis IX's sanctity. See Chester Jordan, *Louis IX and the Challenge of the Crusade*, 117, and Vauchez, *Sainthood*, 305, who has explained this by the need to make bishop saints entirely religious. For original sources mentioning Philip's crusading activities, see Guillaume de Nangis, *Vie et vertus de Saint Louis*, 79; Matthew Paris, *Chronica majora*, IV, 490.

127 His *vita* also records that he was patient at the time of adversities and infirmities, as well as in bodily afflictions, but more significance is given to other adversities and quarrels. *Vita s. Philippi archiepiscopi Bituricensis*, ed. Martene and Durand, col. 1930.

128 BAV, MS Vat. lat. 4019, fol. 45r-v: 'semper uidit ipsam intrare lectum et jacentem indutum uno corseto, et credit quod ita indutus iacebat propterque in quadam infirmitate.'

129 BAV, MS Vat. lat. 4019, fol. 38r-v: 'Dicens iste qui loquitur quod frequenter dicebat dictus Archiepiscopus talia uerba, "Hic ure, hic seca" et maxime in ultima infirmitate.' The *curator* Johannes's testimony is in BAV, MS Vat. lat. 4019, fol. 41r.

ure, hic seca is a phrase attributed to St. Augustine, for example in Peter Lombard's (d. 1160) commentary on Psalm 6:1, although not identifiable in his writings.[130] The point is the beneficial effect of infirmity and the saint asking God to chastise him even more. This is a common theme, appearing in many hagiographic documents, albeit most often as a reference to Paul's statement 'Cum infirmor potens sum' ('When I am weak, then I am strong').[131] So, for these particular witnesses, Philip's infirmity was indeed a vital element in his saintly patience; why so few of the witnesses mentioned it is at least partly explainable by the general emphasis on other aspects common to bishop saints.

In Thomas Cantilupe's case, those in favour of his canonization primarily constructed his *patientia* by his attitude towards his famous dispute with Archbishop John Peckham, his disagreement with Count Gilbert of Gloucester, and some disputes during his university career.[132] As André Vauchez puts it, 'several witnesses, mostly clerics, went so far as to describe the bishop as a "martyr" because of the difficulties he had experienced at the end of his life'.[133] Therefore, these (mostly elite male) witnesses constructed this element of his holiness not in corporeal terms but by the problems related to his rule. At the same time, a few of his servants and clerics did interpret his attitude towards infirmities in the same light, as signs of *patientia*. The witness accounts of *dominus* Ricardus de Kymberle, Thomas's follower Bishop Richard Swinefield (d. 1317) and his servant Robertus Deynte give the impression of a chronic or recurrent infirmity, which Robertus also interpreted as fatal,[134] but they mentioned 'colic' or other stomach ailments as the primary diagnosis.[135]

130 See Diekstra (ed.), *The Middle English 'Weye of Paradys'*, 439; Peter Lombard's text is in *Patrologiae cursus completus: series latina* 191, ed. Migne, col. 105.

131 See pp. 170, 179 for other examples.

132 See e.g. BAV MS Vat. lat. 4015, fols. 60r, 76r, 96r-v, 101r, 118v. The dispute with Peckham led to Thomas Cantilupe's excommunication, which in turn resulted in his setting out for Rome to bring the matter before the pope. During this journey he got ill and died at San Severo, near Orvieto. The canonization inquest could not be opened before the question of whether or not he had been absolved before his death was settled, which required an inquest documented and preserved in Vatican Library manuscript Vat. lat. 4016. See Finucane, *Miracles and Pilgrims*, 176; Vauchez, *Sainthood*, 78.

133 Vauchez, *Sainthood*, 171. See e.g. BAV, MS Vat. lat. 4015, fols. 98v, 117v-118v.

134 BAV, MS Vat. lat. 4015, fol. 37v: 'Item respondit quod habuerat infirmitates corporales multas et celebras, et frequenter habebat torsiones in ventre'; MS Vat. lat. 4015, fol. 109v: 'et quod obierat [...] ex febre et ex dicta colica passione'; MS Vat. lat. 4015, fol. 118v: 'Subiciens quod aduersitate siue graui infirmitate ex dolore uiscerum seu iliaca passione et dolore stomachi per multos annos prius quam esset factus episcopus, et postquam diu uixit extitit molestatus'.

135 BAV, MS Vat. lat. 4015, fols. 94r, 97v.

Although those close to the bishop thus interpreted his infirmities in the light of his sanctity, it is not surprising that in the overall construction of Thomas Cantilupe's holiness, his bodily troubles received little emphasis, although we may reasonably assume that they were a part of his and his followers' lived experience. The same can, to some extent, be said about Philip of Bourges. Masculinity in general was constructed through interaction with other men, so that male patience and not losing one's temper during disputes with them is a frequent theme in (lay) male saints' hagiographies.[136] The male witnesses testifying about Thomas's life certainly had internalized this. Furthermore, in the case of holy bishops, it was of crucial importance to refer to their firmness and opposition to any infringements; in Thomas Cantilupe's case this is visible in the various lawsuits and other conflicts which he eventually won – arguably these victorious conflicts laid the foundation for his holy reputation.[137]

These examples do not mean, however, that a saintly bishop's patience could not have been later reconstructed using a bodily ailment, or that it could not have been a strong feature in the communal memory or oral and written tradition. The canonization inquest of Bishop Brynolf of Skara (*c.*1248-1317) from 1417[138] demonstrates this. Besides referring to more typical aspects of the *patientia* of a saintly bishop, like battles against the persecutions of princes and others,[139] the articles record that Brynolf was 'wonderfully patient': he was poisoned as an infant, and thereafter had worms in his stomach for the rest of his life, which 'greatly tormented' him. The same detail is also used to define his *caritas*. According to the text, his wet nurse was the person responsible for the infestation, and she did the same to Brynolf's sister, who died. As a bishop, he provided the wet nurse with an honest living,[140] which is again an example of a saint's benevolence towards a servant who failed in her duty. The witness statements show that the incident was a common part of his *fama*, and it was actively transmitted

136 Weissenberg, 'What man are you?', 112-13; Karras, *From Boys to Men*, 151-52. As pointed out by Heinonen, 'Henry Suso and the Divine Knighthood', 85-86, one reason for this gendered *patientia* is that only men – mendicants included – could actively participate in the world and have the chance to experience such problems.

137 Vauchez, *Sainthood*, 294.

138 For the hearing, see Fröjmark, 'Canonization Process of Brynolf Algotsson'. It is a relatively condensed document, but it records the main elements of his *vita*.

139 *Vita s. Brynolphi episc. Scarensis, com processu euis canonizationis*, ed. Annerstedt (PC Brynolf of Skara), 142.

140 PC Brynolf of Skara, 142. Some witnesses however said they knew nothing about it; see e.g. PC Brynolf of Skara, 152.

at a communal level by elderly clerics,[141] books of the church of Skara,[142] and what the contemporary bishop of Skara had heard about the matter from his grandmother.[143] There was some variation in the description of the symptoms from croaking frogs to worms and to the wet nurse poisoning him because of the habits of her unspecified homeland.[144] Despite their vagueness, these testimonies show that the community of devotees – those conducting the inquiry and those testifying in it – could also define a holy bishop's *patientia* largely in corporeal terms, and a physical infirmity could survive as an important element of it for decades.

Old Age and Infirmity

In observing, negotiating, and redefining a holy person's infirmity, their community members and those conducting the canonization inquests gave varying meanings to the saint's age. Article 56 in St. Clare of Montefalco's process (1318-19) records a conversation where she reportedly was not only infirm but also 'of advanced age' ('provecte etatis'),[145] although she was only 40 years old at the time of her death. At the same time, the witnesses to Nicholas of Tolentino's ailing health did not make a clear connection with his ageing, although he was some ten years older than Clare at the time of his death.[146] Furthermore, the connection between John Buoni's infirmity and old age (he died when he was 80) appears somewhat vague in the testimonies.

141 PC Brynolf of Skara, 148, 153, 161, 162.
142 PC Brynolf of Skara, 158.
143 PC Brynolf of Skara, 155-56; see also 158.
144 PC Brynolf of Skara, 150: 'et quod rane co[a]xabant in stomacho eiusdem beati Brynolphi'; see also 165, 167. Having been poisoned as an infant is an extraordinary diagnosis for any hagiographic material, and although worms occasionally appear in miracle accounts, they are by no means a standard infirmity either. For miracles including worms, see *Processus seu negocium canonizacionis b. Katerine de Vadstenis*, ed. Collijn (PC Catherine of Vadstena), 78-79; *Processus canonizationis s. Ludovici ep. Tolosani*, ed. Collegio S. Bonaventura (PC Louis of Toulouse), 165; *Miracula sancti Stanislai*, ed. Kętrzyński, 314; Frohne and Kuuliala, 'The Trauma of Pain', 233-34; for worms as the cause of illness and death, see Haas, *The Renaissance Man and his Children*, 163-64.
145 *Il processo di canonizzazione di Chiara da Montefalco*, ed. Menestò (PC Clare of Montefalco), 8; for Clare and her canonization process, see pp. 85-87 below.
146 Death at that age could be considered untimely. Shahar, *Growing Old in the Middle Ages*, 22. There is some variation in the scheme of the ages of man at the time; for example, according to Isidore of Seville, both Clare of Montefalco and Nicholas of Tolentino belonged to the group of *iuventus* which lasted from 28 to the fiftieth year. Burrow, *Ages of Man*, 82. In the scheme of 'four ages of man', old age, *senectus*, started at 38 or 40. Sears, *The Ages of Man*, 30.

A remarkably clear time frame and diagnosis of a saint's infirmity was given in the canonization hearing of Dauphine of Puimichel, although overall her sanctity was not reconstructed in a significantly corporeal way, despite her association with the Franciscan order from an early age.[147] Her canonization inquest provides an exceptional window into the views of people of very high social standing who had known the saint personally, often for a long time – the proportion of witnesses with noble or otherwise elite social standing is unusually high in this document.[148] Article 33 of the hearing clearly documents the type of infirmity she had and connected it with her *patientia*. According to the text, 'lady Dauphine, when she was alive among humans, had suffered for several years and for a long time of her life from various infirmities of fevers and dropsy in her body' and that she tolerated these 'passions and infirmities' with great patience.[149]

As in the case of Dauphine's illness at the beginning of her marriage, the witnesses who testified to the article belonged to her innermost circle; as usual, the general public was not consulted about such details. Those testifying were Bertrandus Iusberti,[150] Durandus Andree, Bertranda Bartholomea, and Philippe de Cabassole (1305-1372), the bishop of Cavaillon and the titular patriarch of Jerusalem who later became a cardinal.[151] Furthermore, Catherina de Podio, who had lived with Dauphine for several years, testified to the infirmity under an earlier article concerning Dauphine's penitentiary practices. Most detailed information about the physical side of things came, quite unsurprisingly, from Durandus Andree, who, as mentioned above, was Dauphine's physician and confessor. In addition to fever and dropsy, Durandus added that he had witnessed Dauphine having tremors in her

147 See Andenna, 'Women at the Angevin Court', 47-51, for Franciscan influence in Dauphine's life.

148 See Kuuliala, 'Nobility, Community and Physical Infirmity'.

149 PC Dauphine of Puimichel, 52: 'Item, quod publica vox et fama et communis opinio, communis assercio et reputacio in partibus regni Sicilie et in partibus Provincie et alibi, ac eciam verum et notorium est et fuit quod dicta domina Dalphina, dum in humanis agebat, per multos annos et longa tempora vite sue habuit et passa fuit varias sui corporis infirmitates febrium et ydropisis; et ipsas passiones et infirmitates cum magna paciencia sustinuit et tolleravit'.

150 He was also among the witnesses in St. Elzéar of Sabran's inquest. 'Le sommaire de l'enquete pour la canonisation de s. Elzear de Sabran, TOF (d. 1323)', ed. Cambell.

151 Philippe de Cabassole is nowadays best known for his intimate and long-lasting friendship with Petrarch. Visiting Philippe's villa in Vaucluse greatly influenced the poet's decision to settle there. Petrarch later dedicated his *De vita solitaria* to Philippe. See Enenkel, 'Vorwort zur Textausgabe', 12-14. The edition records Philippe's testimony as concerning article 32, which records Dauphine's deeds on behalf of the sick and the poor. The contents, however, strongly suggest that he is giving testimony to the thirty-third article. PC Dauphine of Puimichel, 538.

heart and other 'hidden and secret infirmities in her secret body parts'.[152] Bertrandus Iusberti was also able to call on his first-hand knowledge, stating that he saw Dauphine's stomach swollen because of the infirmity.[153] Catherina de Podio mentioned 'secret infirmities' and stomach issues as well, adding pain in the tibiae to the list.[154]

The most important informant in the matter was, however, Bertranda. The commissioners clearly considered her an important and trustworthy witness, as she gave a very detailed account of Dauphine's life and miracles.[155] As one of the women who had lived with Dauphine since she renounced her wealth and earthly status after Elzéar's death, Bertranda appears to have been one of the key distributors of the details about her life among her devotees; for example, Bertrandus Iusberti named her as one of those giving details of Dauphine's infirmity. The commissioners asked her about its duration; according to her, it had lasted 'for thirty years', getting worse towards the end of her life.[156] This would make Dauphine around 40 at the onset of her condition, which would have begun around or at the time Elzéar's death. According to the statements, some details of Dauphine's ailments were quite widely known, at least geographically. Philippe de Cabassole was asked where he had seen Dauphine infirm. He replied that in Naples, Apt, Cavaillon, L'Isle-sur-la-Sorgue, and Châteauneuf-de-Gadagne.[157] Dauphine was close to Queen Sancia of Majorca (*c.*1285-1345), whose lady-in-waiting she became when Elzéar de Sabran went to King Robert of Anjou's (1275-1343) court in 1314. She also spent a large part of her life in Naples after Elzéar's death, making her vow of poverty there in 1333 before returning to Provence in 1343.[158] Therefore it is entirely plausible that some of these issues were a part of Dauphine's *fama* at the court of Naples as well.[159]

152 PC Dauphine of Puimichel, 264-65: 'Et vidit dictam dominam Dalphinam pacientem ydropismim, prout in articulo continetur, et eciam habentem tremorem cordis et alias occultas et secretas infirmitates in partibus secretis sui corporis.'

153 PC Dauphine of Puimichel, 229.

154 PC Dauphine of Puimichel, 394: 'dixit quod paciebatur tam in ventre quam in tibiis et maxime in una, et habebat alias infirmitates secretas.'

155 PC Dauphine of Puimichel, 303-42.

156 PC Dauphine of Puimichel, 333: 'Interrogata per quot annos habuit dictas passiones et infirmitates, dixit quod bene per XXX annos ante obitum ipsius domine Dalphine inceperunt et duraverunt sibi crescendo usque ad obitum suum.'

157 PC Dauphine of Puimichel, 538.

158 At that time King Robert made Elzéar the counsellor of his son Charles, who was married to Catherine of Austria. Andenna, 'Women at the Angevin Court', 47-49.

159 According to Dauphine's Occitan *Vie*, she stayed in Naples from 1326 to 1336 and then in Provence until 1340, when Queen Sancia asked her to return there for the last time. PC Dauphine of Puimichel, 541, n. 2. Philippe de Cabassole testified that the queen asked her there because

Although Dauphine had renounced her earthly wealth and status, for the community around Apt, where she spent the last two decades of her life, she continued to have a reputation as a person resolving quarrels and discord.[160] An article and the corresponding witness accounts given by her long-time associates and venerators use her infirmity and disability to underline the significance of this activity, showing her willingness to undertake such tasks despite the physical difficulty it caused her. According to these statements, she had herself carried to the required location because she was unable to walk or ride due to the 'impediment of old age and infirmity'.[161] This article referred to 'perilous quarrels' between Count Hugo II de Baucio (or Hugues de Baux, 1311-1351) and Raimundo II de Agunto. Bertrandus Iusberti explained that Dauphine was at that time *infirma et debilis* so that she could neither walk nor ride a horse, and she had herself carried to Cabaillon. This was based on hearsay, as Bertrandus had not been present but heard about the matter from *magister* Nicholas Loarenchi. Nicholas was the postulator and procurator of the hearing, having already acted as the procurator of St. Elzéar's canonization inquest.[162] He appears to have been a keen distributor of Dauphine's *fama*, and if he highlighted Dauphine's infirmity in this enterprise, he must have considered it important, perhaps also from the inquisitorial point of view.

The time frame of these events appears to have been significant for the commissioners, who sought to find out the onset of Dauphine's infirmity in several places, presumably precisely because it was used in so many situations to enhance Dauphine's saintly deeds. Bertrandus explained that all this occurred before the time of the 'first mortality' ('prime mortalitatis'), when he was living in Dauphine's household.[163] This refers to 1348, when the

of her own illness; PC Dauphine of Puimichel, 541. Sancia was widowed in 1343, and a year later renounced her regency and became a nun, when Philippe de Cabassole became a member of the Council of Regency. She finally died only eighteen months later in a convent, at the age of 60. Greatly influenced by the Spiritual Franciscans, throughout her life Sancia of Majorca had wished to become a cloistered nun. Nevertheless, she led a public life as the queen consort of King Robert, and had an active role at the Neapolitan court, becoming also the mentor of Robert's daughter and heir to the throne, Joan I of Naples. See Loconte, 'Constructing Female Sanctity in Late Medieval Naples'. Robert also played an important role in Elzéar's canonization, as requested by the Franciscan friar Francis de Meyronnes (or Francesco de Marone), who took Elzéar's final confession, and who was close to the king. Vauchez, *Sainthood*, 80, n. 65; 'Vita s. Elzearii de Sabrano, conf.', *AASS*, Sept. VII, 592.

160 See also Archambeau, 'Remembering Countess Delphine's Books', esp. 35.

161 PC Dauphine of Puimichel, 55: 'se propterea transferebat, licet nec equitare nec peditare posset propter senectutis et infirmitatum suarum impedimenta.'

162 PC Dauphine of Puimichel, 233-35; see also the testimony of Durandus Andree on 269.

163 PC Dauphine of Puimichel, 234.

first wave of the plague had arrived in Provence; the witnesses in Dauphine's hearing often used this as a reference point.[164] Bertranda Bartholomea, on the other hand, said this occurred *after* the first mortality; while in her testimony to another article she said that at the time of the first plague, Dauphine was not yet 'oppressed by infirmities or old age'.[165] This suggests that the aggravation of Dauphine's infirmity occurred quite suddenly. However, this was not relevant for the canonization inquiry; her persistence in helping her community when physically disabled was the crucial issue.

In the eyes of the devotees, different types of public acts could be coloured and made more significant by the holy person's visible infirmity, connected with old age. This appears very pronounced in the mid-fifteenth-century process of St. Vincent Ferrer. He was primarily known as a preacher, and his saintly *fama* developed largely during the final years of his life. His outstanding preaching skills and their popularity and effect play a crucial role in the testimonies about his long life.[166] Concerning his final years, many witnesses described his bodily weakness due to his old age, and how, when he preached or celebrated the Mass, he appeared to have the strength of a 30-year-old man.[167] Some used the common way of delineating a physical disability in hagiographic texts by referring to him as hardly able to walk or get to his pulpit without the help of others.[168] These remarks connect Vincent's frail body, continuing preaching activities, and saintly character in a very tangible manner, as a sign of the concept of the Holy Spirit's influence on his preaching.[169]

It is worth pointing out, however, that precisely the testimonies recorded in Naples and Toulouse focus on Vincent as a preacher, while the ones recorded in Brittany focus on his miracle-working abilities (no documents of the inquest conducted in Avignon have survived). This again demonstrates the influence of the selection of witnesses and the differences between

164 Archambeau, 'Healing Options during the Plague', esp. 536.

165 PC Dauphine of Puimichel, 329: 'Interrogata de tempore quo vidit et audivit predicta, dixit quod a tempore prime mortalitatis citra, [...] videlicet tempore quo non fuit dicta domina Dalphina gravata infirmitatibus vel senio'; PC Dauphine of Puimichel, 337: 'Et interrogate quando hoc fuit, dixit quod post primam mortalitatem'.

166 Vincent's cult, *fama*, and canonization, have been extensively analysed by Laura A. Smoller in several works; see *The Saint and the Chopped-Up Baby*; 'Miracle, Memory, and Meaning'; 'Defining the Boundaries of the Natural'; and 'Northern and Southern Sanctity'.

167 *Procès de la canonisation de saint Vincent Ferrier*, ed. Fages (PC Vincent Ferrer), 6, 10, 15, 32, 64, 246, 343, 345, 356, 390.

168 PC Vincent Ferrer, 205: 'qui vis sine alterius adjutorio ambulare, et habitacula in quibus predicabat ascendere poterat'.

169 Smoller, *The Saint and the Chopped-Up Baby*, 21, 100.

individual processes. Vincent's hearings and their characteristics have been extensively analysed by Laura Ackerman Smoller. For example, the *articuli* in the Naples and Toulouse hearings as well as the elite status of witnesses has resulted in the emphasis on Vincent's professional activities, while in Brittany no articles were used and the commissioners and subcommissioners sought to interrogate as many people as possible, so the social diversity of witnesses is much greater. The portrayal of Vincent's life is very uniform in the Brittany testimonies, describing him as 'a new apostle', without detailing his professional activities, whereas those recorded in Toulouse and Naples have more variation.[170] One of the most exceptional testimonies concerning Vincent's preaching activities and infirmity was given in Toulouse by *frater* Petrus de Colomberio. He reported Vincent's popularity as a preacher without referring to his infirmity. When testifying about his *patientia*, he however told of having seen Vincent falling from his donkey but suffering no injury. This he perceived as the work of God rather than that of humans, 'because he suffered from a certain infirmity in his tibia, which he had had a long time ago, and for which reason he rode a donkey'.[171] Petrus was the only witness to refer to any long-term infirmity in Vincent's leg. Whether or not he really had such impairment cannot be deduced from this one deposition nor is it essential for the current discussion. Rather, Petrus's testimony again illustrates that for individual community members the appearance and significance of a holy person's infirmity or bodily characteristics could vary.[172]

170 Smoller, 'Northern and Southern Sanctity'.

171 PC Vincent Ferrer, 285: 'Item dixit quantum ad patientiam, quod nunquam vidit eum impatientem, licet bina vice vidit ipsum cadentem cum asino in terra, tamen nullam lesionem suscipientem: de quo omnes mirabantur, et plus reputabant esse divinum opus quam humanum, cum pateretur in tibia quandam infirmitatem quam longo ante habuerat, occasione cujus asinu equitabat.'

172 This is also nicely illustrated in the testimonies recorded regarding St. Frances of Rome's and St. Bernardino of Siena's use of eyeglasses when reading. In Bernardino's case they became an established part of his iconography, while in the case of Frances, they are not shown, although she is often portrayed with a book. Ilardi, *Renaissance Vision from Spectacles to Telescopes*, 169-71. The testimonies in Frances's hearing that refer to the visual aids do not connect them to low vision in any manner but refer to them in passing, stating that the witnesses had seen Francesca reading with eyeglasses. See PC Frances of Rome, 55: 'sepius consueverat orare et scripturas divinas in vulgari sermone legere cum oculariis, in eius minibus tenendo dictas scripturas'; PC Frances of Rome, 279: 'Agnes Pauli Lelli [...] presens fuit et vidit quod b. F^{a} eundo per vineam offitium cum ocularibus ex libro dixit.' (I cannot help wondering to what extent these statements question the remarks that she was not particularly literate; see Cohen, *The Modulated Scream*, 189-90, 308, n. 86.) Eyeglasses were no longer a rarity by this time, but undoubtedly they were a mark of some loss of vision. Nevertheless, the witnesses referring to them did not interpret them in that manner.

The connection of infirmity and preaching is also visible in the famous preacher St. Bernardino of Siena's third canonization hearing, conducted in 1448-49,[173] but here the witnesses, who were clerics or elite laymen, emphasized the preacher's infirmity less than in the hearings of St. Vincent. The twenty-seventh article, which discusses the saint's *patientia* records that he endured many tribulations 'patiently and preaching the word of God'.[174] Given St. Bernardino's importance as a preacher, and that preaching was a primary element of his *fama sanctitatis*, it is only natural that the articles directed the witness statements to see also his infirmities in this light. One of the witnesses, the Sienese nobleman Leonardus Bartholomei de Benvolientibus, specified that the saint suffered from *maxime fluxum ventris* for fourteen years but never gave up preaching.[175] Some other witnesses gave similar statements, some of them adding *malo* or *infirmitas arenule* or *podagra* (possibly gout) to the list of infirmities.[176] However, in all witness statements regarding his *vita*, St. Bernardino's other tribulations, especially the reproach he faced from the Augustinian friars Gabriele de Spoleto and Andrea de Mediolano, receive significantly more attention.[177] This attention is related to the masculinity of holiness in a similar manner to the testimonies about the *patientia* of St. Thomas Cantilupe, although Bernardino refused to be made the bishop of Siena – only in Bernardino's case the hardships mostly refer to the other friars who disapproved of his actions and the public enthusiasm he engendered, or other incidents that occurred during his preaching.[178]

The witnesses who testified in the hearings of St. Vincent and St. Bernardino about the glory of an aging, saintly preacher facing adversities had a model in earlier hagiography. There was a view that old age could

173 St. Bernardino of Siena (1380-1444), an Observang Franciscan and a popular preacher, is one of the best-known late medieval Italian saints. The scholarship on him is vast. For his cult and canonization, see e.g. Mormando, *The Preacher's Demons*; Pellegrini, 'Introduzione'; Pellegrini, 'La sainteté au XVème siècle'; Pellegrini, 'Sui miracoli di Bernardino da Siena'; Krafft, *Papsturkunde und Heiligsprechung*, 954-65.

174 *Il processo di canonizzazione di Bernardino da Siena (1445-1450)*, ed. Pellegrini (PC Bernardino of Siena), 333: 'Item quod multos et varios labores et incommoditates, tam diurnos quam nocturnos, ac eciam persecuciones, pacienter passus est predicando Dei verbum et alia pia et sancta opera exercendo inter christianos propter fidem Christi.'

175 PC Bernardino of Siena, 352: 'est passus magnas incommoditates, circuendo huc et illuc cum variis infirmitatibus et maxime fluxu ventris, quem per annos XIII continuos passus fuit; nec propter hunc opus predicacionis dimictebat.'

176 PC Bernardino of Siena, 357, 362, 372, 375, 394, 401.

177 See e.g. PC Bernardino of Siena, 352-53, 357-58, 372-73, 391, 401.

178 For this dispute, see Mormando, *The Preacher's Demons*, 28, and for the attack he received when preaching against sodomy, 109-64; Rocke, *Forbidden Friendships*, 36-44.

increase the soul's vigour in devotion to God, even though it weakened bodily strength. Whether or not this happened depended on God and the person in question.[179] The anonymous *vita* of St. William of Bourges (*c.*1155-1209) records how infirm he was when giving his last sermon, and how it gave strength to his inner spirit. The author quotes 2 Corinthians 12:10.[180] Similarly, the *vita* of Bishop Hugh of Grenoble (1053-1132), also known as Hugh of Châteauneuf, records that when the effects of old age and illness began to take hold, Hugh asked for permission to leave his position. Pope Honorius II refused this request, as he thought that the authority and holy manner of life of the weak and ill man was a better example for the diocese than that of someone else who would be robust and healthy.[181] Especially concerning old age and lay priests, this view is also important in the canon law regulations. According to the *Decretum Gratiani*, old age in itself or a minor bodily debility was not a sufficient reason for retirement. The law text also directly quotes 2 Corinthians 12:10, stating that 'as the apostle says, when I am infirm, then I am strong'.[182]

Although old age could *cause* bodily infirmity, old age and illness did not invariably have causality in testimonies about saints' lives. In this, they reflect the contemporary medical and theological ideas. There were medical views about the marasmus of old age and its illnesslike pathology, which derived mainly from Galen and other ancient authorities.[183] However, Irina Metzler has written that medieval attitude towards the bodily consequences of old age differed markedly from ours in the sense that it did not pathologize them. Old age could be considered an advantage or a very unfortunate state, but it was not a disease, the concern of doctors, or a deviation from

179 Shahar, *Growing Old in the Middle Ages*, 54-55.

180 'Vita, Guilielmus Archiepiscopus Bituricensis, in Gallia (s.)', *AASS*, Ian. I, 633. William was canonized by Honorius III in 1218. He was considered a model archbishop, who had the benefit of the church in his interests, supporting papal policy and reforms as well as increasing ecclesiastical resources. Kroll and Bachrach, *The Mystic Mind*, 108. William was the uncle of Philip of Bourges, which was significant for the latter's *fama*. On the hagiographers' habit of emphasizing the saints' good family and stressing their even more desirable qualities, see Bartlett, *Why Can the Dead Do Such Great Things?*, 525.

181 'Vita, Hugo Episcopus Gratianopolitanus, in Gallia (s.)', *AASS*, Apr. I, 44: 'Creditum est enim, quod sola auctoritate et sanctae conversationis exemplo plus posset plebi prodesse subjectae debilis et aegrotus, quam quivis alius, robustus licet et sanus.'

182 See Salonen, 'What Happened to Aged Priests', 185-86. The law text is at lib. 1, tit. 9, cap. 4: 'pro talibus enim de se dicit Apostolus: cum infirmor, tunc fortior sum: quia nonnunquam corporis infirmitas fortitudinem cordis augmentat'. UCLA Digital Library Program, http://digital.library.ucla.edu/canonlaw/librarian?ITEMPAGE=CJC2_B01&NEXT (accessed 20 May 2019).

183 Schäfer, 'More than a Fading Flame', esp. 257.

the normalized body.[184] Attitudes to old people had varied considerably in ancient societies,[185] and continued to vary in the Middle Ages. Medieval writers recognized, admitted, and pondered the negative aspects of old age, being fully aware that it led to physical weakness and loss of vigour; after all, old age was a burden of mankind produced by the original sin.[186] Perhaps the best-known medieval negative conception related to old people is that of a *vetula*, an old woman considered to be ridiculous or even dangerous.[187] Old people might be ridiculed for their old age and its consequences, but they might equally be respected for their wisdom. If an old person (usually a man, as the image of old women was much more negative) retained his mental capacity, his age could even become an advantage.[188]

This gendered view of old age is barely detectable in the descriptions of saints' infirmities. The descriptions of old age concern mostly saints with a clerical status and are related to the activities they undertook in their office, but it is possible that the references to Clare of Montefalco's 'old age', connected with her reign as an abbess (discussed shortly), also derive from these ideas. If so, her holy infirmity was viewed as both feminine in its mystical elements and masculine as it underlined her excellence in taking care of her office. Furthermore, as we have seen, Dauphine of Puimichel's role in settling quarrels – despite the weakness of old age – was praised. However, one testimony suggests that her infirmity and old age might have been seen in a negative light more widely than the records reveal. Alasacia de Mesellano, a draper's widow from Apt, testified about Dauphine's begging activities and the ridicule she faced because of them. The commissioners asked her what words had been said, to which she responded that when Dauphine was asking for alms, paupers, murmuring among themselves, said: 'That *vetula* asks for alms and she has a big stomach, and she is being given two pieces of bread; and we are not given anything but a little coin!'[189] The paupers were obviously unaware of or did not agree with Dauphine's saintly *fama* or the dropsy that made her stomach swell, so they saw the old beggar woman

184 Metzler, *A Social History of Disability*, 93.

185 See e.g. Harlow and Laurence, 'Age, Agency and Disability'.

186 Metzler, *A Social History of Disability*, 93-96; Shahar, *Growing Old in the Middle Ages*, 38.

187 See e.g. Miller, *Medieval Monstrosity and the Female Body*; Pratt, '*De vetula*'.

188 Gordon, 'Representations of Aging and Disability', 421-36; Metzler, *Disability in The Middle Ages*, 163-65; Metzler, *A Social History of Disability*, 105-15.

189 PC Dauphine of Puimichel, 438: 'dixit quod per pauperes, quando querebat elemosinas dicta domina Dalphina, dicebatur sibi deridendo eam et murmurando contra eam: "Ista vetula querit elemosinas et habet grossum ventrem, et dantur sibi duos panes; et nobis non datur nisi una pecia modica!"' See also pp. 149-50 below for the ridicule Dauphine and other begging saints faced.

through their cultural lens as the stereotypical, deceptive, and ridiculous *vetula*. Yet the mention of her old age in the context of her good deeds in her community and the spiritual guidance she gave places it in the category a 'good' or respectable old age. Just as saints' bodies were exceptional in many ways, so too were the reactions to their ageing. The effects of old age on their bodies were first and foremost defined in the light of their sainthood and its most important aspects. For saints, old age and its infirmities became an ability, not a disability. The ailing and ageing body of a saint became a tool for showing an example to others as well as acting as a proof of the sanctity itself.

Infirmity, Raptures, and the Marks of Passion

In the corporality of female saints, the various types of bodily suffering such as self-chastisement, physical illness, and painful, mystic experiences often intermingled as an extreme way to practise *imitatio Christi*.[190] As already mentioned, there are indications that in general, hagiography became more and more corporeal in the later Middle Ages, and as saints' *vitae* were circulating widely, they provided models not just for those wishing to follow in earlier saints' footsteps, but also for their devotees.[191] At the same time, it appears that the faithful were more prone to accept very corporeal forms of *imitatio Christi* than the majority of churchmen, who did not normally approve of any deification of the human body, although laypeople were often aware of its dangers as well.[192] In the canonization testimonies concerning saints known for their raptures and mystical experiences, it was thus necessary to distinguish physical infirmity from other forms of *imitatio Christi*.[193]

As the examples discussed above have demonstrated, in most cases the details of a holy person's infirmity were primarily the concern of their innermost circle – or at least, it was they who most often testified about them. When it comes to more spiritual manifestations of bodily suffering

190 For example Bynum, *Holy Feast and Holy Fast*, 114.

191 See Klaniczay, *Uses of Supernatural Power*, 95-110, and also Gaposchkin, *The Making of Saint Louis*, 27-28.

192 Vauchez, *Sainthood*, 440; Bynum, *Holy Feast and Holy Fast*, 86-87.

193 Citing Bynum, Sarah Alison Miller writes that 'there was no clear division between illness, asceticism, mortification and self-torture', which were all means to imitate Christ's passion. Miller, *Medieval Monstrosity and the Female Body*, 104. However, in the context of 'official', proven sanctity this does not hold true, but as the canonization documents demonstrate, in the vast majority of cases there was a need to make a distinction, and the devotees were also able to make this distinction, even if they needed some guidance from the questions posed.

and *imitatio Christi*, especially in case of female saints, it usually became a more widely emphasized aspect of holiness, but still the witness statements were given by those expected to have accurate knowledge of the holy person's body.[194] The most illuminating example of this is the inquest into the bodily manifestations of Clare of Montefalco's sanctity.

Clare was born around 1268 into a wealthy family. Her father, Damiano Vengente, had built a hermitage, where Clare's older sister Iohanna lived with another woman as Tertiary Franciscans. When Clare was 6 years old, Iohanna obtained permission from the pope to receive more sisters, and Clare also joined the hermitage. The growing number of sisters resulted in the need to build a bigger establishment. In 1290, the sisters wished to make their lives more strictly monastic, and the bishop of Spoleto founded their monastery, which was to follow the Rule of St. Augustine, as the Tertiary Order of St. Francis was not yet established. After Iohanna's death in 1291, Clare became the abbess.[195]

The extraordinary events after Clare's death on 18 August 1308 have been well documented and analysed in research. The nuns, who wished to embalm Clare's body, famously discovered the symbols of Christ's passion (the crucifix, crown of thorns, the whip, column, sponge, and rod) inside her heart and some days later three gallstones in her bladder, taken as a sign of the trinity. The news of the discovery arose some suspicion among local authorities, and the *podestà*, or chief magistrate, of Montefalco with his officials examined the authenticity of the objects. Soon afterwards Bérenger de Saint-Affrique, vicar of the bishop of Spoleto in 1308-10, investigated the matter in order to reveal a fraud.[196] The result of the investigation was that the nuns could not have placed the objects in Clare's heart. This made Bérenger obtain permission from the bishop to open a diocesan inquiry into Clare's life and virtues.[197] Bérenger's work continued until 1315, and

194 The problematic nature of such experiences is clearly visible in the securing of the cult of St. Catherine of Siena, one of the best-known 'suffering saints' canonized in our period. The most notable, corporeal manifestation of her sanctity – the claims of her having been stigmatized – made her canonization a problematic issue. Klaniczay, 'The Power of the Saints', 131-32. By this time, stigmatization had become almost exclusively a phenomenon of female ecstatic religiosity. Klaniczay, 'On the Stigmatization of Saint Margaret of Hungary', 280. For the Processo Castellano and its lack of critical voices, see Ferzoco, 'Processo Castellano and the Canonization of Catherine of Siena', esp. 192-94.

195 Later on, Spiritual Franciscans have claimed that Clare was a part of their organization; on their connection, see Burr, *Spiritual Franciscans*, 316-20.

196 Menestò, 'La biografia di Chiara', 166-67.

197 Barone, 'Il processo di canonizzazione di Chiara da Montefalco', 182-83. Enrico Menestò writes that Bérenger de Saint-Affrique had no 'hagiographic background'; instead he had experience in church administration and possibly also in juridical culture. Bérenger wrote her biography largely

he finally went to present the results of the inquiry to the pope in autumn 1316.[198] After a verification of Bérenger's investigation in the curia, the pope opened an official canonization inquest, the documents of which survive only in fragments.[199] It was held between September 1318 and July 1319. Verifying the documents took ten years, but the final verdict was in support of Clare's canonization; why this did not happen is not known.[200] The process was resumed once in 1737 with no result, and for the third time in the nineteenth century, which finally resulted in the official canonization in 1881 by Leo XIII.[201]

In addition to her numerous miracles showing her importance as a thaumaturge, for Clare's community of devotees – including the nuns and the conductors and promoters of her canonization – her sanctity was very corporeal to begin with. In this, medical knowledge, communication, and precision appear extremely important.[202] Bérenger de Saint-Affrique mentioned in Clare's *vita* that the nuns had opened the gall bladder on medical advice,[203] which was undoubtedly a way of quelling any suspicion

based on the documents of the diocesan investigation. It is possible that these depositions were incorporated into the apostolic proceedings. Menestò, 'The Apostolic Canonization Proceedings of Clare of Montefalco', 108. See also Menestò, 'La biografia di Chiara', 165, 169. For the marks of the passion in Clare's heart, see Elliott, *Proving Woman*, 146-48, 164-65; Park, 'The Criminal and Saintly Body'; Park, 'Relics of a Fertile Heart'.

198 Menestò, 'La biografia di Chiara', 169.

199 They contain about two-thirds of the articles, that is, nos. 13-222, the depositions of witnesses 1 (partly), and 38-238 (the total number of witnesses was 486), and the beginning of the *relatio*. On the manuscripts, see Menestò, 'The Apostolic Canonization Proceedings of Clare of Montefalco', 107-8; Menestò, 'Introduzione'.

200 One possible explanation is the occasional allusion to the heresy of the Free Spirit in the process and in Clare's spiritual ideas, although Clare is known to have denounced the teachings of Bentivenga da Gubbio, the leader of the movement. Menestò, 'La biografia di Chiara', 178-79. Clare's visions and mystical experiences, which conflict with the theory of visions of Pope John XXII, may provide another explanation. See Barone, 'Il processo di canonizzazione di Chiara da Montefalco', 184-85.

201 Barone, 'Il processo di canonizzazione di Chiara da Montefalco', 189-90; Menestò, 'The Apostolic Canonization Proceedings of Clare of Montefalco', 105-6.

202 This is emphasized by the frequent references to Simon de Spoleto, who was the physician of the monastery and the town of Montefalco. He was present at Clare's death, and afterwards the nuns inquired of him whether the marvels discovered could have been caused by a natural infirmity. Simon stated that this was in no way possible, which was heard by several people. Unfortunately, Simon's own testimony is among the lost ones. PC Clare of Montefalco, 88, 90, 249, 341. See also Elliott, *Proving Woman*, 146-48. Virginia Langum has recently argued that of the medieval mystics, at least Julian of Norwich and Margery Kempe, used their medical knowledge to define their mystical experiences and differentiate them from their illnesses. Langum, 'Medicine, Female Mystics and Illness Experience'.

203 Park, 'Relics of a Fertile Heart', 119; *Vita sanctae Clarae de Cruce*, ed. Semenza, 60-61.

their actions had aroused, but it also reflects the interaction between devotees. Sister Francescha, who testified in the hearing, was the daughter of physician Gualterius de Montefalco, who attended Clare during her infirmities,[204] and also happened to be the sister who had the most important role in the dissection of Clare's body.[205] As argued by Katharine Park, the nuns' actions as well as the importance of their discoveries is related to the emergence of the dissection as a practice in Latin Europe in the late thirteenth and early fourteenth centuries, and to its growing importance as an element of legal practice, medical study, and public health procedures.[206] The views of Clare's saintly corporality that have been preserved to this day are thus a combination of the nuns' veneration of her, the medical culture of the time, and Bérenger's intervention, in which he 'sought to obtain from the historical memory of the witnesses confirmation of a legend that was itself taking shape and structure through his direct intervention'.[207]

The importance of medical culture does not, however, show clearly in most of the (preserved) articles that Bérenger wrote. When reporting that Clare's ill health limited her ascetic practices or how she instructed younger nuns to be active in their penitence when she was 'burned with infirmities', he made no mention of any precise diagnoses.[208] The same pertains to other articles where he referred to Clare's infirmity. In this respect, the way Clare's ill health is treated in the hearing is similar to other inquests of the period. As for the nuns testifying to these articles, there are differences in their eagerness to give diagnoses. In testifying about Clare's *patientia*, Sister Francescha and Sister Thomassa, for example, mentioned that Clare was grateful for her tribulations and infirmities and that she said she was not worthy of them. Sister Thomassa also wondered how Clare could sustain her infirmities, which she defined as 'stomach pain and colic', without complaints.[209] Here again we encounter the benefits of infirmities expressed

204 Her testimony is in PC Clare of Montefalco, 329-48.

205 Park, 'Relics of a Fertile Heart', 119.

206 Park, 'Relics of a Fertile Heart', esp. 117-19.

207 Menestò, 'The Apostolic Canonization Proceedings of Clare of Montefalco', 109-10.

208 PC Clare of Montefalco, 3; as for instructing on penitence, Clare reportedly said that if she had their bodily strength, she would never lie in bed, PC Clare of Montefalco, 8, see also 197.

209 PC Clare of Montefalco, 181: 'vidit dicta testis ipsam s. Claram multis et diversis temporibus infirmam variis infirmitatibus, et maxime de dolore stomachy et doloribus yliatis, et quod nunquam potuit ipsa testis perpendere, ut dicit, quod ipsa sancta Clara huiusmodi infirmitatibus conquereretur seu murmuraret; immo, ut ipsa testis audivit, gratias Deo referendo, dicebat hec et similia verba: "O quantus fuit dolor quem Dominus meus Yhesus Christus substinuit pro me! Ego sum digna, si plus possem portare doloribus et infirmitatibus maioribus, omnia habere!"' PC Clare of Montefalco,

by a holy person and reported by a devotee. Although the testimonies do not specifically refer to any biblical passage, there is a clear resemblance to 2 Corinthians 12:10 ('Cum infirmor potens sum').[210] Sister Thomassa and abbess Iohanna returned to the topic of 'colic' also later when they were testifying to articles related to the events before Clare's death, including her battles with demons and lack of pain in final illness.[211] In this instance the commissioners appear to have been more eager to get a proper diagnosis.[212] This probably relates to the hagiographic importance of the saint's death, and possibly also to the battles with demons, similarly to the hearing of St. Nicholas of Tolentino.

For the nuns Clare's period as an abbess and her ability to be a good one when poor health prevented her from carrying out physical duties were of crucial importance. Sister Marina, for example, testified about all the chores Clare did in serving other sisters and how, when she was so weak or infirm that she could no longer do them, she helped the sisters with her words.[213] This example, as well as the other instances where the nuns told of Clare's rule with or without referring to infirmity, can be compared with those concerning Clare of Assisi discussed above. Occasionally the sisters could emphasize these merits even more than Clare's corporality, as the same Sister Marina did when testifying about her *patientia*. Instead of referring to any infirmity, she related Clare's patience when some local men attacked the monastery and insulted the sisters.[214] As another example of Clare's qualities considered important, her brother's testimony includes a lengthy paragraph about her extraordinary intelligence as well as her skill in teaching the younger sisters.[215] The importance of saintly abbesses' rule in office was a significant element of their *fama*, albeit often neglected in research.[216] Even if in the 'official' saintly corporality of female saints was

332-33: 'dixit se scire quia ipsa dicebat quod non erat dingna habere ipsas tribulationes et infirmitates et indigentias, sed quod diligebat habere tribulationes et infirmitates et indigentias'.

210 See note 131 (p. 73).

211 PC Clare of Montefalco, 78-79, 237.

212 On demons present at the saint's death, see e.g. G. Adams, *Visions in Late Medieval England*, 96-100, 116. On community and saint's final illness, see pp. 152-54 below.

213 PC Clare of Montefalco, 107: 'quando erat adeo debilis vel infirma quod non posset fatigari, iuvabat dictas sorores in consiliis et dulcibus verbis.'

214 PC Clare of Montefalco, 109-10, and Sister Thomassa's deposition on 181.

215 PC Clare of Montefalco, 276-78.

216 Burr, *Spiritual Franciscans*, 316, judges Clare of Montefalco to have been a 'good abbess' and writes regarding her raptures that she 'combined them with wise spiritual direction of her charges and, perhaps more surprisingly, sound decisions concerning internal organization'. For an overview of an abbess's duties, see Bodawré, 'Abbesses', 1-4.

often emphasized more than it was with men, Clare's example shows clearly that they too had various saintly roles. Although Clare's reign was most important to the other nuns and her interaction with her other devotees was very limited, her qualities as an abbess were recognized by members of the lay community as well. This is shown in the deposition of Petructius Thomassii, Clare's notary for five years, who mentioned the spiritual consolations he had received from her.[217]

There is more precision in investigating corporeal symptoms in the articles and corresponding testimonies, which directly address Clare's bodily symptoms as a sign of her *imitatio Christi*, the objects discovered in her heart, or her raptures. This is hardly surprising, given the suspicions they awoke and their importance for the cult. Sister Thomassa told the commissioners how Clare often told the nuns about Christ's passion, instructing them to meditate on it with tears, compassion, and devotion.[218] As noted by Monique Scheer, emotions as practices are transferred between people,[219] or as written by Damien Boquet and Piroska Nagy, emotions, that an affected person shares, are passed on.[220] Here the community of nuns were socialized into a culturally established way of meditating on Christ's passion with specific sentiments and reactions. Simultaneously, their veneration of 'their' saint, and their observance of the characteristics of her sainthood grew stronger.

Unlike in most processes, the articles in Clare's hearing refer to her imitation of Christ's suffering, stating that Clare felt the cross in her heart and often showed signs of pain.[221] In mystical consolation literature the presence of God often brought deep pain as well as pleasure,[222] the pain Clare felt being one example of this. Connecting Clare's compassion with the discovery of the objects of passion after her death was thus undoubtedly a conscious choice of Bérenger de Saint-Affrique, but the nuns were also aware of the care that was needed in testifying about such issues. Sister Thomassa's detailed testimony on the matter shows that she considered both Clare's words and the corporeal manifestations important. According to her, Clare often spoke about the issue, suffering with Christ, and when she heard Christ's death being related or preached about, she cried a lot and it 'caused

217 PC Clare of Montefalco, 391-92.

218 PC Clare of Montefalco, 193.

219 Scheer, 'Are Emotions a Kind of Practice?', esp. 218.

220 Boquet and Nagy, *Medieval Sensibilities*, 217.

221 PC Clare of Montefalco, 7: 'Item quod ipsa sancta Clara retulit, dum vivebat, quod Deus revelaverat ei passionem Christi et quod ipsa viderat per revelationem Dei passionem Christi plene, sicut si fuisset presens quando Christus fuit crucifixus.'

222 Rittgers, *The Reformation of Suffering*, 78.

her pain which was visible externally'.[223] For them, the *imitatio Christi* and the pain it caused was evident in Clare's tears, a reaction considered the road to salvation,[224] and in the external signs of her infirmity, even if not specified by the witnesses.

As Nancy Caciola wrote in the introduction to her book *Discerning Spirits*, medieval interpretations of spiritual influence, whether possession or raptures and visions, 'always pulse back and forth between the two poles of interior and exterior'.[225] Therefore, although the nuns and other witnesses to Clare's life sought to transmit her inner spiritual experience to the commissioners, its outer manifestations were of crucial importance. When giving a testimony about Clare's frequent spiritual raptures and elevations, the commissioners inquired of Sister Marina as to whether Clare had 'women's infirmities, defects of body or heart, or falling sickness', which could leave her 'insensible'. She replied 'no' to all these questions.[226] Sister Thomassa's testimony elicited similar questions, to which she responded that towards the end of her life, Clare experienced some pain in the female parts, but not so much that it would have left her insensible.[227]

The questions the commissioners posed derive from the view of many important theologians that rapturelike states could be caused by demons or bodily and mental illnesses. Some of them had similarly critical views of visions.[228] Therefore, from the fourteenth century onwards, the commis-

223 PC Clare of Montefalco, 193: 'quandoque audiebat legi de passione Christi, vel predicam de morte Christi vel alias loqui de morte Christi, lacrimabatur multum de ipsa morte Christi et affligebatur fortiter sicut exterius apparebat.' See also 120 for Sister Marina's testimony on the matter.

224 See Cohen, *The Modulated Scream*, 29.

225 Caciola, *Discerning Spirits*, 19-20.

226 PC Clare of Montefalco, 118: 'Interrogata de infirmitate matricis et defectus corporis et cordis et de morbo caducho, utrum dicta sancta Clara pateretur dictas infirmitates que reddunt infirmas nec aliquando quasi sicut extra se et insemsibiles, dixit quod nunquam habuit dictas infirmitates nec aliquam earum dicta sancta Clara.'

227 PC Clare of Montefalco, 191: 'Interrogata de infirmitate matricis, de defectu cordis et de caduco morbo, utrum pateretur dictas infirmitates, dixit quod non, nisi quod aliquando circha finem vite sue visa fuit aliquantulum <pati> de dolore matricis, sed non taliter quod rederet eam insensibilem, nisi quod eam aliqualiter affligebat.'

228 See Dinzelbacher, *Mystik und Natur*, 64-65; Elliott, 'The Physiology of Rapture and Female Spirituality', 141-49; Elliott, *Proving Woman*, 273-75; Goodich, *Miracles and Wonders*, 69-70. The hagiographers could also make use of the various mechanisms behind rapturelike symptoms. For instance, the anonymous author of the *Miracoli* of St. Catherine of Siena, written in 1374 when the holy woman was still alive, records one of her visions in August 1374 and writes that during them, she was 'mortally ill' but had no symptoms of the plague. Instead, '[s]he became totally numb, not in the manner when in contemplation she was enraptured to the heavens, but through an illness of the body'. 'The *Miracoli* of Catherine of Siena', ed. and trans. Lehmijoki-Gardner, 102; see 87-89 on the text.

sioners sought to delineate the reasons for the experience the witnesses interpreted as raptures, and increasingly investigated and interpreted them in medicalized terms.[229] This is one example of late medieval medicalization, where authority was not necessarily given to medical professionals, but various parties use medical vocabulary and knowledge.[230] The concern over the cause of raptures is most pronounced in the canonization processes of female saints, since women were considered more prone to both demonic possession and spiritual raptures; in Clare of Montefalco's case also because she was one of the first and most prominent examples of the new female religious movement.[231] This is one of the few instances where it is possible to identify when a change occurred in canonization inquests, as those for female saints in the thirteenth century are not yet really concerned with this issue.

Although those venerating a saint were quick to separate raptures, visions, and the pain of *imitatio Christi* from somatic conditions, there certainly were voices of doubt as well. It is just that they are rarely recorded in the canonization inquests. Clare of Montefalco's process includes one very critical deposition, that of the Franciscan friar Thomas Boni de Fulgineo, who outspokenly rejected her sanctity. Among his views were that the objects of passion were a fraud, and he accused her of associating with heretic clergymen who had links with the Free Spirit movement.[232] He also stated that Clare often fell to the ground, but he could not tell whether or not this was caused by a 'good spirit'.[233] As no further inquiries about this matter are recorded, the meaning of this 'diagnosis' is left somewhat unclear, but it is quite possible that the statement implied epilepsy, an illness considered to cause rapturelike states.[234] Clare's process also includes a punishment miracle, which interlinks the voices of doubt and the corporeal signs of her

229 See also Elliott, 'The Physiology of Rapture and Female Spirituality', 157, 161-64; Elliott, *Proving Woman*, 211.

230 See Singer, *Blindness and Therapy*, 8-9.

231 Park, 'Relics of a Fertile Heart', 120-21.

232 PC Clare of Montefalco, 434-36. On this witness account, see Elliott, *Proving Woman*, 147-48; Klaniczay 'The Inquisition of Miracles', 63-64; Vauchez, *Santi, profeti e visionari*, 239-41.

233 PC Clare of Montefalco, 435-36: 'utrum procederet a spiritu bono vel non, dixit se nescire.'

234 For example, Margery Kempe's reactions to the images of Christ were interpreted as epilepsy by some, and Prophet Mohammed's vision of the archangel was, among other things, explained as an attack of epilepsy by several medieval writers. See Claassens, 'Jacob van Maerlant on Muhammed and Islam', 219-20; Pearman, *Women and Disability in Medieval Literature*, 116. Some modern scholars have also attempted to diagnose Margery, as well as Julian of Norwich, another famous mystic, with different physical and mental illnesses. For this discussion, see Miller, *Medieval Monstrosity and the Female Body*, 105-7; Vuille, 'Maybe I'm Crazy?'.

sainthood.[235] Three witnesses (two of them sons of the *podestà*) narrated an instance where a group of men went to see the objects of passion immediately after Clare's death. One of the men, Symon ser Gilii, started to ridicule them. Immediately his nose began to bleed profusely, to the point that he was so weak that the others had to support him. The *sacerdos* placed Clare's heart right above the repentant Symon's face, which cured him. Afterwards he venerated Clare and became a great friend of the monastery, visiting it often.[236] A case like this was of course an obvious sign of the veracity of the objects, and must have helped in disseminating their *fama* within the local community.

Punishment miracles are generally quite rare in late medieval canonization inquests, and one so closely connected to a corporeal feature of sainthood is even more exceptional. That of Symon ser Gilii, however, gives a glimpse of the interaction that occurred around the particular signs of holiness. Mystic experiences and their corporality had to be communally negotiated, and presumably they were also discussed somewhat critically, which is visible also in other types of hagiographic texts.[237] The few examples included in canonization documents concern elite members of society, like another one recorded in St. Birgitta of Sweden's canonization inquest.[238] Petrus Olavi, the prior of the Cistercian monastery in Alvastra, recorded Birgitta's visions. He was at first reluctant to take the task appointed by Christ, partly due to his suspicion that they were a demonic trick. Suddenly he acquired a grave infirmity, which forced him to lie in bed 'half-dead' ('semi mortuus') for a night, and he realized the error in his thinking.[239] Again, this disciplinary miracle illustrates a particular – and immensely important – aspect of Birgitta's sanctity through her interpreter's body,[240] but it was also of crucial importance for Petrus, whose career was at stake and depended on the success of Birgitta's canonization.[241] Petrus also testified to having been present when a monk of the same monastery had told Birgitta in the late 1340s that she did not have a 'healthy brain' ('sanum

235 For miracles and 'voices of doubt' more generally, see Goodich, *Miracles and Wonders*, 47-68. For punishment miracles, see Klaniczay, 'Miracoli di punizione e *maleficia*'.

236 PC Clare of Montefalco, 459-60, 461, 484.

237 For examples, see Cohen, *The Modulated Scream*, 122-23.

238 See also Elliott, 'The Physiology of Rapture and Female Spirituality', 157, 161-64.

239 PC Birgitta of Sweden, 510-11.

240 Birgitta's canonization inquest includes a relatively high number of punishment miracles (of various types) that her blasphemers faced. Sahlin, *Birgitta of Sweden and the Voice of Prophecy*, 154-55.

241 See Salmesvuori, *Power and Sainthood*, 43, 47.

cerebrum') but that she was prone to fantasies, and about an instance when a knight suggested that Birgitta should lessen her asceticism, which caused her raptures.[242] It is intriguing, however, that the testimonies to Birgitta's raptures and other such states rarely include any references to somatic conditions as their potential cause. Then again, as mentioned above, Birgitta is one of those female saints in whose *fama* physical suffering did not play a major role. This may explain why such explanations for her raptures and visions were not as topical as for Clare.

Very corporeal, trancelike contemplation of Christ's suffering was also part of the *fama* of St. Frances of Rome, and in her process it was also investigated and interpreted in both medical and non-medical terms. In addition to recording the tears she shed, the sixth article in her first canonization hearings describes how Frances's contemplation made her suffer equally, remain insensible in her body, and have her legs as if attached to a cross, making her unable to walk. Furthermore, the contemplation of the wounds of Christ's body made a waterlike liquid run from the same side of her body. The testimonies to this article recorded in 1440 and 1443 were given by Frances's confessor and hagiographer Johannes Matteotti and *frater* Petrus, the prior of the monastery of Santa Sabina, as well as Frances's spiritual daughters Rita Covelli, Agnes Pauli Lelli, and Jacobella de Brunomonte. The only person who mentioned that Frances held her legs in the manner of a victim of crucifixion was Johannes Matteotti, and he connected the episode with Frances's reception of the Eucharist from his hands.[243] Katharine Park has observed that male hagiographers tended to translate 'internal mystical experiences of their female subjects into externally perceptible corporeal signs, like *stigmata*, bleeding wounds, and other paramystical phenomena'.[244] Similarly, Amy Hollywood has written that the late medieval female mystics stressed their visions while their hagiographers insisted on

242 PC Birgitta of Sweden, 488, 493. Dyan Elliott has translated the statement that Birgitta would not have had *sanum cerebrum* as 'brain damage'. Elliott, 'The Physiology of Rapture and Female Spirituality', 164. It is hard to interpret exactly what type of a diagnosis the friar had in his mind; he could also refer to lack of reason in general, caused by some form of madness. This was certainly one of Jean Gerson's arguments in his doubts regarding revelations. Jean Gerson, *Distinguishing True from False Revelations*, 345-46. As pointed out by Langum, *Medicine and the Seven Deadly Sins*, 149-50, his arguments are highly medicalized throughout, which is one indication of the importance of medicine for delineating embodiment of the holy. See also Pfau, 'Madness in the Realm', 169-72; Sahlin, *Birgitta of Sweden and the Voice of Prophecy*, 163-68. For Jean Gerson's critique of Birgitta's canonization, see Elliott, *Proving Woman*, 282-83, and for the criticism she faced from her contemporaries, Sahlin, *Birgitta of Sweden and the Voice of Prophecy*, 147-48, 228.
243 PC Frances of Rome, 18-19.
244 Park, 'Relics of a Fertile Heart', 122.

external marks.[245] Johannes clearly found this important, as he recorded the wound in Frances's *vita*,[246] and according to Agnes Pauli Lelli, he also performed tests to see if Frances's imperceptible state was true.[247]

It is difficult to ascertain how much of the witnesses' testimonies was left out, and whether the spiritual daughters referred to the outer expressions of Frances's raptures as well. What their testimonies do reveal is that the raptures and the liquid were a crucial, communal memory for them. Referring to a mid-fourteenth century *Zouche Hours*, Michael Camille has stated that Christ's body interacted with that of his viewers, and his blood intermingled with the milk that squirts from his mother's breast. Thus, all senses were included in the devotional urge.[248] The spiritual daughters' testimonies equally give a picture of Frances as a 'mediator' between them and Christ's passion, in the same manner as in the testimonies of the nuns in Clare of Montefalco's monastery. The role of physical pain is, however, less obvious. In the testimonies from 1443 it is mainly referred to in symbolic terms and in the witnesses' descriptions of Frances stating that after her rapture, when receiving the Eucharist, she was 'healed',[249] whereas the additions of 1453 give a more explicit description, especially the testimony of Frances's daughter-in-law Mabilia. She testified that many thought Frances might die of the pain that her contemplations caused.[250] The interplay between communality and the personal is especially evident in the testimony of Agnes Pauli Lelli. She was the *principalis et mater spiritualis* of Frances's congregation, had known Frances from around 1410, and lived in the same *cellula* with her. From this perspective, it is no wonder that she is the most often cited witness in the hearing.[251] Her testimony from 1443 gives the impression that the liquid flowed often, as she testified to having seen Frances's tears oftentimes, as well as to wiping the liquid from her breast and washing and managing the cloths.[252] For her, taking part in this manifestation of sainthood was a tangible and concrete experience.

Frances's raptures were also investigated in the hearing of 1451, which was the most organized of the three inquests.[253] It offers an intriguing opportunity to investigate how different the witness accounts of an event

245 Hollywood, *Soul as Virgin Wife*, 27-36.

246 'Acta Francisca Romana vidua', *AASS*, Mar. II, 182.

247 PC Frances of Rome, 61. See also Cohen, *The Modulated Scream*, 123.

248 Camille, 'The Image and the Self', 77.

249 PC Frances of Rome, 19-20.

250 PC Frances of Rome, 21.

251 Esch, 'Die Zeugenaussagen', 144.

252 PC Frances of Rome, 20-21.

253 Esch, 'I processi medioevali', 41-43, 47-48; Lugano, 'Introduzione', pp. xvi-xviii.

can be almost a decade after the previous hearing, when examined by different people who formed their questions differently. Twelve testimonies were recorded to article 14 on Frances's 'devotion and the elevation of her mind' ('De eius devotione et mentis elevatione');[254] from those who had testified in the 1430 and 1433 hearings, Agnes Pauli Lelli and *frater* Ypolitus testified again. This time neither the article nor the testimonies mention the position of Frances's hands and legs or liquid running from her chest. Instead, *domina* Agnes, *frater* Ypolitus, and many others stated they had seen her raptures many times in her house in Trastevere, as well as when receiving the Eucharist. Furthermore, some witnesses specifically testified that they had seen her in such a state at the time of the death of Vannotzia, her sister-in-law, who had lived a holy life.[255]

The commissioners of this hearing asked Agnes Pauli Lelli, *frater* Ypolitus, and *domna* Rensia, another oblate, if signs of any infirmity appeared at the time of the extasies and immobility. All of them replied 'no', as expected.[256] They inquired of Frances's daughter-in-law Mabilia more specifically whether Frances's immobility was due to *infirmitate mentis*, and she clearly stated that there was 'no sign of infirmity'.[257] From *domna* Ceccha Nucii the commissioners inquired if she believed Frances's rapture was caused by pain, *dementia* (or madness), or another debility or infirmity.[258] *Dementia* was thought to be caused by an imbalance in the four humours affecting the anterior of the brain, and this could cause loss of control, perception, and sensation.[259] These were precisely the visible symptoms that Frances was described as having during her raptures. Exactly why these questions were posed (or recorded) to these witnesses is impossible to know. Nevertheless, for the women, and undoubtedly for the clerics testifying in Frances's process, the more mystical side of her *imitatio Christi* was its strongest memory, but they were able to interpret it in medical terms when asked to do so.

The complexity of interplay between the hagiographers, conductors of a hearing, and other devotees of a holy woman is perhaps even more obvious

254 The article and the witness accounts are in PC Frances of Rome, 229-32.

255 For Vannotzia, whose saintlike life paralleled that of Frances in many ways, see Esposito, 'St. Francesca and the Female Religious Communities', 199-200.

256 PC Frances of Rome, 230-32.

257 PC Frances of Rome, 230-31: 'testis dixit quod credit ipsam fuisse raptam quia contemplando divina rapiebatur in extasin, et non ex infirmitate fuisse alienatam; quia nullum in ea apparuit signum infirmitatis tempore hiusmodi extasis, neque ante neque post.'

258 PC Frances of Rome, 231: 'Interrogata si credit ipsam in extasi raptam fuisse aut ex dolore vel dementia vel ex aliqua alia debilitate et infirmitate fuisse immobilem.'

259 Turner, *Care and Custody*, 52-53.

in the case of Dorothea of Montau, who met her confessor Johannes Marienwerder around three years before her death.[260] The narrations about her mystic experiences, especially how God, according to the articles, 'imprinted bleeding and painful wounds on her' are one of a kind in the canonization processes.[261] As the procurator, Johannes Marienwerder formulated the articles, it became explicit that though Dorothea fiercely chastised her own flesh, her suffering was ultimately brought upon her by God precisely to prove her sanctity.[262] Most of the witnesses to the wounds were clerics who had known Dorothea personally, and the same goes for her raptures, about which the only suspicion the commissioners raised was whether she was asleep.[263] It is remarkable, however, that *patientia* was not a core element of her wounds.[264] One of the longest testimonies about the wounds was given by Johannes Reyman, a canon lawyer who had known Dorothea's mother personally and who had been taking notes about Dorothea's life before she became an anchoress.[265] According to him, because of these 'wounds of the soul', Dorothea often appeared 'exhausted and infirm' ('marcida et infirma'), 'as if she had been afflicted by corporeal wounds'. The possibility that these wounds were of mundane origin was not recorded,[266] but he used somatic infirmity as a metaphor to describe the bodily effect of these God-sent wounds.

The testimony of Sister Katherina of the Teutonic Order gives a glimpse of the interplay between the confessor and other devotees of Dorothea in

260 Elliott, 'Authorizing a Life', 169-71.
261 PC Dorothea of Montau, 15: 'In locis predictis fuit et est publica vox et fama, quod, dum dicta Dorothea vitam ageret in humanis, pluribus vicibus Deus ipsam afflixit seu affligi fecit vulneribus ad eius sanctitatem melius approbandam et confirmandam.' PC Dorothea of Montau, 19-20: 'Jhesus Cristus [...] ipsi Dorothee dupliciter vulnera impressit, interius scilicet et exterius in corpore, [...] qua in sanguinis effusione ac multiplici afflixione eam sibi disposuerat desponsare. Quedam vulnera per annos 40 duraverunt.' See also Classen, 'Wounding the Body and Freeing the Spirit', 419.
262 This is related to the ideals regarding moderation in abstinence. See pp. 121-37 below for further discussion on the matter.
263 For some reason, the testimony of Nicolaus von Hohenstein, who had been Dorothea's confessor in Gdansk, only includes a very brief witness account of the corporality of her sanctity, making no mention of the wounds. PC Dorothea of Montau, 80. See PC Dorothea of Montau, 257, for Johannes Marienwerder's testimony on raptures.
264 See, however, PC Dorothea of Montau, 280: 'a iuventute sua admirabilis patiente fuit, quia omnia sibi illata a Deo, utputa gravia vulnera, libenter suscepit'; Johannes Marienwerder also mentioned the diabolic temptations and her patience towards them. Johannes Mönch's testimony is in PC Dorothea of Montau, 411-12; he specified that Dorothea herself had told him that she never had any *impatientia* because of the (childhood) wounds, even though they made her very infirm.
265 None of these writings have survived. Hartmann, 'Bridal Mysticism', 103.
266 PC Dorothea of Montau, 195-200.

interpreting the corporeal signs of her sainthood.[267] Because Katherina had been Dorothea's cohabitant, the commissioners considered it worthwhile to interrogate her more closely. Katherina testified that Johannes had told her that Dorothea had an 'apostema'. Katherina, for her part, asked Dorothea if that was the case, and eventually Dorothea showed her 'a terrible wound' under her left arm. Dorothea told her that she had had it since Rome – apparently referring to her pilgrimage to Rome during the papal Jubilee of 1390, when she was reportedly gravely infirm.[268] Katherina was asked how she knew that God imprinted the wounds on Dorothea, to which she replied that He is powerful enough to do so, but this is the only reference to the matter in her long testimony.[269] The commissioners then moved on to interrogate her about Dorothea's other wounds, which Katherina had seen in her thighs, and, as a reply to a question about their type, Katherina explained that the 'scabies'[270] were caused by self-chastisement. It is hard to tell what effect the structure of the written statement and its relatively summarized nature has had on our version of Katherina's testimony, but it seems that she had an idea either that there were two explanations for the wounds *or* that their being imprinted by God and caused by self-chastisement were more or less the same thing. No attempt by the commissioners to make any distinction was recorded in the statement.

Among the female and non-clerical witnesses to Dorothea's life, Katherina is an exception because of her close acquaintanceship with the saint, and she was one of the key informants for the details of Dorothea's life among the elite witnesses in the process. It is more difficult to decide which aspects of Dorothea's life were most prominent for the larger community of devotees. The canonization protocols portray her primarily as a thaumaturge. This is a contrast with the *Vita germanica* by Johannes Marienwerder intended for the propagation of her cult, which largely focuses on her wounds and her brutal husband[271] – an aspect of suffering that gets relatively little emphasis in the

267 Her testimony on the wounds is in PC Dorothea of Montau, 139-40.

268 See pp. 176-77 below for further discussion on the pilgrimage.

269 Her testimony to the article about the childhood accident is very brief. PC Dorothea of Montau, 144.

270 In medieval medicine, *scabies* was used to denote an itching skin disease. The term was commonly associated with leprosy, but not synonymous with it. It was rather something that could develop into *lepra*. Demaitre, *Leprosy in Premodern Medicine*, 89, 191-92, 218; Demaitre, *Medieval Medicine*, 108-9. In Katherina's testimony, however, it appears to have been used to mean an unspecified skin condition.

271 Heß, *Heilige machen*, 245-46, 256-64. According to Almut Suerbaum, Johannes's motive for composing the vernacular *vita* was to reach a lay audience who might adopt some of main characteristics of Dorothea's life; not her extreme ascetic practices, but the principle of Eucharistic

canonization records.[272] Johannes testified that, in addition to Dorothea herself, his other informants on Dorothea's life were 'some women' in Gdansk,[273] who were presumably spreading Dorothea's *fama* more widely in the city. The few laywomen who gave testimonies about Dorothea's life based their knowledge on Johannes's writings, sermons, or actual aquaintance with him, but one, Margaretha Creuczeburgische, had apparently known Dorothea personally and heard her say that God inflicted great wounds upon her. Interestingly, according to Margaretha's own words, she did not desire to hear more about them because she was not 'competent' to hear such good things at the time.[274]

A larger audience also had access to the corporality of Dorothea's sanctity after her death. The usual informants Johannes Marienwerder and Sister Katherina testified about the many scars on Dorothea's body that they and some other people had witnessed,[275] while Bishop Johannes Mönch stated that there was a huge crowd of people present after Dorothea's death, which *prevented* him from seeing the scars.[276] Johannes Rote, a *camerarius* of Bishop

devotion. The vernacular version also centres on the association of suffering with spiritual raptures. In the Latin texts, he stresses the biblical justification for Dorothea's asceticism, especially its significance in overcoming the world. Suerbaum, 'An Urban Housewife as a Saint', 184-85, 187. As a topic Dorothea's Eucharistic devotion is beyond the scope of this study; however, it is worth pointing out that this could also have very corporeal characteristics. Johannes Marienwerder testified about Dorothea's craving for the said sacrament and its very tangible physical pain. PC Dorothea of Montau, 270-71. He was closely involved in Dorothea's devotion to the Eucharist, since he was the person authorizing her to take it frequently, instead of once a year as was common for laypeople. Kieckhefer, *Unquiet Souls*, 30; Bynum, *Holy Feast and Holy Fast*, 55.

272 Using Dorothea as a model example, Barbara G. Newman writes about the *topos* of saintly women who 'bear their husbands' abuse with enough patience to win a martyr's crown in heaven'. B. Newman, *From Virile Woman*, 115. On the marital violence in Dorothea's vernacular *vita*, see Hartmann, 'Bridal Mysticism', 106-8; Heß, *Heilige machen*, 245-46; for marital violence in hagiographic texts, see e.g. Goodich, 'Miseries of Dulcia St. Chartier (1266) and Cristina of Wellington (1294)'. As an interesting aside to the current discussion, in the German *Life* Johannes explains Adalbert's behaviour partly by his being 'choleric' by nature but also by his 'arthritis'. In *Vita Lindana* Adalbert is described as easily agitated, due to bodily complexion and the infirmity of paralysis. Choleric temperament meant that one was prone to anger, but Johannes appears to have seen his infirmity as one reason for Adalbert's behaviour. See 'Vita b. Dorotheae Lindana', *AASS*, Oct. XIII, 514; Hartmann, 'Bridal Mysticism', 106; Lamberg, 'Anger as a Spiritual, Social and Mental Disorder', 70-71.

273 PC Dorothea of Montau, 259.

274 PC Dorothea of Montau, 96: 'quod Deponens cum Dorothea converstata fuit, aliquotiens audivit Dorotheam sibi dicere, quod homines essent, quibus Deus inferret vulnera gratie, divina et magna. De quibus ipsa deponens non curavit protunc aliqua audire; credit, quod non fuit capax tunc tanti boni.'

275 PC Dorothea of Montau, 139-40, 260-63.

276 PC Dorothea of Montau, 416: 'Et in die obitus eius libenter vidisset vulnera eius; sed ad feretrum per multitudine populi non poterat accedere, quia tota nocte eius corpus custodiebant cum maxima devotione.'

Johannes replied to the commissioners' question that he had not seen any wounds when Dorothea was alive, but he saw them after her death when her corpse was visible for eighteen weeks.[277] For some (elite) witnesses, the scars were a manifestation of self-chastisement rather than a sign of the divine wounds.[278] Undoubtedly different interpretations of the wounds' origins were possible, depending on the devotee's status and the information they had or considered important. These scars were, nevertheless, a tangible proof of the physical marks left by the divine power, and as such one of the characteristics in the embodiment of the cult of saints.

Above we have seen examples of the interlinking of infirmity and mystic experiences in female saints' canonization inquests. As discussed by several scholars, mysticism, especially when combined with self-inflicted pain and other extreme, bodily manifestations, was largely a female phenomenon.[279] However, this does not mean that a male saint would not have similar experiences, that a male saint's mystical experience would not have been corporeal, or that a male saint's devotees would not have considered them important.[280] In any particular community, male and female mystic experience and corporality may have been notionally the same, and medieval idea of a holy person's body did not necessarily conform to any general pattern identified or conceived by modern scholarship. After all, the most famous stigmatic was a male saint, and as we have seen, in the case of some male saints like St. Louis IX, extreme suffering could be one of the deepest manifestations of their sanctity. Furthermore, even if intense *imitatio Christi* was considered primarily a female phenomenon, in late medieval culture it held positive connotations and was not only a matter of women. Men and women could express their religious sensibilities in a similar manner.[281]

Of the saints whose cults were investigated in a canonization inquest, St. Elzéar of Sabran is the most traditional example of a male mystic, and the only male saint of the period with truly mystic gifts. The descriptions of his mystic experiences recorded in his *vita* are very similar to those of female saints, including his carrying of Christ's passion in his heart and rejoicing in

277 PC Dorothea of Montau, 401.

278 See e.g. the testimony of *magister* Bertrandus, PC Dorothea of Montau, 387: 'domina Dorothea corpus suum diversis modis afflixit iam nova vulnera infligendo et inveterate renovando'.

279 Hildegard of Bingen even connected her visionary abilities with the illness she had; Miller, *Medieval Monstrosity and the Female Body*, 104-5.

280 Traditionally male saints' mysticism has been considered more literary or intellectual than that of women. See e.g. Heinonen, 'Henry Suso and the Divine Knighthood', 79-80, on the dangers of making overly courageous generalizations on gender and mysticism.

281 Boquet and Nagy, *Medieval Sensibilities*, 206-8; see also pp. 18-19 above.

his adversities.[282] Due to the disappearance of the records of that inquest, it is not known how his mystic experiences would have been handled during the interrogations. The *vita* however records that his household members suspected that his states had a physical origin. Once he was left speechless and unable to eat because of the visions, which prompted his uncle to ask if he suffered from an infirmity.[283] In another instance, a physician was invited to 'liberate' him, but upon his arrival, the *medicus* found the count at the window both 'immobile and insensible', twice failing to react when he addressed him. The third time he did return to himself, closing his open eyes with pain and difficulty. It seemed to the physician that the eyes were full of grains of sand.[284]

Despite the different source genre, the mechanisms of interpreting the authenticity and corporeality of Elzéar's mystic experience resembled those of our female saints, with the exception that those investigating the matter were physicians and a male relative. As seen in the canonization inquest of Charles of Blois, in the household of a secular ruler, servants were one group of people whose information on the bodily manifestations of sainthood was relied on; possibly this was the situation with Elzéar as well. In any case, his *imitatio Christi* was of a very tangible kind, and there was some drawing of the line between a spiritual rapture and a physical infirmity. The *vita* can also be read as the household's attempt to interpret the count's physicality and its meanings, but undoubtedly, the reference to the physician also served as a proof of the visibility and significance of the phenomenon.

The Saint and the Suffering Family

The features of saints' lives discussed above primarily relate to their religious or secular elite status. Although they were meaningful for at least some of the devotees, who also saw infirmity as a way to highlight and even

282 Vauchez, *Sainthood*, 362; 'Vita s. Elzearii de Sabrano, conf.', *AASS*, Sept. VII, 580: 'Et ibi tantum fuit cum Christo crucifixo confixus, quod non solum ejus passionem & mortem continue portabat in corde, verum pro Christo mori summo peroptabat ardore. Et ex tunc non solum injurias & tribulationes & pericula & damna patienter ferebat, imo de quibuscumque adversis gaudebat'.

283 'Vita s. Elzearii de Sabrano, conf.', *AASS*, Sept. VII, 581.

284 'Vita s. Elzearii de Sabrano, conf.', *AASS*, Sept. VII, 580: 'tunc medicus liberorum dicti regis adveniens, et aulam ingrediens, atque eum in fenestra immobiliter et insensibiliter stantem reperiens, accessit, et bis advocans eum, nihil respondit. Tandem tertio vocatus, ad se rediit, et oculos, quos continue apertos tenuerat, cum difficultate et dolore clausit: videbatur enim sibi, quod haberet eos arena minuta plenos.'

construct these elements, a large majority of them could not necessarily relate to these aspects of saints' lives in their own everyday lives. However, occasionally canonization inquests also investigated matters such as the loss of family and household members or their illnesses, which the living saints sought to alleviate. In a society where infant mortality rate was high and life precarious in many ways, these features of *fama* provided their own sort of comfort. In the last section of this chapter, our focus will thus be turned to the saint as a carer, a family member, and a friend; the main focus will be on how family members' infirmities were used to construct sanctity.

A saint's patient attitude towards the death of family members or friends is a hagiographic *topos*. The witnesses either reported that the holy person took such losses without complaints, or if he or she had shed tears, the witnesses were able to give appropriate explanations for them. As we have seen, the feature occasionally comes up in the narrations about male saints, especially in the case of the two military leaders, St. Louis IX and Charles of Blois, who took losses of the soldiers in their armies with patience. Otherwise the descriptions mostly concern female saints. One of the nuns testified that when St. Clare of Montefalco was asked for a reason for her tears when her sister died, since it was believed that Iohanna's soul was in paradise, Clare responded that she cried for herself because Iohanna had always provided her with an example and words about God.[285] Similar remarks concerning the death of family members, or children when the saint was a mother, are recorded elsewhere.[286] This is especially the case in the documents concerning St. Frances of Rome, whose cult echoes many Marian themes.[287] Appropriately, her loss of two children plays an important role in this imagery, and Johannes Matteotti's narration relates her grief while referring to that of the Virgin Mary, characteristic of all maternity.[288] As female saints were extraordinary women and mothers, their attitude towards children's deaths could not be like that of other mothers, and succumbing to God's will when facing a mother's deepest sorrow has an established position in the genre.[289] In Frances's case, besides *patientia* the

285 PC Clare of Montefalco, 181.

286 *Il processo Castellano*, ed. Laurent, 59; PC Birgitta of Sweden, 17-18; the witnesses in Birgitta's process testifying to this article appropriately reported her serene behaviour. For example, *dominus* Elzearius, a cardinal, reported that at the time of Karl's death, she did not cry but appeared to be in deep contemplation, and told another woman that she much preferred him being with God. PC Birgitta of Sweden, 249; see also 261.

287 Boanas and Roper, 'Feminine Piety in Fifteenth-Century Rome', 180.

288 See Atkinson, *The Oldest Vocation*, 162; Lett, *L'Enfant des miracles*, 201.

289 Bartolomei Romagnoli, 'Vita di santa Francesca Romana', 106-7.

saintliness of her sorrow was emphasized by her vision of her son after his death – although it is interesting that these cases were not recorded in her canonization inquests.[290]

Besides losing children, facing infirmities and loss of a spouse were a feature of some female saints' *fama*. Lay male saints could obviously face a similar fate, but there are no such examples among our saints, whose wives outlived them; furthermore, like the sorrows of motherhood, the nurturing role of a wife appears a gendered phenomenon. In most cases, the same witnesses who reported the female saints' abhorrence of their marriage also reported the emotional side of loss and uncertainty at the time of the husband's illness or death. It can be argued, following Barbara Hanawalt's terminology regarding medieval English peasant families, that in the case of Elizabeth of Hungary and Louis IV, Dauphine of Puimichel and Elzéar of Sabran, as well as Frances of Rome and Lorenzo Ponziani, we can see an aristocratic, sanctified version of 'partnership marriage'.[291] Marita von Weissenberg, who has developed a similar notion, calls this 'community marriage'.[292]

Although the context and depicted lived reality of these saintly couples may differ from those of their common lay devotees, the principle behind marital life remains the same: acting together for a common goal. The four handmaids' testimonies portray St. Elizabeth's marriage with Louis as a happy one, but do not touch on the issue of infirmity and marriage, although, unusually in hagiographic texts, they record Elizabeth's great sorrow at the time of his death.[293] In the case of Dauphine and Elzéar, their need to conceal their chosen lifestyle was recorded in Dauphine's canonization inquest.[294] Unlike other sources about them, the part of Dauphine's Occitan *Vie* describing her *patientia* narrates how this decision led to a situation interpreted as an infirmity by their family. Elzéar's parents, for whom an heir would have been of crucial importance, wanted the couple to find treatment for their childlessness, and had them taken to Marseille to be examined by the famous physician Arnaldus de Villa Nova (*c*.1240-1311). Arnaldus was,

290 However, Bartolomei Romagnoli, 'Vita di santa Francesca Romana', 107, points out that the narrations of the incidents in Matteotti's *vitae* are detailed and personal, and he undoubtedly gathered the information from Frances herself.

291 See Hanawalt, *Ties that Bound*, 219.

292 Weissenberg, 'Men, Marriage, and Masculinity', 88.

293 See e.g. Elliott, *Proving Woman*, 58; PC Elizabeth of Hungary, 124-25.

294 PC Dauphine of Puimichel, 41; see also 318-19, for Bertranda Bartholomea's testimony on the matter. Ysnardus Risi, who had been Dauphine's confessor, stated that the reason for the secrecy was Elzéar's parents' wish for grandchildren. PC Dauphine of Puimichel, 193.

however, told about the couple's decision, and did not reveal their secret but pretended to treat them for two weeks, in the end pronouncing that he had found four deficiencies in Dauphine and three in Elzéar. He even presented his findings to a gathering of physicians, who agreed with him, and the couple could happily return home.[295] That this incident only appears in Dauphine's *Vie* may be partially explained by the gendered expectations. Sterility in marriage was more often considered to be the woman's fault, although both medical and hagiographic texts show that the matter was not black and white; there was an understanding – as demonstrated in Arnaldus's fake diagnosis – that a man could be sterile as well.[296]

As mentioned above, the double *Vie* was supposedly intended for a lay audience, who could also relate to the fertility issues. In the part of Elzéar's *Vie*, it narrates that he had been severely ill before the final illness that killed him. After his recovery, people asked if he had been afraid to die, to which he replied that he had not, and that he would be glad to suffer any type of death God decided to send him.[297] This incident is especially interesting from the viewpoint of Elzéar's two *Lives*, since the Latin version does not refer to that illness, but in its place records his fearlessness when endangered at sea.[298] For some reason the anonymous author of the Occitan *Vie* decided to change the way Elzéar's trust in God was reconstructed. Considering the text's lay audience, it may be that a grave illness was more effective for this purpose, being something everyone had to face one way or another. Although that particular bout of illness did not kill him, the author seems to connect the mentality around it with the fatal one, as he made a point of the short time period and formulated it stating that after being cured, Elzéar did not live for a longer time than a year.[299]

295 *Vie, Dauphine*, 158-64. In addition to the physician's examination, some women were placed in their bedroom to keep an eye on the couple's nightly activities, but Dauphine tricked them too. *Vie, Dauphine*, 165. Green, *Making Women's Medicine Masculine*, 87, points out that although this episode might be read just as hagiographic exaggeration, there are actually seven texts pertaining to infertility circulating in Montpellier in the fourteenth century, five of which bear Arnaldus's name, and although there is a lot of fantasy in the attributions, they depict Montpellier as the most important centre for the study of infertility. The most likely text actually to have been written by Arnaldus is a table listing impediments to conception.

296 The scholarship on medieval ideas about sterility is vast. See Cadden, *Meanings of Sex Difference*, 228-53; Finucane, *Rescue of the Innocents*, 17-23; Green, *Making Women's Medicine Masculine*, 87-91.

297 *Vie, Elzéar*, 114-15.

298 See *Vie, Elzéar*, 115, n. 88. The dangerous situation at sea is described in 'Vita s. Elzearii de Sabrano, conf.', *AASS*, Sept. VII, 591-92.

299 *Vie, Elzéar*, 114-15.

For the procurator of Dauphine's process, Elzéar's death when the couple were residing in Naples was clearly an important aspect of Dauphine's sainthood. This is understandable because it was the event that shaped her future life in poverty and therefore her saintly career. This is explicitly stated in the document. According to the articles, Dauphine grieved over the death of her husband, whom she 'loved very much' ('valde diligebat'), and which she foresaw before the official announcement by King Robert and Queen Sancia. According to article 19, Dauphine reflected upon Elzéar's presence and spiritual consolation, and as a consequence could not hold back her tears but remained for a long time in 'continuous pain/sorrow and tears' ('in continuis dolore et lacrimis per longum tempus permansisset'), with no remedy. This lasted until her husband appeared to her and, quoting Psalm 123:7, said: 'The snare is broken, and we are free'. The article then explains how the meaning of these words was later explained to Dauphine in a vision. For Elzéar they meant that he was freed from earthly dangers and snares so that he could be in the glory of paradise. For her they signified that she was now free from everything mundane and could devote her life entirely to God, as Elzéar had been the only earthly thing she had loved. This made Dauphine very happy and she decided to give up all her earthly possessions, and had no more pain or sorrow over her husband's death.[300]

It is questionable how widely the events described in the protocols and Dauphine's inner experiences were known. Few witnesses testified to the article, and of those Durandus Andree said that he did not know or hear if it was a public *fama*, while according to Bertranda Bartholomea, the matter was known in the countess's household.[301] Bertrandus Iusberti stated that when Elzéar had been alive, it had 'impeded her from serving God as she should'.[302] Dauphine's sorrow and recovery were thus adapted to the conventions of sainthood. By emphasizing her *dolor*, as well as by using vocabulary related to infirmity and healing, the text portrays Dauphine's sorrow as a 'condition' for which God brought a miraculous cure by granting her the vision. Only after she recovered from it could she completely fulfil her destiny as a saint.

The context of spousal relations and their connection with infirmity were much more tightly linked with communal realities in the hearing of

300 PC Dauphine of Puimichel, 43-44. Her Occitan *Vie* records the same events, mentioning her sorrow, constant tears, and lack of a cure, as well as God's mercy in giving her the revelation and the happiness of her being freed from her marriage. *Vie, Dauphine*, 180-83.

301 PC Dauphine of Puimichel, 255, 323.

302 PC Dauphine of Puimichel, 219: 'dum ipse vivebat, impediebat ipsam quandoque, videlicet quod non poterat servire Deo sicut debebat'.

St. Frances of Rome. As pointed out by Guy Boanas and Lyndal Roper, her final success in achieving a non-sexual marriage and having a protective attitude towards her husband (which will be addressed below) portray her marriage as a rather unconventional one, at least from the point of view of the 'official' ideal of an obedient and fecund wife.[303] The sources for Frances's sainthood give an impression of a 'happy marriage', despite her reluctance to engage in sexual relations. To begin with, as pointed out by Alessandra Bartolomei Romagnoli, Lorenzo Ponziani's tolerance towards his wife's religious lifestyle is a point to be taken into account. The sources also give an impression that Frances never put her spiritual needs above those of her family.[304]

When it comes to Frances's marriage, from the viewpoint of this study the most interesting detail is Lorenzo's injury and infirmity at the time of one of the armed occupations of Rome (1408-09 or 1413-14). Although it has a minor role in the inquest and other hagiographic writings, Lorenzo's infirmity has a clear purpose and significance. As Bartolomei Romagnoli writes, Frances's tribulations at the time of the war, including Lorenzo's injury, are examples of an actual, historical situation in a hagiographic context. In the *vita*, but also in the canonization testimonies, they 'symbolically foreshadow the drama of a city being oppressed by tyranny'.[305]

The testimonies recorded in 1440, 1443, and 1453 group several tribulations Frances and the family faced during the occupations, including her brother and son being captured, and the family losing an essential source of its wealth, the cattle. Lorenzo, who fought with the troops of the Orsini family against King Ladislaus of Naples, was severely wounded and exiled. The witnesses testified to the article reporting these events and Frances 'rejoicing with Job' together with an article recording her patience over over the death of her children and the infirmity of her husband, referring to Paul's view of the glory in infirmities.[306] As discussed above, usually such a reference to the Bible was attached to descriptions of the saints' own

303 Boanas and Roper, 'Feminine Piety in Fifteenth-Century Rome', 191.

304 Bartolomei Romagnoli, 'Vita di santa Francesca Romana', 105.

305 Bartolomei Romagnoli, 'Vita di santa Francesca Romana', 102: 'viene adombrato simbolicamente anche il dramma di una città oppressa dalla tirannia.' Similar connotations are noticeable in the diocesan hearing of St. Catherine of Siena. It is known that in July 1374 the saint's brother and his several children died of the plague. Her patient attitude to these deaths, described by the devotees, was very much connected with the dangers and disease around them, acting as a means of consolation and encouragement. *Il processo Castellano*, ed. Laurent, 59, n. 49.

306 PC Frances of Rome, 46: 'mortem filiorum et filiarum et infirmitates mariti et cognati ita patienter et quasi incredibili patientia tolerabat, totum illud Pauli apostolic posset sibi ascribe, scilicet, libenter igitur gloriabor in infirmitatibus meis ut inhabitet in me virtus Christi.'

ailments, but here the article parallels a saint's own bodily sufferings with those of the family, or even merges the two into one.

As usual, clerics close to Frances and her female associates testified, specifying how Frances always thanked the Highest in these tribulations. The joint witness account of 1440 also states that at the time of her children's death and during the infirmity of her husband, she was so patient and tolerant 'that nobody would believe it if they had not seen it', and she appeared to be glad rather than sad.[307] In the more detailed individual depositions of 1443, Johannes Matteotti described Lorenzo's 'mortal wounds', and her persuading him to save the assassins.[308] The documents are vague about the possible long-term consequences of the wounds. Interestingly, the most detailed information we have about the duration of Lorenzo's (final) infirmity comes from Matteotti's recording of Frances's battles with demons, dictated to him.[309] The first of these narrations concerns year 1430 and portrays Frances taking care of her ailing husband but being disturbed in this task by the demons. In another case, from 1431, the demons forcefully beat Lorenzo, whereas in 1432 Lorenzo went to bed 'cum magno labore' after returning from a distant location, when a malign spirit threw lice into the bed.[310]

Frances's actions and her attitude towards family members' suffering were something the witnesses, and most likely the whole community, could easily relate to. It appears rather curious that this issue comes up so often in the descriptions of the demonic attacks, but presumably Lorenzo's infirm state and Frances's ideal actions as the carer had something to do with this, since the depictions of the battles against demons, among other things, contrast their maliciousness with her goodness and his weakness.[311]

307 PC Frances of Rome, 46-47: 'ita patientem et tollerabilem quod nemo posset credere si non vidisset'.

308 PC Frances of Rome, 47; see also Rita Covelli's testimony on 47. *Frater* Bartholomeus mentioned her patience at the time of Lorenzo's wounding, and *frater* Ypolitus testified that he once saw her crying at the grave of her child, but she was crying for her sins. PC Frances of Rome, 48.

309 Esther Cohen points out that Frances's visions of hell show that her knowledge of its topography was rather weak; she was not very educated or intellectual. Cohen, *The Modulated Scream*, 190.

310 Matteotti, *Vita s. Francesca Romana*, 770, 795-96; 'Acta Francisca Romana vidua', *AASS*, Mar. II, 153, 159. Matteotti also records two other instances of Frances taking care of her husband. In 1433 Lorenzo was lying in bed gravely infirm, and when Frances left the room to warm his bedcovers, three malign spirits dressed up as popes attacked her. Similarly, in another instance when she wanted to warm the covers a demon took the form of a serpent and said that it wanted to place itself on the side of the husband. Matteotti, *Vita s. Francesca Romana*, 788; 'Acta Francisca Romana vidua', *AASS*, Mar. II, 160-61.

311 Boanas and Roper, 'Feminine Piety in Fifteenth-Century Rome', 187-88, write that according to the texts, he provided no support or comfort for her during any of her battles with the demons – a

At the same time, although the demonic attacks were investigated in the canonization inquests, the instances recorded do not include those occurring while Frances was tending Lorenzo.[312] In a way, the topic is treated in the canonization documents and in the *vitae* similarly to most of the infirmities of saints; it was enough to record the infirmity and to emphasize the saint's reaction towards it, but more detailed information was not considered necessary.

Frances's role as a carer intermingles with her communal role as someone with *fama sanctitatis* and a figure of an exemplary wife and mother in a city facing troubled times.[313] The descriptions of her actions can also be read in the framework of the originally Roman concept *maritalis affectio*, which includes the ideal of tender care shown towards an ailing spouse.[314] It was seen to derive from intimacy, mutuality, and familiarity, but medieval writers emphasized that it must not be confused with *amor*.[315] Usually it did, however, include the marital debt,[316] which Frances finally avoided with her husband's consent. Taking care of Lorenzo added to Frances's virtues by emphasizing this kind of marital obligation. There have been different views on the matter, however. Caroline Walker Bynum uses Frances as an example of those saints who 'hated their marriage'.[317] This impression mostly relates to the hagiographic construction of the beginning of her marriage. Robert Bartlett goes further and interprets Frances's attitude to

description which would have gained piquancy from the well-known facts of her husband's noble rank and career. On the other hand, his supporting her would have diminished her saintliness and resistance. No matter what their status, saints faced demons and the devil alone.

312 PC Frances of Rome, 50-57, 246-48.

313 For women's role as care-takers, see Hanawalt, '*Of Good and Ill Repute*', 164-65; Katajala-Peltomaa, *Gender, Miracles, and Daily Life*, *passim*; Lett, *L'Enfant des miracles*, 141. In his study on Renaissance families, Louis Haas has, however, pointed out that when a child was sick, it was both parents' duty to find treatment. Haas, *Renaissance Man and his Children*, 162. As for specifically mid-fifteenth-century Italy, St. Bernardino of Siena wrote in a sermon from 1424 concerning 'taking a wife' that 'if you fall sick, she looks after you with faith, love and charity for both your body and your soul'. Rusconi, 'St. Bernardino of Siena, the Wife, and Possessions', 182. In the case of Frances and Lorenzo, all this occurred in an exemplary way, especially considering her battles with the demons that were threatening also his well-being.

314 See e.g. Sheehan, '*Maritalis Affectio* Revisited'. This view is most visible in the decretal *Perveniens* of Pope Alexander III (1159-1181). The letter, addressed to the Archbishop of Canterbury, discusses the problem of lepers abandoned by their spouses. The pope advised the archbishop to urge a husband or wife to follow their sick spouse and to 'minister to them with conjugal affection'. McNamer, *Affective Meditation*, 49; Sheehan, '*Maritalis Affectio* Revisited', esp. 37; the decretal did not concern sexual intercourse but cohabitation and care-taking.

315 Wogan-Browne, 'How to Marry Your Wife with Chastity, Honour, and Fin' Amour', 137.

316 Sheehan, '*Maritalis Affectio* Revisited', 40.

317 Bynum, *Holy Feast and Holy Fast*, 215.

her husband's capture and death as a sign or result of her disgust towards men, and appears to take the notion that her children's deaths gave her joy, not sorrow, to make her a 'less pathetic figure than Elizabeth [of Hungary], although not a more attractive one'.[318] I would, however, be very careful of interpreting the descriptions of her *patientia* as accounts of her 'real' emotions. The conventions of the genre have a powerful influence on their wording, and the later memory and reconstruction of sanctity are the essential information the texts can give us. Furthermore, the holy women's described repugnance towards marriage did not necessarily denote hatred of their chosen spouses, but abhorrence at their inability to fulfil the vows of virginity they had made.[319]

I think it is safe to extend the idea of the dangers of the turbulent political situation in fifteenth-century Rome and their meaning to the hagiographers and devotees to the whole concept of a nurturing wife and saint. Late medieval lay female saints with ailing husbands are not very common, but St. Frances was not the only one. As an example, the *vita* (no canonization process exists) of St. Isabel of Aragon (also known as St. Elizabeth of Portugal, 1271-1336)[320] reports that she took care of her ailing husband King Denis of Portugal (1261-1325) 'for a long period of time'. The beginning of the narrative of this phase in her life states that 'in all her deeds, she always had the service of God before her eyes', which connects her care activities with the acts of mercy. Isabel took care of her husband 'as long as she could and the king permitted', which interestingly hints at some control, or perhaps responsibility, on the husband's part.[321] The *vita* further states that she served him 'just as if she was a domestic servant and a simple woman',[322] which also connects this care role with her humility. Iona McCleery has written that Isabel's *vita* was likely intended to serve as a model for other women of the royal house.[323] This female piety in encountering a suffering husband is, therefore, one characteristic of an ideal woman in this entourage. St. Frances's societal background was quite different, but

318 Bartlett, *Why Can the Dead Do Such Great Things?*, 76-77.

319 A vow of virginity could even be considered a precontract with Christ in the same manner as the vows of nuns. See Salih, *Versions of Virginity*, 234.

320 On her queenship and cult, see McCleery, 'Isabel of Aragon (d. 1336): Model Queen or Model Saint?'

321 'Vita, Elisabetha Regina Portugalliae (s.)', *AASS*, Iul. II, 183: 'Cum vero tempus advenit, quod Rex Don Dionysius incidit in morbum gravem, quo diutius laboravit; Regina ei inserviebat, quatenus poterat, et Rex permittebat, quod in ejus servitio occuparetur.'

322 'Vita, Elisabetha Regina Portugalliae (s.)', *AASS*, Iul. II, 183: 'tamquam ancilla domestica et simplex femina'.

323 McCleery, 'Isabel of Aragon (d. 1336): Model Queen or Model Saint?', 599-60.

vitae had, in general, a didactic purpose, and canonization processes are known to have distributed and spread the established ideas of sanctity among the witnesses.[324]

At the same time, a saintly wife's nurturing role was apparently not always as straightforward as in the case of St. Frances or St. Isabel. Catherine of Vadstena (*c.*1332-1381), St. Birgitta of Sweden's daughter, was married to Eggaret von Kurnen, a young nobleman, at the age of 13, with whom she made a vow of chastity. In all documents, Catherine's sanctity is tightly interlinked with that of her mother's. According to Catherine's *vita*, she felt a great urge to join in her mother's pilgrimage to Rome, to the point where she started to appear *languida*. At this point her brother Karl made threats to Eggaret's life should he let her go. Catherine got hold of his letter and managed to resolve the situation with the help of her maternal uncle. Having been to Rome for a while, Catherine wished to return to Sweden and to her infirm husband. After this, her mother famously had a vision in which Christ explained that the infirmity that Catherine's husband suffered was fatal.[325] Unlike in the *Revelations*, Catherine's own testimony in her mother's inquest does not refer to her wish to return to her husband because of the illness, and the depositions in Catherine's inquiry, held in 1475-77, refer to this testimony.[326] Because of the nature of Catherine's hearing, and the long time between her death and the interrogations, these statements are curt and do not give much extra information, often referring to 'old books', Birgitta's process, or Catherine's *vita* as the source of information,[327] although some oral tradition about Catherine's marriage seems to have been preserved.[328]

Catherine's loyalty – or the lack of it – to her ailing husband has rather different connotations to that of St. Frances, at least at first glance. The husband's infirmity serves the purpose of highlighting his wife's saintly character, but in Catherine's case the duty that it illustrates is towards her mother and their coexistence, which later enhanced Catherine's *fama sanctitatis*.[329] In a way Catherine acted *against* her gendered duties to an

324 See note 69 (p. 62) above.

325 'Vita, Catharina Suedica', *AASS*, Mar. III, 507-8 (edited also in *Vita Katherine*); *Revelations of St. Birgitta of Sweden*, ed. and trans. Searby and Morris, III, 179-80.

326 PC Birgitta of Sweden, 323-24; PC Catherine of Vadstena, 15-16, 34-35, 44, 57, 124. For Catherine's process, see Fröjmark, *Mirakler och helgonkult*, 58-63.

327 The witnesses typically referred to Catherine's *vita* as their source of information. See e.g. PC Catherine of Vadstena, 51: 'quod credit contenta in dicto articulo fore vera referens se ad Vitam'; PC Catherine of Vadstena, 60.

328 PC Catherine of Vadstena, 57; see also 68-69.

329 The relationship between Birgitta and Catherine has raised some discussion. See e.g. Elliott, *Spiritual Marriage*, 277-80; Nieuwland, 'Motherhood and sanctity in the life of Saint Birgitta of

infirm husband in following the much more powerful calls of her mother and Christ, but the testimonies in her hearing keep repeating that she did this with her husband's consent, which most likely made her actions more acceptable and understandable in the eyes of the witnesses. All this got its reward, however, in Birgitta's vision showing that infirmity and death were Eggaret's recompense for his sacrifice.[330] Eggaret's final illness and death thus receive very hagiographic overtones, for Christ revealed to Birgitta that '[i]t is fitting for him on his way to the Almighty to have his accounts in hand and it is good for him to be away from carnal acts'.[331] After all, Birgitta taught her devotees that caring too much for one's family members made one care less about those in need.[332] Perhaps here we can see a similarity with the hagiography of Frances of Rome. Although the latter was portrayed as a devoted wife and mother, her life as a saint surpassed all that, and her caring attitude towards her ailing husband had the air of spirituality and abstinence. The same goes for Elizabeth of Hungary and Dauphine of Puimichel, whose husbands' deaths made it possible for them to donate their possessions to help others.[333]

Sweden', 311-12.

330 See Elliott, *Spiritual Marriage*, 278.

331 *The Revelations of St. Birgitta of Sweden*, ed. and trans. Searby and Morris, III, 179.

332 Salmesvuori, *Power and Sainthood*, 31.

333 For the excessive charity of female saints, see e.g. Cullum, 'Gendering Charity'.

Abstinence, Devotional Practices, and Social Control

Abstract

Abstinence from earthly pleasures – such as fasting, using a hair shirt, and ascetic sleeping conditions – as well as devotional practices were vital aspects of a holy life. They were frequently reported in canonization testimonies and other hagiographic texts. An important feature in this was discretion; a holy person was supposed to exceed the limits of common human endurance but not practice excessive self-harm. This chapter discusses infirmity as a delineating factor that allowed and required discretion in asceticism and devotional practices. At the same time, various members of a saint's community were presented as taking part in delineating their ascetic practices as well as interpreting and even emotionally partaking in it.

Keywords: sainthood, asceticism, austerity, devotional practices, social control

There have already been a few references to saints' ascetic practices and how it interlinks, to a varying degree, with the testimonies of their infirmities. When it comes to saints' lives, in addition to *patientia*, *abstinentia* appears fundamental in all late medieval canonization hearings. Fasting,[1] rough sleeping conditions,[2] and wearing a hair shirt or an iron breastplate were frequently investigated and reported. To a point they delineated late

1 Abstinence from food was the most fundamental way of self-denial for a saintly candidate, and so by the later Middle Ages had become one of the requirements of saints investigated in all canonization inquests, men and women alike. Bynum, *Holy Feast and Holy Fast*, 82; Vauchez, *Sainthood*, 301. See also Pincikowski, *Bodies of Pain*, 13.

2 Ascetic sleeping habits is another hagiographic trope, but here the need to relax the regimen at the time of infirmity was not of crucial importance; having an ascetic bed at the time of death was also a *topos*. Gaposchkin, *The Making of Saint Louis*, 27.

Kuuliala, Jenni, *Saints, Infirmity, and Community in the Late Middle Ages*.
Taylor & Francis Group 2020
DOI: 10.5117/9789462983373_ABSTI

medieval sainthood, because there existed the idea that the more ascetic one's life was, the more pleasing it was to God, and that mortifying one's body gave access to the divine.[3] Furthermore, penitential and devotional acts like excessive prayers and vigils or taking care of the sick, were a crucial feature of a saintly life.[4] In medieval thinking, asceticism can be viewed as a set of practices or a transformative process, which purifies and improves the ascetic's spiritual health and functions as a method to avoid sin. Penance, on the other hand, was motivated by sin, which it amends.[5] Physical discomfort and even pain was a logical, evident aspect of the two practices, but in canonization testimonies its role appears to be similar, regardless of whether the witness was describing the saint's asceticism or penitence. Because sainthood was always negotiated within a community, the descriptions of *abstinentia*, penitence, devotion, and their connection with *infirmitas* provide a window onto the ways various community members aimed at exerting influence over the lifestyles and physical regimen of saints.

Harmful *penitentia* and Discretion

The level of asceticism that was appropriate for and expected of saints was subject to constant negotiation, especially as regards its bodily consequences. The same goes for devotional acts, although their corporality appears more subdued than it does with asceticism in most processes. These practices received varying emphases in the inquests, and often the witnesses reported them as a whole. *Infirmitas* plays a crucial role in the depositions, occasionally as a result of extreme austerity or at least being aggravated by it, but more often acting as a delineating and defining factor that could underline the holy person's penitence as well as his or her discretion.

In the writings of late medieval German mystics, analysed by Ronald K. Rittgers, suffering that was inflicted by the divine was of the greatest value, but self-inflicted suffering was also necessary.[6] Canonization testimonies do not directly address the question of the relative value of the two, but some gradation is detectable in them. As discussed elsewhere in this book, saints reportedly praised and thanked God for infirmities which were either God-sent or which had no apparent origins, and the witnesses

3 See e.g. Hughes-Edwards, *Reading Medieval Anchoritism*, 71; Vauchez, *Sainthood*, 191

4 Klaniczay, *Holy Rulers and Blessed Princesses*, 270; Vauchez, *Sainthood*, 510-11.

5 Hughes-Edwards, *Reading Medieval Anchoritism*, 59-61.

6 Rittgers, *The Reformation of Suffering*, 76.

were unanimous in the glory of their subjects' patience when facing such hardships. When it comes to infirmities that were caused or aggravated by asceticism and penitentiary practices, the situation is more multifaceted. Although the witnesses praised holy men and women for their self-torture, discretion (*discretio*) was a central theme in depositions regarding asceticism, penitence, and infirmity.

The need for discretion was central, and the witnesses were aware of its importance. It was emphasized by many thirteenth-century spiritual leaders; for example, Thomas Aquinas was of the opinion that to make one's body ill by fasting would make a person lose their 'dignity'.[7] Excessive abstinence could signal hypocrisy and the mere outward appearance of sanctity, but it could also make one so weak that the devil found a way to influence one. Furthermore, self-desctruction could even be considered a form of suicide and therefore a mortal sin.[8] At the same time, the descriptions in *vitae* of fasting especially become more extreme in the fourteenth and fifteenth centuries, above all in the case of female saints.[9] The same can be said with some reservations about the canonization protocols, mostly because they tended to become more organized and detailed in every respect, and because there was a growing tendency to highlight the legendary, more extraordinary, characteristics of sainthood.[10] The conductors of the hearings and the witnesses thus needed to find a balance between their detailed, often even graphic descriptions of the holy persons' self-torment and the proofs of discretion.

Saints' devotees had cultural models for their interpretation of extreme asceticism, but often the lines between proper and improper austerity and harming of their own bodies, as well as miraculous survival of the same practices, were fluid.[11] Survival from extreme asceticism and *penitentia* was only possible by the grace of God and therefore reserved only for the few who were

7 Bynum, *Holy Feast and Holy Fast*, 239. Already the monastic rules of late antiquity considered fasting to be important, *but* only to the point permitted by one's health; Crislip, *From Monastery to Hospital*, 30, 74-75; Kuuliala, '*Infirmitas* in Monastic Rules'; Schulenburg, *Forgetful of their Sex*, 374-89.

8 Hughes-Edwards, *Reading Medieval Anchoritism*, 72-73; Bynum, *Holy Feast and Holy Fast*, 42-46, 84-85, 196, 239; Vauchez, *Sainthood*, 340, 350. Vauchez, *Sainthood*, 333, suggests that extreme asceticism might be one reason why so few eremitical saints received official canonization.

9 Bynum, *Holy Feast and Holy Fast*, 146.

10 Vauchez, *Sainthood*, 527-34. Of the thirteenth-century inquests, St. Margaret of Hungary's was among those reporting the extreme asceticism of a saint's eating habits, but the testimonies still focus more on other sides of her holiness. PC Margaret of Hungary, 154-55, 406-7.

11 See also Hughes-Edwards, *Reading Medieval Anchoritism*, 73, for this 'fine line' in medieval *vitae*.

worthy of it.[12] This concept is clearly visible in the inquest testimonies where witnesses marvel at a holy person's endurance. A brother testifying in John Buoni's hearing, for instance, said that the Holy Ghost must have fed him or he would not have stayed alive.[13] Occasionally the witnesses specifically referred to the lack of infirmity as a point of comparison when speaking about the saint's endurance. The canon Johannes Reyman recounted the miraculous stamina of Dorothea of Montau's body, making a point that she was 'not impeded by infirmities' ('infirmitate non impedita') despite her austerity.[14] Furthermore, when testifying about Clare of Montefalco's abstinence, Sister Thomassa stated that 'all sisters' were greatly astonished that she could survive.[15]

As mentioned above, the voices of doubt regarding saints' lives are rare in canonization processes, but an instance recorded in Bérenger's *vita* of St. Clare of Montefalco gives a glimpse of the doubts this kind of miraculous survival could raise. A physician called Phylippus (or Philippus) de Spoleto went to see Clare, who was infirm. He heard that she often spent long periods of time eating hardly anything and was incredulous about her ability to survive this. On his way back home, beautiful weather suddenly gave way to storm and thunder, so that he arrived in Spoleto 'almost dead' ('semivivus'). When he fell asleep at home, he heard Clare's voice saying that all this happened because of his incredulity, and so he changed his mind.[16] As Bérenger's *vita* is based on the diocesan hearing, Phylippus most likely testified about the incident there, but possibly also in the canonization inquiry; he is listed as a witness, although his testimony has not been preserved. Furthermore, notary Petructius Thomassii referred to him as an informant regarding Clare's raptures, during which she 'appeared as if dead' ('videbatur mortua') and did not eat or drink, and her survival seemed miraculous.[17] The miraculous 'conversion' the physician faced was surely a powerful way of demonstrating the extraordinary nature of Clare's asceticism as well as her superhuman endurance. That the doubter in this case was a physician is an important detail for, as will be discussed shortly, they had an important role in interpreting and giving proofs of saints' corporeal marks.

12 Vauchez, *Sainthood*, 192.

13 'Processus apostolici, de b. Joanne Buono', *AASS*, Oct. IX, 830.

14 PC Dorothea of Montau, 195-200. Similarly, Johannes Marienwerder testified that once she no longer slept alongside her husband, Dorothea slept on the bare ground and sometimes on stones, sometimes leaning her head against a wall or stones. According to Johannes, she did this for sixteen years without being 'impeded by infirmity'. PC Dorothea of Montau, 273.

15 PC Clare of Montefalco, 186.

16 *Vita sanctae Clarae de Cruce*, ed. Semenza, 26.

17 PC Clare of Montefalco, 392.

Clare of Montefalco's case is also interesting from the viewpoint of drawing the line between a self-inflicted and a non-self-inflicted infirmity, for besides the notions of her miraculous survival, the witnesses testified that her austerity led to infirmity. The articles report in detail her dietary practices and how she fasted 'almost always' ('quasi continue'), and only when she was 'very infirm' ('tantum infirmata') did she eat more, because the physicians, her confessor, and the abbess told her to.[18] Sister Thomassa added that her penitence was so great that the infirmities became major, but her testimony does not specify their origins.[19] At the same time, Sister Francescha's testimony about Clare's two final years reports that her state of infirmity was caused by her austerity, which Francescha had heard of from the nuns who had lived longer in the monastery.[20] When we think about the testimonies discussed above concerning Clare's painful and corporeal *imitatio Christi* and her gratitude for her infirmities, the process gives a somewhat contradictory image of the origins of her bodily tribulations. Neither the *articuli* nor the testimony of Clare's brother Franciscus refer to her asceticism or penitence as causing or aggravating infirmity.[21] Statements of the causation thus came from the nuns who lived in close contact with her and for whom it presumably was more natural or even beneficial to come to such a conclusion after living under the holy woman's influence, often for a long period of time. Especially the nuns who entered the monastery after Clare had received her fame as a living saint were socialized into seeing her in a certain light and interpreting her corporeal experiences as a sign of her holiness. It is also possible that this causality was problematic from the theological point of view precisely because of the importance of *discretio*, emphasized in the articles, especially in the case of a female saint whose holiness had such mystic and corporeal forms.

Close contact with the living saint is evident also in the testimonies concerning the sainthood of Margaret of Hungary, showing that the way a cloistered nun's sainthood was constructed was perhaps more intensely communal than in the case of saints living in the secular world. Wilfully causing long-term bodily harm to oneself also came up in some of the testimonies, where their source was prayer and devotion. The cantrix Catharina testified that Margaret 'destroyed' her face and body due to her many prayers: her face was 'deformata', her head was stiff or numb from

18 PC Clare of Montefalco, 4-5.
19 PC Clare of Montefalco, 174.
20 PC Clare of Montefalco, 332.
21 PC Clare of Montefalco, 4-5, 267-68.

shedding so many tears, and for many years she kept her head 'rolled back', but after her death her face was beautiful again.[22] Similarly, Sister Judith testified that Margaret had a swollen knee due to her many genuflects, and that Margaret often said to her in secret that she had pain in that knee.[23] Here the holy woman's own reference to pain highlights her sainthood in a private setting, while the sisters simultaneously valourized the pain and subdued it by the saint's wish, presumably in order to maintain her discretion. The testimony of Margaretha, from the house of Árpád,[24] is among those with most references to the corporality of Margaret's sainthood. She testified that when Margaret's arms were too weak to flog herself for around four years before her death, she had another nun, Sister Sabina, do that for her. Interestingly, Sabina did not mention Margaret's infirmity, although she confirmed the flogging.[25] The same goes for another nun, Elisabeth, who Margaret asked to perform this task. It is revealing that Elisabeth testified that because she was her 'only close friend' ('sola privata socia'), she agreed to do so.[26] According to these witnesses, the flogging was done in secret, but the testimonies do not reveal whether its details were known already before Margaret's death. Here again there were witness accounts underlining discretion. *Domina* Agnes testified that already in her childhood, Margaret had given her a belt she used for self-disciplining purposes to keep for her while she was infirm, and when she was healthy, she asked her to return it.[27]

22 PC Margaret of Hungary, 382-83: 'propter multas orationes ista sancta Margaretha taliter destruxerat corpus suum et faciem, quod quasi deformata erat in facie, et ita habebat caput rigidatum propter sparsionem multarum lacrymarum, et ipsa portabat in capite multos per annos revolutos, (?) sed quando mortua fuit, habuit pulchriorem faciem, quam in vita sua.'

23 PC Margaret of Hungary, 324-25. Furthermore, the process records an instance when St. Margaret was praying all night, and dislocated her shoulder, which caused her great pain. The prioress and other sisters were searching for medicine, while another nun named Margaretha derided the wish for medical treatment. Immediately her own shoulder started to hurt and was only cured after she confessed her thoughts to St. Margaret. PC Margaret of Hungary, 184-87, 214-15. The point of this testimony is the punishment miracle, and the connection with the corporeal consequences of Margaret's vigils is left somewhat vague, but it implies that the praying somehow caused the dislocation. See also Klaniczay, *Holy Rulers and Blessed Princesses*, 275-76, for this miracle and other disciplinary miracles in Margaret's process.

24 Margaretha is named as the daughter of Anne, sister of the wife of King Stephen V in the document. The editors of Margaret's process point out that Anne was actually the daughter of Stephen and Margaret's sister Anne. PC Margaret of Hungary, 181, n. 46.

25 PC Margaret of Hungary, 184-85, 246-47. As for other saints of the period, St. Hedwig of Silesia is also reported as having had her servants scourge her. Klaniczay, *Holy Rulers and Blessed Princesses*, 266.

26 PC Margaret of Hungary, 238-39.

27 PC Margaret of Hungary, 352-55.

The witness accounts of Margaret's self-torture, like many of those concerning Clare of Montefalco, show that in the case of nuns, some members of their community had more intimate knowledge not only about their religious customs but also their corporeal manifestations, and that personal relationships played a major role in distributing information about these matters. It is also plausible, following Laura Ackerman Smoller's train of thought regarding witnesses' tendency to highlight their own role in miracle narratives,[28] that mentioning details of a holy person's corporality was a way for the witnesses to emphasize their own intimacy with her (or him), and consequently, the importance of their own role within the community of devotees.[29] Furthermore, Robert Mills has written that there was a belief that a bodily sensation, such as pain, could, at least imaginatively, transfer from body to body; that is, by their *imitatio Christi* saints sensed Christ's suffering, which was then transferred to the bodies of the devotees.[30] Canonization testimonies hardly reflect or discuss such views, but presumably especially those living in close proximity to the saint, whose suffering may or may not have been self-inflicted, held similar views and considered themselves to be fusing with the body of 'their' saint as well as that of Christ.

In addition to these female saints, rigorous austerity and penitence to the point of harming one's body is clearly visible in the inquests of many male saints. This is the case especially with testimonies concerning hermits, but strict penitentiary practices were important to the *fama* of male saints who belonged to religious orders or were bishops or rulers as well.[31] Among the most striking examples are the testimonies in the process of Italian Benedictine monk and hermit Lawrence of Subiaco, also known as Lawrence Loricatus (conducted in Subiaco, 1244).[32] They include rather gruesome descriptions of his habits. As usual, the witnesses to his life were clerics and elite laymen, while the ordinary laypeople of the area testified about his miracles. The document includes no *articuli*, so we do not know how the question regarding his penitentiary practices was put to the witnesses. In addition to eating only bread and water, they reported his wearing an iron breastplate and iron rings around his head, arms, legs, and neck, which gave him his byname Loricatus; the witnesses reported that pus was discharged

28 Smoller, 'Miracle, Memory, and Meaning', 434-40.

29 For women's, especially nuns', friendship in the Middle Ages, see Classen, 'Introduction', 82-87.

30 Mills, *Suspended Animation*, esp. 162.

31 Vauchez, *Sainthood*, 193.

32 For Lawrence and the canonization process, see Goodich, *Vita perfecta*, 40, 132; Vauchez, *Sainthood*, 192, 282, 330, 334-35.

from the wounds the rings caused, and that he had a great number of lice on his head and 'boundless fissures' ('infinita foramina').[33] Lawrence was from Apulia and was therefore influenced by the Eastern tradition. The habit of torturing oneself with an iron breastplate was an anomaly among the western holy figures rather than a norm.[34] As in the above example, for the witnesses in his inquest, this kind of extreme asceticism was a significant, personal observation; for example *miles* Maginardus specified when testifying about the topic that he was 'greatly acquinted' with the hermit.[35]

Although the descriptions of the bodily consequences of Lawrence's austerity are quite extreme, the conductors of bishops', priests', and rulers' canonization inquests and the witnesses in them gave similar reports. Some ways of emphasizing extreme austerity, like lice as a result of a hair shirt, appear *topos*like examples of the witnesses using certain expressions to highlight their message. These accounts also show that although there are differences between the processes and individual testimonies in how infirmity and sainthood were connected, certain expressions and interpretations were universal regardless of the saint's 'type'. For example, Johannes Bute testified in Thomas Cantilupe's inquiry that the hair shirt infected the bishop's skin, and many saw lice in the garment.[36] The servants of Charles of Blois and Yves of Tréguier made similar remarks.[37] In addition to the lice, Charles's servants noticed the lesions and wounds as well as the duke's 'inflated eyes' ('oculos inflatos') in the mornings.[38] Like the nuns in Clare of Montefalco's or Margaret of Hungary's monasteries, those living in his household paid close attention to bodily signs, which they then interpreted as manifestations of penitence and, consequently, sainthood. Undoubtedly Charles's holiness was a personal affair for his servants, who had witnessed

33 PC Lawrence Loricatus, 690, 692.

34 Vauchez, *Sainthood*, 192-93. The 1306-7 canonization process records of pope Celestine V, also known as Peter of Morrone (1215-1296, papacy lasted for five months in 1294), include few testimonies about his life, but in them his ascetic habits are quite extreme as well; *frater* Bartholomeus de Trasaco, for example, testified that in addition to a hair shirt, he also wore an iron chain under his clothes. *Il processo di canonizzazione di Celestino V*, ed. Bartolomei Romagnoli and Marini (PC Celestine V), II, 300-1. For the saint and his canonization, see Marini, 'Introduzione'.

35 PC Lawrence Loricatus, 663: 'quod maximam familiaritatem cum dicto fratre habebat'.

36 BAV, MS Vat. lat. 4015, fols. 103v, 107v, 108r.

37 BAV, MS Vat. lat. 4025, fols. 14v, 32v; PC Charles of Blois, 34, 79; PC Yves of Tréguier, 39. See also pp. 124-25 below for Louis IX's use of a hair shirt and PC Margaret of Hungary, 184-85 for a similar statement.

38 BAV, MS Vat. lat. 4025, fols. 14v, 32v, 36v, 50r, 67r; PC Charles of Blois, 34, 79, 86, 121, 163.

his life in close proximity and participated in it. In some other cases there was some disagreement about the usage of a hair shirt and its consequences. Thomas Cantilupe's nephew Willelmus de Cantilupo testified that he had never seen his uncle use a hair shirt, even though he had helped him to dress for years.[39] These statements obviously do not tell a modern reader about how these holy men *actually* lived their penitentiary practices but rather about the meanings and significances given to them within the religious community that observed them. It is worth emphasizing that in a majority of cases, the information about the extreme usage of a hair shirt came from servants and other people who knew the saint personally. The *fama* of the behaviour could spread, but the details appear to have remained in a close circle.

While penitence itself was a practice that manifested itself corporally to the household members, infirmity was the factor which the witnesses most often used to delineate the *discretio* and sobriety of austerity, for male and female saints alike. The need of *discretio* was thus neither a gendered phenomenon nor related to the holy person's status, although its manifestations and extent could vary. Often discretion was a result of a demand or request made by a specific person, a topic discussed below, but quite often the witnesses also reported infirmity as a delineator of austerity but also of piety and devotion simply as a matter of fact,[40] almost as if it was an entity of its own that could regulate the holy person's behaviour. In these statements infirmity was an obvious, natural part of human life that could – and should – regulate even the most holy acts. In many miracle accounts illnesses and impairments are referred to as 'arriving', 'tormenting', or 'taking over' their victim; perhaps the matter-of-fact statements about their role as it related to saints' lives stem from the same way of thinking.[41] There were witnesses in the hearings of Charles of Blois, Thomas Cantilupe, and Philip of Bourges who reported how each of them followed a strict dietary regimen unless they were infirm.[42] Similar references to *discretio* were made even in the

39 Vauchez, *Sainthood*, 302. The testimony is on BAV, MS Vat. lat. 4015, fols. 57v-59v.

40 An exception is Johannes of Marienwerder's testimony, in which he stated that Dorothea's way of chastising herself was not caused by vainglory but by *caritas* and her willingness to be the 'perfect imitator' of Christ's passion. PC Dorothea of Montau, 258-60. He clearly recognized the importance of *discretio*, undoubtedly knowing how extreme his description of her penitence was, but chose not to use infirmity as a reference point.

41 Gentilcore, *Healers and Healing*, 182; I have discussed this in relation to Dorothea of Montau's canonization process in Kuuliala, 'Disability and Religious Practices'.

42 BAV, MS Vat. lat. 4015, fol. 34r; BAV, MS Vat. lat. 4025, fols. 5v, 13v; PC Charles of Blois, 13, 32; BAV, MS Vat. lat. 4019, fol. 33r. See also Vauchez, *Sainthood*, 301, on Philip's fasting. One witness in Vincent Ferrer's hearing directly stated that Vincent was very *sobrius* and that he used a hair

hearings of hermits; the witnesses to Lawrence of Subiaco's *vita* specified that when his bodily state became so bad that he could no longer get up from bed, he relaxed his dietary regimen.[43]

Although sobriety comes up in most processes when they investigated saints' austerity, devotion, and infirmity, there are exceptions to the pattern. According to one Dominican brother, St. Dominic, for instance, did not give up his fasting at the time of severe infirmity.[44] Exactly where these contradictory statements derived from is difficult to ascertain, especially in early hearings such as that of St. Dominic which were recorded in a very summarized form, but certainly individual memories and views played a crucial role here. Contradictory statements were, however, most often given regarding sleeping habits, regardless of the saint's gender or status, possibly because harsh sleeping conditions were not considered to pose as great a risk to one's health as a severe diet or infesting oneself with lice and wounds. Furthermore, austere sleeping conditions at the time of the saint's final illness were repeated in several processes,[45] but even this was not an absolute norm. Vincent Ferrer reportedly only slept in a bed when he was ill, some witnesses specifying that he did so only during the final illness,[46] and Dauphine of Puimichel's hearing records that she used a sack and a woollen rug as bedclothes until 'great bodily infirmity weighed her down'.[47]

Even in the case of those saints who reportedly were 'discreet', the witnesses did not always portray *discretio* as an easy process. Rather, austerity and penitence were acts that the saints' communities not only observed and interpreted but also attempted to control, drawing the line between what was admirable and beneficial, and what was too harmful. Sarah Kay and Miri Rubin have written that 'authority over the body was contested between physicians and priests, between the clergy and the laity, and between men and women'.[48] While this statement can be attested in the whole field of interpreting and reconstructing saints' bodies, it is particularly fitting when it comes to their infirmity, asceticism, and devotional practices. The

shirt in health, and when infirm an *estamina*, a more comfortable woollen shirt later considered a relic. PC Vincent Ferrer, 23.

43 PC Lawrence Loricatus, 663-64, 690, 691, 692, 693.

44 *Processus canonizationis s. Dominici*, ed. Waltz (PC Dominic of Caleruega), 134.

45 BAV, MS Vat. lat. 4025, fol. 11v; PC Charles of Blois, 27-28; PC Clare of Montefalco, 4, 331; PC Dominic of Caleruega, 7, 182; PC Yves of Tréguier, 53, 110.

46 PC Vincent Ferrer, 24, 60.

47 PC Dauphine of Puimichel, 45: 'et hoc quousque magne infirmitates corporis eandem gravaverunt'; PC Dauphine of Puimichel, 306.

48 Kay and Rubin, 'Introduction', 5.

demand of *discretio* in austerity and penitence was widely internalized but producing and constructing it was not always a straightforward process. The witnesses to saints' lives wanted to show that the holy figures were discreet in their austerity but also to make sure that their message about the saints' exceptional, even miraculous self-chastisement came across clearly. Already in the examples discussed above there have been some references to the roles of various community members in controlling the saint's austerity. These narrations show, on the one hand, how abstinence and self-chastisement were communally negotiated, and on the other hand, what meanings the witnesses and commissioners of canonization inquests gave to these situations. As will be shown below, often infirmity was an important reason and tool in these interventions.

Controlling Austerity

In the attempts to control a holy person's austerity and devotional practices, the role of certain groups of people appears prominent. The witnesses mention most often the confessor. Since the ordinance of the Fourth Lateran Council in 1215 regulating that every Christian of age must confess at least once a year, the role of (auricular) confession had become prominent within western Christendom. Confession responded to several spiritual concerns, of which particularly the fight against heresies and personal piety pertain directly to sainthood.[49]

The role of individual confessors is well-known in hagiographic research, most often referred to in studies of female saints' *vitae*.[50] As we have already seen in the discussion of Dorothea of Montau and Frances of Rome, confessors often had the role of formulating the saintly role and reputation of 'their' saints.[51] They also had the power to regulate the holy women's lifestyles, including penitentiary practices and attitudes towards the body, but they

49 Elliott, *Proving Woman*, 9-12; for the culture of confession in general, see Rusconi, *L'Ordine dei peccati*.

50 The model of 'pairing' religious reformers and elite ladies has its predecessors already in antiquity, for example in St. Jerome and the pious women he advised. In the twelfth century, the model was defined by Robert d'Arbrissel's abbey Fontevrault and Abelard's designs for Héloise's monastery. The spiritual guardian quickly became a major influence in saintly women's lives. Klaniczay, *The Uses of Supernatural Power*, 106. On medieval holy women and their confessors, see Coakley, 'Friars as Confidants'; Coackley, *Women, Men, and Spiritual Power*; Mooney (ed.), *Gendered Voices*.

51 This was especially crucial for a lay saint. Lehmijoki-Gardner, *Worldly Saints*, 54.

could also be their admirers, pupils, and even friends.[52] Among the saints and confessors discussed in this study, St. Elizabeth's confessor Conrad of Marburg had the most brutal role in punishing the saint and promoting extreme asceticism; other confessors were significantly gentler.[53] The testimonies to St. Elizabeth's life given by her handmaids are not entirely comparable to testimonies in later processes. The testimony of Irmingard is telling, however, as regards the significance given to Conrad's actions. Irmingard testified about an incident where he punished Elizabeth and her by beating. According to Irmingard, her wounds took three weeks to heal, while Elizabeth's lasted longer because her punishment had been greater.[54] Elizabeth's obedience to Conrad was a central aspect of her piety, as well as an 'exemplar used to combat heresy',[55] which Irmingard's account of the longevity of the wounds highlights.[56] This was not, however, the norm, and this kind of narrative cannot be seen as acceptance and submission to contemporary misogynism. As concluded by Caroline Walker Bynum, it appears that 'women's religiosity was a reaction against the moderation urged by church leaders, against new efforts to make a place – but a secondary place – for women and for the laity within a Christian universe'.[57]

Usually the witness accounts show the confessor restricting an ascetic woman's behaviour rather than encouraging it, but obedience to the confessor also highlighted holiness. These testimonies gave the witnesses a chance to admire the saints' austerity as well as their obedience to a spiritual father – which continued to work as a way for the church to fight heresies. Among the most famous narratives regarding obedience and a confessor promoting discretion are those included in St. Clare of Assisi's canonization protocols. Clare's *fama* included the view that she had made herself infirm by her (dietary) austerity.[58] A sister named Pacifica de Gelfutio testified that St. Francis of Assisi and the bishop of Assisi ordered that Clare should eat

52 Coakley, *Women, Men, and Spiritual Power*, 2; Elliott, *Spiritual Marriage*, 205-8.

53 Klaniczay, *The Uses of Supernatural Power*, 107. Another confessor who strongly favoured extreme asceticism was Catherine of Siena's confessor Raymond of Capua. He wrote biographies, not only of Catherine but also of other female saints associated with fasting and miraculous feeding. Bynum, *Holy Feast and Holy Fast*, 166. For Catherine and Raymond, see also Coakley, *Women, Men, and Spiritual Power*, 170-92; Matter, 'Undebated Debate'; Scott, 'Mystical Death'. As we have seen, also Johannes Marienwerder praised Dorothea of Montau's extreme austerity.

54 PC Elizabeth of Hungary, 135-36; for English translation, *Dicta quatuor ancillarum*, ed. and trans. Wolf, 212-13.

55 Elliott, *Proving Woman*, 5.

56 On this incident and Elizabeth's obedience, see Elliott, *Proving Woman*, 101-2.

57 Bynum, *Holy Feast and Holy Fast*, 237-44; for the quotation, see 238

58 Bynum, *Holy Feast and Holy Fast*, 99-100; see also p. 61 above.

at least half a lump of bread on three weekdays.[59] A sister named Agnese testified that when Clare became *infirmata*, she started to use a straw mattress by order of St. Francis.[60] St. Francis was one of those influential thirteenth-century writers in favour of controlling and moderating asceticism, his intervention in Clare's fasting and sleeping being one practical example.[61] At the same time, obedience to the regulations of one's order was one of the virtues that saints living in a monastic setting were supposed to have.[62] Clare's obedience and personal relationship with Francis were central to her *fama*, of which the nuns were undoubtedly aware, but given Francis's importance to their order, his role must also have been a vivid memory in their community.

A more thorough investigation into a female saint's obedience towards her confessor, in which infirmity served as a point where intervention was needed, was conducted in St. Frances of Rome's hearings. As Frances was an exceptional female saint in her activities, it seems plausible that for the conductors of the hearing and the witnesses alike, moderation in her penitence and austerity, and especially her obedience, were so important that they chose to underline this aspect of her sanctity. The hearing of 1440 dedicated its ninth article to Frances's obedience to her confessors. As proof of this it records an instance where Frances was gravely infirm ('gravi infirmitate detenta') and her first confessor, Antonius de Monte Sabelli, ordered her to drink wine. Frances obeyed but immediately vomited it up. The witnesses to the article confirmed this.[63] Her mind thus followed the ideals of *discretio* but her body turned an inability to do so into a proof of sanctity. Furthermore, the 1451 hearing, which investigated Frances's habit of sleeping in linen clothes or a hair shirt 'in infirmity and in health', underlined her obedience. Sister Anastasia testified that after Frances acquired her infirmity, she gave up the habit and her flagellation 'propter obedientiam' on the order of Johannes Matteotti. Agnes Pauli Lelli said that Frances used a hair shirt until the last four years before her death, when she gave it up as a result of the confessor's order because of 'the debility of old age' ('propter

59 PC Clare of Assisi, 444.

60 PC Clare of Assisi, 475: 'da poi che fo infirmata, per comandamento de sancto Francescho teneva uno sacchone de paglia'. Two other sisters reported the incident as well; PC Clare of Assisi, 449, 460.

61 Vauchez, *Sainthood*, 340, 350. Possibly his teachings had some effect as well, since in her letter Clare warned St. Agnes of Bohemia about excessive self-denial. Klaniczay, *Holy Rulers and Blessed Princesses*, 266.

62 Menestò, 'Apostolic Canonization Proceedings of Clare of Montefalco', 112.

63 PC Frances of Rome, 26-27.

ipsius debilitatem senectutis') but slept in linen cloths until her death.[64] The two women thus made a point of mentioning the reason why Frances moderated her austerity. This also gave a practical reason to the confessor's demands, making both parties appear to be reasonable and to be acting in a way that led to *fama sanctitatis*. Given that both Anastasia and Agnes were members of Frances's Order, they had witnessed her ways from close proximity and presumably also had an opinion about how to build her *fama*. Furthermore, Agnes' leading role as the *gubernatrix oblatorum* gave her authority in transmitting knowledge of the saint's activities.

Although research has primarily focused on the relationship between female saints and mystics and their confessors, canonization process records and other hagiographic texts show that in late medieval culture male saints' confessors were important as well. In many of these narrations the holy man's obedience is not as straightforward as in the case of female saints, yet the confessors were reported as having a controlling role even when the saint belonged to the uppermost clerical or secular elite. The emphasis on contrition and penance in later medieval culture had made confessors indispensable and influential members of each court and noble household.[65] In delineating the holy persons' indiscretion and bodily discomfort, they could quite literally make their bodily state better as well as increase their chances of being recognized as saints by making their behaviour more discreet – or at least giving proofs of this kind of behaviour. Guillaume de Saint-Pathus's *Vie* of St. Louis IX does not refer to any restrictions made by a confessor,[66] but when recording Louis's use of a hair shirt, Geoffrey de Beaulieu's *vita* states that his confessor instructed him that this kind of excessive penitence was not suitable for a man in his position. Louis then 'humbly admitted to his confessor that a hair shirt of this sort was extremely painful to his delicate skin'.[67] It is probable that Geoffrey, who was Louis's confessor for twenty years, is referring to his own conversation with the saintly king.[68] The 'sensitivity' of the king's skin again demonstrates the

64 PC Frances of Rome, 240-41.

65 Lawrence, *The Friars*, 170.

66 He depicted Louis's penitence according to the tradition and mentioned Geoffrey as the confessor. Guillaume de Saint-Pathus, *Vie de saint Louis*, 119-23.

67 Sometimes the king still wore a hair belt next to his skin, and as compensation for this concession, told the confessor to distribute alms among the poor on every Friday at Advent. 'Geoffrey of Beaulieu's *Life and Saintly Comportment of Louis, Former King of Franks, of Pious Memory*', transl. L. F. Field, ed. Gaposchkin and S. L. Field, 89. For the Latin text, see 'Vita, Ludovicus Francorum rex', *AASS*, Aug. V, 547-48: 'Tandem confessori suo humiliter recognovit, quod hujusmodi cilicium carnis ejus teneritudinem supra modum gravabat.'

68 Gaposchkin and Field, 'Introduction', 19-20.

shifting meanings given to saintly candidates' various corporeal characteristics. In the narrative, Louis IX's status as the king gives his bodily 'weakness' a different meaning than the same weakness would have for the female saints and probably also for male saints who were not rulers, although the role of suffering in Louis's cult resembles the Franciscan ideals. At least in the case of female saints, bishops, and hermits the aggravation of the discomfort because of the skin's sensitivity would most likely have added to the glory of their penitence.

The role of a confessor appears more complex in the canonization inquest of St. Peter of Luxembourg (1369-1387), held in Avignon in 1389-90. Among his other prestigious offices, Peter was elected the cardinal deacon of (anti)pope Clement VII,[69] but throughout the document there are witness statements referring to his wish to devote his life to prayer and *penitentia*.[70] Article 50 of the hearing mentions that there were suspicions that Peter might have shortened his life because of his asceticism and that his confessors advised him to moderate his practices. According to the article, Peter listened to them 'gladly and humbly' ('libenter & humiliter') but did not follow the orders.[71] The Augustinian friar Aegidius de Aurelianis was one of Peter's confessors and was, according to his own testimony, often the one trying to rein him in because he had doubts about his excessiveness and indiscretion, seeing that he was young and weak ('juvenis & debilis') in body. He also testified that he had reprehended Peter for his habit of using a knotted cord until he could no longer see it. However, at the time of Peter's death there were wounds and scars on his body that revealed its usage, which were visible to many.[72] Although again the wider public did not testify about Peter's life, Aegidius' statement can be compared with the narrations of Dorothea of Montau's scars, visible after her death and responsible for transmitting knowledge of her exceptional asceticism. Several high-ranking witnesses in Peter's hearing testified regarding attempts to regulate his behaviour.[73] Nicolaus Clacquin, the canon of Cambrai, and the chaplain of Peter and his mother Countess Mathilde (or Mahaut) de Châtillon (1335-78), for instance, testified that after his and the servants' attempts had proven to be in vain,

69 Before becoming a cardinal, during his short life Peter was elected as a canon of the cathedral chapter of Notre Dame de Paris in 1379, an Archdeachon of Dreux and Archdeacon of Cambrai, and the bishop of Metz. For an outline of his life, see Kieckhefer, *Unquiet Souls*, 33-44.

70 Peter's extreme penitence and its bodily consequences are also reported in the anonymous, contemporary *vita*; see 'Vita, Petrus de Luxemburgo S. R. E. Cardinalis', *AASS*, Iul. I, 513.

71 'Processus de vita & miraculis b. Petri de Luxemburgo', *AASS*, Iul. I, 535.

72 'Processus de vita & miraculis b. Petri de Luxemburgo', *AASS*, Iul. I, 537.

73 See e.g. 'Processus de vita & miraculis b. Petri de Luxemburgo', *AASS*, Iul. I, 535, 537.

they particularly asked Aegidius as well as the cardinal of Saluzzo (possibly Amedeo di Saluzzo, d. 1419) to do the same.[74] The other elite clerical witnesses in the hearing made similar remarks, mentioning that the young cardinal hid the cord from the confessor. It seems evident that at the time the household members and other high-ranking clerics saw his behaviour as a problem, but eventually turned problematic incidents into proofs of Peter's saintly habits.

Extreme asceticism could be seen as a situation so problematic that someone from the very uppermost level of the clerical hierarchy intervened. An article and corresponding depositions record that Clement VII, who also used Peter of Luxembourg's *fama* in his claims for papacy during the Western Schism,[75] attempted to restrain his asceticism, and ordered him to follow the physicians' orders because of his *infirmitas*.[76] Andreas de Luxemburgo, bishop of Cambrai, even testified that Clement VII ordered this under threat of excommunicating Peter – unlike in the case of the confessors, here Peter reportedly agreed to follow the order.[77] In Philip of Bourges' canonization process two witnesses, Philip's servant and *frater* Johannes, mentioned that Innocent IV (papacy 1243-54) pleaded that Philip ease his asceticism. Johannes stated that this was because Philip would then be better able to take care of his duties.[78] These incidents presumably were known to a restricted audience – at least Peter of Luxembourg's chaplain testified that Clement's actions were known among Peter's *familiares*.[79] They were, however, included in the two saints' *vitae*, and were thus distributed to a much larger audience as a sign of their extreme asceticism and *discretio*.[80]

The testimonies reflect the conflicting aspects of a prelate's sainthood, in which the characteristics of a hermit monk were 'more or less harmoniously superimposed' on a temporal and religious leader.[81] In the processes, their lives had to be reconstructed in a manner suitable for a saint, but it is obvious that from the point of view of the church a bishop or cardinal who, in his search for a saintly lifestyle, rendered himself incapable of fulfilling

74 'Processus de vita & miraculis b. Petri de Luxemburgo', *AASS*, Iul. I, 537.

75 Blumenfeld-Kosinski, *Poets, Saints, and Visionaries*, 76.

76 'Processus de vita & miraculis b. Petri de Luxemburgo', *AASS*, Iul. I, 535

77 'Processus de vita & miraculis b. Petri de Luxemburgo', *AASS*, Iul. I, 536; see also 537 for a shorter testimony on the matter. Clement's worry is also reported in Peter's fifteenth-century *vita*; 'Vita, Petrus de Luxemburgo', *AASS*, Iul. I, 513.

78 BAV, MS Vat. lat. 4019, fols. 43r, 47v. See also Vauchez, *Sainthood*, 301.

79 'Processus de vita & miraculis b. Petri de Luxemburgo', *AASS*, Iul. I, 537.

80 'Processus de vita & miraculis b. Petri de Luxemburgo', *AASS*, Iul. I, 513; *Vita s. Philippi Archiepiscopi Bituricensis*, ed. Martene and Durand, col. 1921.

81 See Vauchez, *Sainthood*, 304.

the duties of his office was a problem.[82] Yet, even those testifying about the sainthood of hermits could report an order of a high-ranking cleric. *Miles* Maginardus testified that Cardinal Ugolino (later Gregory IX) visited Lawrence of Subiaco some ten years before his death. Finding the holy man *graviter afflictum* due to his extreme asceticism, the cardinal persuaded him to lead a more discreet life and modify his austerity. For some reason only one witness reported the cardinal's visit, but it was recorded in the chronicles of Subiaco.[83] It is not entirely clear why the cardinal took an interest in Lawrence's case, unless he was asked to do so by his companions.[84] The Rule of St. Benedict, which regulated who could become a hermit, includes some concern about the potentially divisive nature of excessive asceticism but leaves a lot to the individual's own judgement.[85] Overtly ascetic behaviour could even be a sign of pride, and monastic life was supposed to nurture and promote humility. Furthermore, medieval society was well aware of the dangers of confusing piety with pride.[86] All three popes mentioned as regulating excessive asceticism were also active in the campaigns against heresies, some of whose followers practised rigorous asceticism, especially the Cathar perfects.[87] Their overall suspicious attitude towards any kind of extremism may also have played a role here, and controlling saints' asceticism was one way of fighting heresies,[88] in a same manner as female saints' obedience was.

As mentioned above, a witness reported that Clement VII referred to physicians when reprimanding Peter of Luxembourg. The growing importance of medical professionals and medical science in medieval canonization processes

82 Gratian's *Decretum* regulated that a bishop or prelate could not be replaced even when he was ill and infirm, but in those cases a *coadiutor* should be found, and he should take care of the daily duties. However, this was not the definitive rule in the later Middle Ages, as Raymond of Penyaforte's set of laws, written in 1230s, became more popular. Penyaforte's *Decretals* state that the reason for finding stewards to replace infirm bishops and prelates is that their sickness may discourage others, and therefore it might be more difficult to find people able to fight for the church. Trembinski, 'An Infirm Man', 276-77; she discusses the influence of these regulations on the life of St. Francis of Assisi, coming to the conclusion that Francis was forced to leave his position as the leader of his Order because of his increasing disabilities. See also Trembinski, 'Illness and Authority', 113-15. For priests' bodily infirmities and the concept of *defectus corporalis*, Salonen and Hanska, *Entering a Clerical Career*, 122-29.

83 PC Lawrence Loricatus, 663-64; Jannuccelli, *Memorie di Subiaco e sua badia*, 179-80.

84 See PC Lawrence Loricatus, 663-64, 692, for the companions' attempts to delineate his asceticism.

85 Hughes-Edwards, *Reading Medieval Anchoritism*, 61-62.

86 See e.g. Bynum, *Holy Feast and Holy Fast*, 86, 97; Jotischky, *Hermit's Cookbook*, 48.

87 See Moore, *War on Heresy*, 278-82, for the basic details. Innocent III's actions in this field are discussed in Bolton, '*Vita ascetica:* A Papal Quandary'.

88 See Hughes-Edwards, *Reading Medieval Anchoritism*, 72.

is a known phenomenon, studied especially in the context of miracles. In testimonies about miraculous cures, witnesses often referred to the diagnoses, verdicts, and futile treatments of physicians, occasionally also of surgeons. Especially in southern European inquests, the *medici* also gave testimonies about their patients' miraculous healings, providing scientific proof of the incurability of a condition by medical means and, consequently, that the cure had to be a miracle.[89] Although primarily originating in the requirements of the inquisitorial process, these statements also demonstrate the interplay between lived religion and medical science, which largely complemented each other.

The role of medical science is not as important in late medieval depositions on saints' lives as it is to miracles, but the presence of medical men in these testimonies as well as their own depositions made up part of the same phenomenon. As already seen in the discussion of the signs of passion in Clare of Montefalco's heart, medical professionals could have a crucial role in interpreting the corporeal phenomena of sainthood, and especially the acceptable limits of asceticism. Most often witnesses simply mentioned that a holy person eased up on their diet or ascetic sleeping habits because of a physician's advice.[90] References to physicians gave weight to the witnesses' views when they were constructing sanctity – or doubting it – according to various tropes and internalized ideas about sainthood. Judging from the canonization testimonies, the saints' devotees saw their role as rather uncomplicated, but the biggest contradictions or conflicts they reported were between medical men and the saints themselves.[91]

As an example of the collaboration between physicians and other members of saints' communities, the confessors who attempted to regulate asceticism reportedly negotiated with them. Although the witnesses saw obedience

89 See e.g. Lett, '*Judicium Medicine* and *Judicium Sanctitatis*'; 'Ziegler, 'Practitioners and Saints'.

90 For example, the Franciscan brother Guillermus de Ansillaco testified that Philip of Bourges usually had no mattress on his bed. After he fell from a horse, he was 'a bit broken/weak' ('aliquantulum fractus'), and, following the physicians' orders, used a mattress for a while. BAV, MS Vat. lat. 4019, fol. 29v. Philip as well as Thomas Cantilupe also eased their diet because of physicians' advice, see BAV, MS Vat. lat. 4015, fol. 108v; BAV, MS Vat. lat. 4019, fol. 33r.

91 There were also irregularities in canonization hearings regarding medical men's role. In St. Nicholas of Tolentino's hearing, his *infirmarius* Iohannucius de Tholentino testified but it appears he was not asked much about Nicholas of Tolentino's infirmity. The same can be said about Petrus Iohannis, *medicus*, who had attended Nicholas at the time of his illness. PC Nicholas of Tolentino, 487, 489. If Iohannucius de Tholentino was indeed the infirmarian of the establishment, he was a very young one, since he testified that he was 10 or 12 years old at the time! See also Lett, *Un procès de canonisation*, 362. In general, infirmarians were very important people in medieval monasteries. They were in charge of the infirmaries, which were often their own establishments. See Lawrence, *Medieval Monasticism*, 111; Mitchell, 'The Infirmaries'.

to a confessor as more important than obedience to a physician, the latter could still give scientific proof of the need of discretion. Furthermore, a proper diet which was neither too overindulgent nor too meagre was one of the nonnaturals and considered essential for a person's health,[92] which explains why physicians were mentioned particularly in testimonies about diet. In addition to Peter of Luxembourg's hearing, the witnesses in Charles of Blois's process also mentioned that physicians controlled his diet in his youth and adulthood.[93] Furthermore, his physician Georgius de Lesnen said that he reproved Charles for his fasting and made his confessor reprove him as well, because it seemed that his bodily strength would wane.[94]

Physicians' presence was common in elite households of the period, which partly explains their important role and acquaintance with the holy person's confessor, but their collaboration was referred to also in other types of settings. Prior Petrus for example testified that St. Birgitta only agreed to take baths, which physicians saw as crucial for the cure of her grave infirmity, after her confessor ordered her to do so in the name of saintly obedience.[95] In the case of St. Clare of Montefalco, her sister the abbess, her confessor, and a physician collaborated in restricting Clare's asceticism.[96] Since late antiquity, the abbot or abbess was the person whose duty it was to control the brothers' and sisters' medical treatment and austerity, as stated in many monastic rules.[97] As Clare's sister and abbess in a cloistered nunnery, Iohanna plays an important part in the articles and testimonies of Clare's hearing. Presumably obedience to her would still not have been proof powerful enough for Bérenger de Saint-Affrique when he penned the articles. At the same time, the presence of all three provides illuminating evidence of the different parties interested in limiting austerity.

92 See Getz, *Medicine in the English Middle Ages*, 87-88; Siraisi, *Medieval and Early Renaissance Medicine*, 137; Rawcliffe, *Medicine and Society*, 39-40.

93 BAV, MS Vat. lat. 4025, fols. 5v, 13v; PC Charles of Blois, 12, 32.

94 BAV, MS Vat. lat 4025, fol. 12r; PC Charles of Blois, 12.

95 PC Birgitta of Sweden, 490. This is among the very rare references to any bodily illness of St. Birgitta. In her testimony about her mother's death, Catherine said that she had 'fevers' for about a year. PC Birgitta of Sweden, 318.

96 PC Clare of Montefalco, 4-5, 176, 180, 185-86.

97 See Crislip, *From Monastery to Hospital*, 74-75; Kuuliala, '*Infirmitas* in Monastic Rules'; Schulenburg, *Forgetful of their Sex*, 374-89; Yearl, 'Medieval Monastic Customaries', 181-84. See also Trembinski, 'An Infirm Man', 285-86, for the requests of St. Francis of Assisi's guardian that he should seek medical treatment. The *magistra* of a novice could have similar authority, as for example *domina* Catherina, the abbess, testified in St. Margaret of Hungary's hearing. Olimpiades, who was her *magistra*, restricted her usage of a hair shirt and her praying. PC Margaret of Hungary, 38-39, and Muessig, 'Learning and Mentoring in the Twelfth Century', 89, for young nuns' training.

In the process records used in this study, there are two instances where the witnesses reported that the saint herself was active in collaborating with a physician. St. Elizabeth of Hungary's handmaid Irmingard stated that Elizabeth sought out a *medicus* to give her a diet that would prevent her from acquiring an infirmity due to her abstinence.[98] This is a quite exceptional testimony about self-regulation, possibly one example of the internalized suspicion towards female piety.[99] The other case is included in the hearing of Dauphine of Puimichel, where an article and corresponding deposition discuss the consequences of the excessive amount of tears she shed due to her devotion. Article 27 records that this caused her vision to deteriorate, she also had 'consumpcione cerebri', consumption of the brain, and many people feared she would become literally blind. This made her look for assistance from a *medicus* because of the pain or damage to her eyes. As the physician in question, Durandus Andree gave a testimony to the article, portraying in an interesting light the interaction between the holy woman and a man who was both her confessor and her physician. Dauphine asked for Durandus's help because of the eye problem, but she asked him to give advice only if he did not prohibit the crying. As the article puts it, she would much rather have destroyed her brain and lost her vision than abstain from shedding tears.[100]

The interaction between Dauphine and her physician-confessor demonstrates one of the cultural meanings blindness could have in the Middle Ages. St. Margaret of Castello, who was born blind and with restricted growth, is described in her *vita* as having the 'divine light' instead of the mundane one.[101] A similar view was expressed by Bonaventure, who wrote in the *vitae* of St. Francis of Assisi that his eye disease was caused by his constant weeping. When the physicians told him to refrain from shedding tears to preserve his eyesight, he replied that he would rather go blind than stop weeping in prayer.[102] At the same time, there are texts comparing blindness

98 PC Elizabeth of Hungary, 137; for English translation, *Dicta quatuor ancillarum*, ed. and trans. Wolf, 213.

99 See Bynum, *Holy Feast and Holy Fast*, 85-87, for discussion on the need of some pious women to hide their asceticism because of clerical suspicion. For example, St. Catherine of Siena claimed that her inability to eat was caused by infirmity rather than her extreme voluntary asceticism.

100 PC Dauphine of Puimichel, 49-50, 259-60. See also Archambeau, 'Remembering Countess Delphine's Books', for this article and the corresponding depositions.

101 *Vita Margaritae de Città de Castello*, ed. Laurent, 121: 'Hec enim oculis corporeis privata nascitur ne mundum videat; que iam lumine divino vescitur, ut in terra stans celum tantum aspiciat.'

102 Trembinski, 'Illness and Authority', 119. In her studies on Francis's infirmities, Trembinski has shown how Francis's hagiographers subdued and modified the bodily consequences of his infirmities as well as their reasons. See also Trembinski, 'An Infirm Man'.

with the *loss* of divine light,[103] and blindness was used as a symbol of pagans and Jews choosing not to 'see' the true religion.[104] These completely opposing views provide clear evidence that no illness or impairment had – or has ever had – purely positive or negative connotations, as they depend on the cultural context and the situation.[105] Durandus agreed to Dauphine's wishes, and suggested a rest from manual labour, reading, and prayers, reassuring the countess that his advice was not against God.[106] This advice or treatment was both religious and medical at the same time, reflecting his two roles. He sought to alleviate her infirmity based on his medical knowledge; according to the theory of non-naturals, lack of sleep and excess of emotions could cause blindness and mental afflictions.[107] At the same time, he accepted her saintly need to suffer.[108]

The topic is one of those where the role of one informant in spreading the information appears crucial. Bertrandus Iusberti testified that he heard about it from Nicholas Loarenchi, who had heard from Durandus Andree that Dauphine was in danger of acquiring 'consumpcione cerebri' due to her tears. This also shows how the information ended up in the articles penned by Nicholas. Bertranda Bartholomea gave a similar testimony.[109] Catherina de Podio, on the other hand, referred to herself and other *familiares* as those in fear of Dauphine getting the illness, but she stated that the contents of the article were known among Dauphine's acquaintances and devotees.[110] All these statements portray different parties' willingness to be intepreters of the marks of sainthood. Rixendis de Insula, a Cistercian nun, gave a somewhat different version of the story. When Dauphine stayed in the convent of the Holy Cross, Rixendis answered her call to clean her table. She saw that Dauphine cried effusively, and the countess told her that it was due to the 'pain and infirmity of the head' ('dolorem et infirmitatem

103 Woolgar, *The Senses in Late Medieval England*, 184.

104 Wheatley, *Stumbling Blocks before the Blind*, 63-72, 76-89. See also Goodich, *Miracles and Wonders*, 22-25.

105 The one illness in whose case this is specifically evident is leprosy. On the religious and cultural ideas concerning it, see Rawcliffe, *Leprosy in Medieval England*, and esp. 110, where she writes that '[a]ttitudes to the sick in any society are rarely monolithic, nor do they change at a uniform rate, however persuasive the arguments of the Church, the state or the medical profession may be.'

106 PC Dauphine of Puimichel, 259-60.

107 See e.g. Siraisi, *Medieval and Early Renaissance Medicine*, 100-1.

108 See also Archambeau, 'Remembering Countess Delphine's Books', 42-43.

109 PC Dauphine of Puimichel, 225, 331.

110 PC Dauphine of Puimichel, 397: 'est publica vox et fama inter familiares et notos et devotos dicte domine Dalphine'.

capitis'). Rixendis suspected that Dauphine had said this so that she would not suspect her of doing it because of penitence and devotion; this apparently was a later conclusion, after Rixendis heard from Dauphine's *familiares* about her penitentiary practices and how it was feared that she would acquire consumption of the brain.[111]

Several witness accounts represent Dauphine as a reluctant saint, which was a proof of her humility.[112] In Rixendis's testimony, her humility interlinks with her physical symptoms. There was a cultural model for interpreting copious tears as a sign of devotion; they were an important aspect of the lives of many later medieval saints, especially emphasized in female saints' *vitae*. They were manifestations of their souls' union with God and a physical sign of the divine will, which worked in the holy person, and were also associated with spiritual cleansing. Even making oneself blind in such a manner was not just an act of humility, but also a way to get closer to God.[113] Rixendis's testimony presents Dauphine as seeking to erase all this from the nun's mind with her reference to infirmity.

Collaboration between household members and the physician-confessor in regard to devotion leading to infirmity is also visible in another instance investigated in Dauphine's hearing. The articles record how she sought new ways of performing penance, when she became *attrita* due to her infirmity, penitence, and old age. This culminated in her excessive reading of saints' lives, and caused mental affliction ('mentis afflictionem'), which 'grew stronger in her now and then due to the infirmity of fever'. For this reason, her household members sometimes hid her books.[114] Bertranda Bartholomea testified that *magister* Nicholas Loarenchi and other *familiares* hid her books, Catherina de Podio that it was done by one of the female companions, and Bertrandus Iusberti had heard that one of the male companions had done it.[115] Based on these testimonies it is impossible to say how gendered the regulation of Dauphine's *penitentia* was. However, this time the testimony of Durandus Andree emphasizes his status as Dauphine's confessor, rather

111 PC Dauphine of Puimichel, 486-87; Archambeau, 'Remembering Countess Delphine's Books', 33-34.

112 Vauchez, *Sainthood*, 411-12.

113 Archambeau, 'Remembering Countess Delphine's Books', 39; Knight, '*Si puose calcina a' propi occhi*', esp. 146-47. Article 27 directly refers to the spiritual benefits of blindness; PC Dauphine of Puimichel, 50. See also Boquet and Nagy, *Medieval Sensibilities*, 46-47, 166, 181, 219-20, for tears and emotions.

114 PC Dauphine of Puimichel, 52-53. See also Archambeau, 'Remembering Countess Delphine's Books', for this article and the corresponding depositions.

115 PC Dauphine of Puimichel, 231, 333-34, 400.

than as a physician. He underlined Dauphine's devotion and piety by saying that her purpose in all this had been to find an example to follow in the lives of the Fathers.[116] As for his own actions, as pointed out by Nicole Archambeau, Durandus was the one who selected appropriate books for the countess, narrowing 'the scope of [her] sanctity to a group of holy people the papal court would find acceptable'.[117] Again, infirmity was recorded in this instance to show the lengths to which Dauphine went with her penitence, which the activities of her household members highlight. At the same time, it is a fine example of the twofold nature of the saintly lifestyle and how individual members or the community could direct holy persons' actions if their behaviour was judged harmful to their body or mind.

There appear to have been some contradictory views about whether or not the use of physicians' help was acceptable for a saint in the first place, or whether abstaining from it was part of their austerity. The critical testimony of friar Thomas Boni de Fulgineo in Clare of Montefalco's inquest is the most illuminating example of this. Thomas questioned whether she led an ascetic lifestyle at all, among other things saying that she enjoyed the best food and had the best physicians.[118] According to him, *not* having access to or using the 'best' physicians and instead enduring illness without alleviation belonged to a saintly lifestyle. At the same time, those in favour of Clare's canonization interpreted and used the physicians' visits in a completely different way – to prove Clare's virginity and purity. Sister Francescha, daughter of physician Gualterius, testified that her father had the saint in his care several times and Clare always fully covered herself.[119] Clare's brother Franciscus, a Franciscan friar, acted as the assessor of the hearing. He testified that he himself took 'one of the best physicians of Italy', who was a devotee of Clare, to see his sister.[120] The status of the physician was important for giving evidence for Clare's purity, viriginity, and seemingly miraculous inability to masturbate, as Franciscus told that the physician found a 'lock' in

116 PC Dauphine of Puimichel, 265. Here her behaviour is described as similar to that of St. Margaret of Hungary who, according to several witnesses in her hearing, often meditated on the lives of various saints like St. Thomas Becket, and was inspired by their legends. See Klaniczay, *The Uses of Supernatural Power*, 108; see also Lewis, 'Male Saints and Devotional Masculinity in Late Medieval England', 122, for the importance of male saints' *vitae* for female readers.

117 Archambeau, 'Remembering Countess Delphine's Books', 43.

118 PC Clare of Montefalco, 435: 'et habebat optimos medicos pro se ipsa.' For Clare's poverty and its differences from the Franciscan ideals, see Burr, *Spiritual Franciscans*, 318-19.

119 PC Clare of Montefalco, 330.

120 PC Clare of Montefalco, 270: 'duxit unum excellentiximum [*sic*] medicum, nomine magistrum Mercatum de Eugubio, de melioribus medicine totius Ytalie, ad dictam s. Claram. Qui medicus eo ipso quod eam vidit, tantam devotionem habuit ad eam'.

Clare's 'secret parts' that even prevented menstruation.[121] Durandus Andree reported a similar instance in his testimony about Dauphine of Puimichel's virginity. He testified that Dauphine's companions Rostagna de Saltu and Huga de Podio gave her medical remedies that Durandus had prescribed for a gynaecological illness and noticed that she was a virgin.[122] Neither one of these women were among the witnesses, and nobody else mentioned the incident. However, in the view of these three people, as well as for those testifying about Clare's virginity, medical treatment functioned as a way to prove purity, so that it became intermingled with their construction of sanctity. Although chastity and virginity were important elements of male sainthood as well,[123] medicalizing it in the manner done in the case of Clare and Dauphine does not appear in canonization processes of males.

Similarly, the reports that the witnesses gave about some saints' reluctance to follow physicians' advice also show the fluctuating role of this behaviour in finding evidence of sanctity.[124] Many of the witnesses in John Buoni's hearing referred to the hermit's refusal to accept any medical treatment. As for his diet, they reported that he only ate meat at a time of infirmity reluctantly when urged by physicians or other brothers to do so.[125] The saint whose refusal to follow physicians' advice concerning his diet – or anything else – appears to have been most successful was St. Nicholas of Tolentino. The fourteenth article states that he refused physicians' advice to eat meat at the time of his infirmity, which was one aspect of his *fama sanctitatis*. A few witnesses confirmed this.[126] The notary Berardus Appillaterre, who

121 Franciscus's testimony regarding this aspect (PC Clare of Montefalco, 270) reads: 'dixit sibi testi quod opportebat quod ipsa reciperet unum summarium quarundam rerum ad quedam loca vel membra naturalia secreta, et hoc quia in se habebat tantam clausuram virginitatis quod non poterat facere vel emictere ea que mulieres communiter faciunt et emictunt, etiam sine opere alicuius alterius creature.' For purity and masturbation, see Elliott, *Fallen Bodies*, 45-52.

122 PC Dauphine of Puimichel, 244.

123 See e.g. Lewis, 'Imitate, too, this king in virtue', 138-39, for the descriptions of chastity in the case of married male saints.

124 An intriguing piece of information concerning Francis of Assisi's medical treatment is given in Bonaventure's *vita*, in which Francis's fellow friars tried to persuade him to seek medical treatment for his eyes. He agreed to have only cauterization, because it was known to be painful and thus allow him to continue suffering during the treatment. Trembinski, 'Illness and Authority', 119. It is surprising that there are no such narratives in the canonization testimonies, since this kind of attitude towards medical advice would enable the saintly figure both to show obedience towards his or her superiors and to continue practising *imitatio Christi*.

125 'Processus apostolici, de b. Joanne Buono', *AASS*, Oct. IX, 816, 818, 832.

126 PC Nicholas of Tolentino, 19; see 221, 401-2, for testimonies to the article. The *relatio* of the process also records this; BAV, MS Vat. lat. 4027, fol. 6v. Although not always so detailed, this information about Nicholas's eating habits had spread among some other members of the local

we have encountered above, gave detailed information about the conflict between the saint and his community members. Berardus and some other men, including the physician of the monastery, went to visit Nicholas to persuade him to ease up on his diet. Nicholas rebuked the visitors, asking if they did not believe that God had enough power in bread, wheat, and oil, so that he could be healed without eating meat. Berardus then rode off to the provincial prior of Nicholas's Order, and asked him to write a letter ordering Nicholas to eat meat as advised by the physician. Nicholas agreed to eat some meat after seeing the letter, and Berardus had some partridge cooked for him. In the end Nicholas ate a tiny amount of the meat, sent the rest to other infirm brothers, and said, rather ironically: 'Oh Berardus, I have obeyed the letter!'[127] Thus the saint managed to stick to his principles regarding fasting and acts of mercy, yet followed the instruction of his superior, which was a sign of obedience.[128]

Most likely the testimony was also a way for Berardus to emphasize his own status as someone close to the holy man within the religious community of the area. At the same time, Nicholas of Tolentino was an ascetic, influential male hermit saint, who was not in a clerical position similar to that of bishops. This might in part explain the references to his ability to refuse physicians' advice, but the witnesses still knew that obeying a superior was of vital importance for his *fama*. In the process of John Buoni, another Italian hermit, the reluctance to follow physicians' treatment was also reported by many witnesses as a sign of his austerity. As for his diet, they reported that, even at a time of infirmity, he only ate meat reluctantly and when urged by physicians or other brothers to do so.[129] It appears that the matter was not always so straightforward, however. The process also records that there was some murmuring among the brothers of his community that rather than being an expression of sanctity, his fasting was caused by a blocked bowel (*strictus budellus*), thus diagnosing his dietary regime as an *infirmitas* that dissuaded him from acting in the manner people commonly did. When John Buoni himself heard about these doubts, he ate a large amount of food

community too, as shown by the witness account of a woman called Iacobucia. She testified that she heard it being said that Nicholas did not eat meat, fish, eggs, or cheese, either at the time of infirmity or at the time of health. PC Nicholas of Tolentino, 232. See also PC Nicholas of Tolentino, 248, 235, 284, 523, for other laypersons' testimonies about his diet.

127 PC Nicholas of Tolentino, 119-20; see 221 for another testimony of the visit.

128 The prior's role and Nicholas's obedience at the time of this infirmity are also referred to in Nicholas's early fourteenth-century *vita*. 'Vita, Nicolaus Tolentinas, ord. eremitarum s. Augustini', *AASS*, Sept. X, 649.

129 'Processus apostolici, de b. Joanne Buono', *AASS*, Oct. IX, 816, 818, 832.

quickly and in public to prove the rumour false.[130] As pointed out by Aviad Kleinberg in his discussion of this case, '[w]hat was the point of behaving like a saint, if it were not recognized as such by others?'[131] The living saints also had to negotiate the communication of their saintly behaviour to their devotees, even if they had very little control over their later reconstruction of it. It is, again, worth pointing out that the voices of doubt came from among his own Order, not from the general public.[132] The other brothers were crucial disseminators of information about John Buoni's cult,[133] and it was above all they who needed to be convinced of his sanctity, including its corporeal aspects.[134]

In general, in addition to the vast majority of witness accounts of saints' lives being given by their household members, members of their monastic order, or other (elite) people close to them, the depositions are typically in close agreement about the sanctity of the person under scrutiny. References like that in John Buoni's inquest or the one given by Thomas Boni de Fulgineo in Clare of Montefalco's hearing are extremely rare. The process of St. Thomas Cantilupe is an exception in that it includes frequent reservations expressed about his holiness, by Franciscans summoned to testify, possibly still irritated by the conflict Thomas had had with the Franciscan archbishop John Peckham.[135] Usually these statements do not mention the bishop's bodily state but refer to his ascetic practices without referring to any infirmities.[136] Punishment miracles, in which a saint chastises someone for

130 'Processus apostolici, de b. Joanne Buono', *AASS*, Oct. IX, 816, 840, 841; see also 838, where a witness is asked about the reason for John Buoni's ascetic diet but does not mention the doubts regarding it.

131 Kleinberg, *Prophets*, 19. This could work in the other direction too. St. Francis of Assisi, who was exasperated by his reputation as a living saint, reportedly informed a crowd coming to his hermitage that during the last Lent he ate food that included pork fat. Vauchez, *Sainthood*, 191, n. 103.

132 See e.g. 'Processus apostolici, de b. Joanne Buono', *AASS*, Oct. IX, 852-56. Although they reported that his fame as a saint had been recognized for years before his death (usually the witnesses said that this was either for seven or for fourteen years before his death) and that many people came to meet him personally, they did not report his bodily state.

133 Some friars even distributed some leaflets recording his miracles *in vita*. This raised criticism in the Order, and when John Buoni himself heard about it, he destroyed the leaflets. See Kleinberg, *Prophets*, 40-62. The relevant witness account is in 'Processus apostolici, de b. Joanne Buono', *AASS*, Oct. IX, 783.

134 This also shows in PC Celestine V, see esp. II, 298-307.

135 Finucane, *Miracles and Pilgrims*, 176; Vauchez, *Sainthood*, 301-3.

136 The testimony of Thomas's nephew Willelmus may be read as an exception, because he stated that Thomas was 'well formed' ('bene compaginatus et bene formatus') but rode bent forward, facing the ground, to show his modesty. Although this description of his posture and

blasphemy, give examples of attitudes that must have been more common than the hearings usually report.[137] Usually the person punished had simply doubted someone's sanctity and miracle-working abilities, but they might also be punished for questioning the corporeal signs of their sainthood. As mentioned above, one man faced Clare of Montefalco's posthumous punishment – a severe nosebleed – after ridiculing the marks of passion found in her heart,[138] and Philip of Bourges' inquest records a case where a diocesan priest acquired *gutta* as a punishment, because he, among other things, said that Philip ate and drank as much as anyone else.[139] These cases place the human body and its ailments at the core of communal ideas and negotiations regarding sanctity.

bodily characteristics does not refer to any infirmity, it does contrast with the attestations of asceticism with a 'well formed' body, which can be seen as synonymous to a 'healthy' or ideal body. BAV, MS Vat. lat. 4015, fol. 59r.

137 Arnold, *Belief and Unbelief*, 221-24.

138 PC Clare of Montefalco, 459-61, 484-85.

139 BAV, MS Vat. lat. 4019, fols. 70v-73v. For a summary of the case, see BAV, MS Vat. lat. 4020, fols. 17v-18r; see also Vauchez, *Sainthood*, 301. A pilgrimage to Philip's shrine on the following day cured him. Interestingly, Gerardus also reported that later on he sometimes suffered from *gutta*, which prayers to Philip always eased. Other depositions to the punishment miracle do not report this aftermath of the incident. On partial cures in canonization processes, see Kuuliala, 'Heavenly Healing or Failure of Faith?'

Holy Infirmity and the Devotees

Abstract
The final chapter of the book focuses on the saintly candidates' devotees and their various encounters with the infirm saint, as well as the attempts and prospects for healing holy infirmity. It also analyses the cultural significances of holy suffering. While the devotees gave varying meanings to saints' infirmities, they did not directly overlap with the documents we have of their own suffering. Saints valued and cherished their own infirmities, but they also helped, even medically, those of their devotees who were ill or suffering. At the same time, it is likely that the culturally internalized narratives of the benefits of infirmity and the valorization of suffering had a therapeutic function in the same way as miracle narratives.

Keywords: sainthood, community, lay piety, medical pluralism, pain, miracles

The communities distributing information about saints' *infirmitates* were not static, but their structures and respective relations changed and were renegotiated. Moreover, the communities of the saints under investigation here, and the group of devotees believing in their holiness or promoting and/or testifying about it, varied greatly. Due to the socio-economic background of the saints, their closest associates tended to be clerics and nuns, often with elite background, or belong to the secular elite. Furthermore, as stated in the Introduction, witnesses belonging to the elite, and especially elite men, were favoured as witnesses to saints' lives. Therefore the image of saintly infirmities as represented in canonization testimonies was primarily born in their circle, and they were also the people who interacted with the infirm saint most intimately on an everyday basis.

Living saints performed miracles, which was one of the prerequisites for canonization, although in most hearings a majority of the miracles

Kuuliala, Jenni, *Saints, Infirmity, and Community in the Late Middle Ages.*
Taylor & Francis Group 2020
DOI: 10.5117/9789462983373_HOLY

investigated were *post mortem*.[1] Often the *miracula in vita* were recorded among the testimonies to the saint's life.[2] Some of the devotees searching for a miraculous intervention came from the social elite as well, but the larger public recorded as having received saintly assistance were townspeople and other persons from the 'middle' social strata.[3] The number of miracles *in vita* that were recorded (as opposed to the number believed by various people to have occurred) varies significantly from hearing to hearing; for ecclesiastical authorities, their status was less straightforward than that of miracles *post mortem*.[4] As an example, all of Louis IX's recorded *miracula* occurred after his death,[5] and a large number of miracles *in vita* were omitted from Bernardino of Siena's hearing.[6] However, the hearings of Nicholas of Tolentino, Dauphine of Puimichel, and especially Frances of Rome include a significant number of miracles done by them when still alive.

This chapter will focus on the (living) saints' interaction with their communities, and the role their and their devotees' bodily infirmity played in negotiating sanctity. As pointed out by Aviad Kleinberg, saints had different roles for each circumstance, and it is thus more fruitful to analyse a 'situation where a person is labelled a saint and his or her behaviour interpreted within the parameters of saintly performance – as the basic unit in the dynamics of sainthood'.[7] How, then, did other members of the community react to the saints' *infirmitates* in different situations and settings, including *miracula in vita*, and in what circumstances did they end up mentioning saints' bodily suffering in their testimonies?

1 Typically the miracles *in vita* were acts of prodigies. Miracles *post mortem* were produced by an intensification of saints' 'beneficial radiation' after their deaths. Vauchez, *Sainthood*, 306, 431, 503-4.

2 Katajala-Peltomaa and Krötzl, 'Approaching Twelfth-Fifteenth-Century Miracles', 4-5.

3 Poor people were generally considered less trustworthy, and their miraculous cures were rarely investigated in canonization inquests. See e.g. Farmer, *Surviving Poverty*, 51-52.

4 Andrić, *Miracles of St. John Capistran*, 194-95; Moore, 'Between Sanctity and Superstition', 58-59, 61-62.

5 This at least partly derives from the fierce campaign for his sanctity initiated by those close to him, rather than from an existing popular lay cult during his lifetime. Such cult beginnings did not, however, necessarily mean that there was a complete absence of miracles *in vita* in the canonization inquests. Charles of Blois's cult appears to have been 'created' only after his death, but there are still sporadic testimonies about him performing miracles – albeit accidentally or reluctantly – during his lifetime. Vauchez, 'Canonisation et politique au XIVe siècle', 383. For examples, see BAV, MS Vat. lat. 4015, fols. 104v, 168r-169v. For promoting cults immediately after the saint's death, see Houts, *Memory and Gender in Medieval Europe*, 47-48; Prudlo, *The Martyred Inquisitor*, 89-96.

6 Pellegrini, 'Testifying to Miracles', 119.

7 Kleinberg, *Prophets*, 7.

Encountering the Infirm Saint

As a communally negotiated phenomenon, sainthood was a very public affair. At the same time, saints were expected to be humble and they often performed both their miracles *in vita* and their most ascetic penitential practices in secret.[8] There were, however, times when even a saint portrayed as most humble and most reluctant could use his body to effect in public, especially for the sake of his community. Louis IX famously turned more towards public acts of charity and piety after his experiences during the crusade.[9] Among the canonization protocols, Charles of Blois's is the one where this kind of behaviour gets most attention. Although the witnesses presented Charles's devoutness and piety as originating in his childhood, according to the trope of *puer sanctus*, some witnesses made it explicit that a change in his habits occurred during his captivity by the English.[10] Perhaps he, like Louis IX, felt responsible for the outcome of the battle he had lost and the ransom paid for him from his subjects' taxes. At any rate, the witnesses formed a picture of a duke who took his piety one step further after his release. One armiger, for instance, reported that he heard from Charles's wife and a servant that he began to use a hair shirt more frequently,[11] and Georgius de Lesnen testified that during his captivity Charles beat himself with a scourge that had small knots in the ends and in which needles had been tied.[12]

Although the duke asked his physician to keep his flagellation secret, he also did very public penance. Several witnesses reported Charles's pilgrimage from the location where he was captured near La Roche-Derrien to the church of Tréguier and the shrine of his favourite saint, St. Yves of Tréguier, whose canonization he had actively promoted.[13] The *cubicularius* Oliverius de Buyguonio testified that Charles had made a vow to Yves when captured by the English, but his testimony gives no further details about the nature

8 St. Hedwig of Silesia's *vita*, for example, credits her for *discretio* and how she did not wish to 'overdo' her penitence and austerity, nor turn it into a public show, and Frances of Rome's hearing reports that she took care to perform her penitentiary practices in secret, despite her being a laywoman and rather public in her other saintly actions. *AASS*, Oct. VIII, 232; PC Frances of Rome, 240-41. See also pp. 132-33 above for Dauphine of Puimichel.

9 On this, see O'Tool, 'Caring for the Blind'.

10 See also Cassard, 'Les coulisses de la sainteté?', 3.

11 BAV, MS Vat. lat. 4025, fol. 26r; PC Charles of Blois, 66.

12 BAV, MS Vat. lat. 4025, fol. 13r; PC Charles of Blois, 31.

13 Cassard, 'Propagande partisane et miracles', 10-11; Goodich, *Miracles and Wonders*, 44-45; Vauchez, *Sainthood*, 312. See BAV, MS Vat. lat. 4025, fols. 34r, 36v-37r, 40r; PC Charles of Blois, 82, 87, 97, for other instances where witnesses mentioned his devotion towards St. Yves.

of the *votum*.[14] Presumably he asked Yves to help with his release, which is a common plea of those unjustly imprisoned or badly treated when captured in medieval hagiographic material.[15] Other witnesses explained the pilgrimage on grounds of Charles's devotion or penitence.[16] The witnesses gave special importance to the pilgrimage's physical consequences. According to Oliverius, Charles walked with bare feet. This happened during winter, and the skin on the soles of Charles's feet peeled off. Oliverius represented all this as an example of Charles's patience, because while his feet were injured, he thanked God.[17] Guillermus Andree also mentioned the icy conditions of the pilgrimage, adding that people put chaffs and cloths on the road to ease Charles's walk, but he did not walk on them. According to Guillermus, Charles's feet were in such bad condition that he was unable to stand on them for fifteen weeks.[18]

Throughout the process, Charles is represented as a somewhat reluctant saint. Some of the beneficiaries of his *miracula in vita*, for example, reported that he asked them to keep the incident a secret.[19] He also did not want

14 BAV, MS Vat. lat. 4025, fol. 13v; PC Charles of Blois, 32. When bringing Yves of Tréguier's case to the papal consistory, Charles and his barons reported miracles done by Yves. One of them concerned the duke's own miraculous cure, after which he made a pilgrimage to Yves's shrine barefoot. Goodich, *Miracles and Wonders*, 44. There is a possibility that this is the same case referred to in the main text.

15 See Goodich, *Violence and Miracle*, 126-29.

16 BAV, MS Vat. lat. 4025, fols. 40v, 52r, 52v; PC Charles of Blois, 97, 127, 135.

17 BAV, MS Vat. lat. 4025, fol. 13v; PC Charles of Blois, 32: 'super quo regraciatus fuit Deo, ac durante infirmitate dictorum pedum dicebat "Laudetur Deus".'

18 BAV, MS Vat. lat. 4025, fol. 40v; PC Charles of Blois, 97. See also BAV, MS Vat. lat. 4025, fols. 51r, 52v, 67; PC Charles of Blois, 124, 135, 164, for reports of the damage to the soles of his feet.

19 Roulandus Murtrarii, a *nuntius*, was accidentally blinded by his master Guy of Brittany (1287-1331; Charles's father-in-law and count of Penthièvre). After the accident, the grieving Guy gave him 15 denars a day as a pension or compensation. One of the witnesses related that after Guy's death, he was riding to the Chateau du Guingamp with Charles when they encountered Roulandus. Roulandus lamented to Charles that the officials did not let him enjoy the said 15 denars a day. Charles told Roulandus that he would set the matter right. Charles also gave Roulandus his gloves to take to a local almshouse. After rubbing his eyes with one of them, Roulandus got his sight back. Charles did not want the miracle to be made public because 'God made him [Roulandus] the grace, and not by his merits'. BAV, MS Vat. lat. 4025, fols. 168r-169v. See Cassard, 'Les coulisses de la sainteté?', 2, for this case as an example of the unequal relationship between a servant and a master. If read in such a manner, Charles's role as a miracle-maker was not just to give Roulandus his sight back but also to correct the ills of his father-in-law. The testimony of Baudetus de Folia recorded in BAV, MS Vat. lat. 4025, fol. 104v, narrates that Charles, riding with his father, encountered a blind pauper asking for alms. Charles gave him his glove and told him to take it to an almshouse situated in their lands and to tell them to give him alms. This blind person also rubbed his eyes with the glove and regained his sight. And similarly, Charles told him not to tell anyone about the incident. This kind of 'accidental' miracle *in vita*

his habit of wearing a hair shirt to be publicly known – which, incidentally, makes the number of witnesses claiming to have first-hand information about it appear rather odd. The pilgrimage to Tréguier and the resulting infirmity must have been a very public penitentiary performance. There clearly was an audience who may have been informed about the pilgrim in advance,[20] and who were ready to interpret it as a sign of saintly behaviour. As worded by Laura Ackerman Smoller, the incident is among those giving Charles 'a reputation of holiness, which, if he did not deliberately cultivate, he at least enjoyed'.[21] Walking barefoot on a pilgrimage was a common practice and a sign of the pilgrim's humility, but that Charles did this in harsh conditions, thus deliberately causing himself as much physical suffering as possible, and that he did it in such a visible manner, indeed indicates a public penance he imposed upon himself.[22] Although a member of the secular elite, Charles's actions here pretty much demonstrate what Robert Maniura has written about pilgrimages being a performance during which a person could 'be good at being Christian'.[23] In the framework of lived religion, this ritualistic act can be seen as a way for him to perform his gender as well as his status as a ruler responsible for his duchy, perhaps to do so in a very open manner that was not possible for him in everyday life. Considering that the distance between La Roche-Derrien and Tréguier is only approximately 6 kilometres, the harsh conditions served an important purpose in creating more labour and injury for the duke.[24]

caused by an item of clothing appears here and there in later medieval canonization hearings. For example, St. Bernardino of Siena's hearing contains the 'accidental' cure of a Spanish leper. Bernardino told the man to keep quiet and leave the area. PC Bernardino of Siena, 417, 500-1.

20 Cassard, 'Propagande partisane et miracles', 12. The performative aspect of pilgrimage has recently received growing attention from scholars. See Dubisch, *In a Different Place*; Maniura, *Pilgrimage to the Images in the Fifteenth Century*, esp. 90-94; Morrison, *Women Pilgrims in Late Medieval England*; Gemi-Iordanou et al. (eds.), *Medicine, Healing and Performance*. Pilgrims are known to have helped each other on the way, and pilgrims were also among those entitled to live by alms. See Webb, *Pilgrims and Pilgrimage in Medieval West*, 89. Such assistance from the masses was, however, a relatively singular phenomenon, undoubtedly available only to those who had special significance for their communities.

21 Smoller, *The Saint and the Chopped-Up Baby*, 27.

22 See Webb, *Pilgrimage in Medieval England*, xiv; Wittmer-Butsch and Rendtel, *Miracula: Wunderheilungen im Mittelalter*, 200, for the humility of pilgrims.

23 See Maniura, *Pilgrimage to the Images in the Fifteenth Century*, 90.

24 In all later medieval hagiography, some pilgrims reportedly travelled significant distances, even if in many cases the local shrine was the one most visited. See Katajala-Peltomaa, 'Devotional Strategies in Eveyday Life', 43, for comparisons between late medieval Sweden and Italy. In the French material, some pilgrims, especially in the miracle collection of St. Louis IX, travelled significant distances as well. See Farmer, *Surviving Poverty*.

Furthermore, the depositions of this spectacle and its corporeal consequences emphasize Charles's habit of venerating Breton saints, following a tradition established by past Breton rulers and legitimizing his own rule despite his non-Breton origins.[25] Susan S. Morrison has written that pilgrimage was an action during which the pilgrim could manipulate his or her audience and at the same time empower it into its own performance.[26] The significance of Charles's pilgrimage was accentuated by the common knowledge of the relatively long *infirmitas* it led to, which the witnesses emphasized by delineating its severity with common hagiographic tropes of the inability to stand on his own feet. For a duke caught up in a political crisis, rendering himself virtually immobile for three months might otherwise have been judged a dereliction of duty, as it prevented him from fulfilling his political and social role. The noble cause turned this temporary disability into a benefit, increasing his status among his subjects.

Saints' physical infirmity or 'inability' could give special glory to their other, more conventional deeds as well. During his lifetime, St. Nicholas of Tolentino was in constant interaction with his community members as a confessor and spiritual and religious role model. In his case we have more statements about his corporality from ordinary community members than is usual. Sari Katajala-Peltomaa pertinently asks if the typically more humble backgrounds of many southern European saints made them more easily approachable for the general laity, and therefore their relationship with the saint more intimate.[27] This difference is observable in the cases of some other living saints under scrutiny here, as Nicholas did not avoid giving his blessings or cures to those believing in his sanctity in the manner of Dauphine of Puimichel, nor did he seek to retreat from the world in the style of the more traditional hermit saints, even though he too often collaborated with his devotees on condition that his deeds would not be publicized before his death.[28]

Many, especially the lay witnesses, referred to the outer signs of Nicholas's infirmity when testifying to his general *memoria*, mostly by mentioning him celebrating the Mass – which was an important aspect of sainthood and the ability to do so an established form of clerical masculinity[29] – while supporting

25 Cassard, 'Propagande partisane et miracles', 10; Charles also venerated other Breton saints for the same purpose.

26 Morrison, *Women Pilgrims in Late Medieval England*, 5. See also Katajala-Peltomaa, 'Gender, Networks, and Collaboration', for various significances of pilgrimage.

27 Katajala-Peltomaa, 'Devotional Strategies in Everyday Life', 41.

28 PC Nicholas of Tolentino, 84; see also Kleinberg, *Prophets*, 43.

29 Cullum 'Feasting not fasting', 188; Vauchez, *Sainthood*, 240, 296.

himself with a cane.[30] Their way of constructing Nicholas's sanctity was, in addition to his thaumaturgic powers, based on the very grassroots-level encounters with him. A woman called Flordalisia specified that she had known Nicholas for thirty years, and that he continuously celebrated the Mass, and did so no matter how *confractus* he was.[31] Similarly, Mercatante Iohannis Adambi de Tholentino said that Nicholas was 'almost always' infirm but still said the Mass every morning.[32] However, apparently even saying the Mass was sometimes prevented by Nicholas's health issues, for Mancinus Fortis de Castro Sancti Angeli testified he did so provided he could walk.[33] The frequent references to Nicholas's infirmity underlined his attendance at Mass, essential for his social and religious role and gender. It is perhaps no surprise that these descriptions tend to come from the lay members of his community, even from the women who were not specifically interrogated about the *articuli* concerning his life but who testified only to Nicholas's *memoria*.[34] As a very common and human phenomenon, his ailing health was something they could easily relate to while giving specific emphasis to his attendance at Mass.

Great importance was also given to Nicholas's infirmity in a miracle account reported by three members of the Appillaterre family: the notary Berardus and his two daughters Berardescha and Ceccha. As a toddler, Ceccha had a swelling in her throat, which the doctors wanted to treat with incisions. Nicholas was severely ill himself, but he sensed Ceccha's mother Margarita's anguish and sorrow, and sent some other brothers to console her. She told them that she feared the operation and the scarring of the girl's throat, which would be a great shame for her.[35] When the other friars

30 PC Nicholas of Tolentino, 209, 219, 248, 272, 273-74.

31 PC Nicholas of Tolentino, 523. *Confractus* is a relatively rare term in medieval hagiography; most often it refers to broken bones, or it is sometimes used as a synonym for *contractus*, which is best translated as 'crippled' or 'lame', sometimes also referring to curvature of the spine. Presumably Flordalisia was referring to the aggravation of Nicholas's infirmity in general here, but the choice of word (at least by the notary) implies some connection with the walking difficulties, or even 'physical impairment' in the modern sense of the word.

32 PC Nicholas of Tolentino, 213: 'quod per dictum tempus, quo cognovit eum, vidit eum quasi communiter infirmum et non dimittebat propterea qui incontinue omni mane diceret missam.' See also the deposition of *domina* Alixa (219), who stated that Nicholas did not fail to say the Mass even when he was infirm.

33 PC Nicholas of Tolentino, 251; see also 399, 409-10.

34 Only one woman, *domina* Angelischa, was interrogated about the *articuli*, although there were many others who had known the saint personally. Angelischa had the reputation of being a 'holy woman' herself, which undoubtedly explains her assumed 'reliability'. Katajala-Peltomaa, *Gender, Miracles, and Daily Life*, 33-36.

35 Such sentiments towards impaired or ill children or people are rare in canonization processes, but when shame or other such notions were recorded, they most often pertained to disfiguring

returned to Nicholas, he told them: 'Go back to her and tell her for me that if I could go to her I would do it willingly; but she knows well that I cannot walk, I am infirm. She should come to me and bring Ceccha, said daughter of hers, and she must not let her be touched by any iron.'[36] Margarita did as instructed, and took her daughter to Nicholas accompanied by a servant. Nicholas told them to visit the shrine of St. Blaise, a known healer of throats,[37] and after the visit, the girl was cured.

The testimonies about this miracle emphasize Nicholas's prophetic abilities and the importance of Margarita as one of his devotees; in addition to Ceccha's case, Nicholas also knew that something was wrong in the case of the family's stillborn child.[38] It is noteworthy concerning the current discussion that Nicholas told the other brothers that Margarita should know that he could not walk because he was *infirmus*, and that Berardus and the two daughters mentioned this in their testimonies. These reports also underlined their status as special devotees of Nicholas. Margarita Appillaterre reportedly had the habit of sending Nicholas food when he was

conditions and sometimes to deafness or blindness, or the inability to earn one's bread due to a physical condition. On facial disfigurement and miracles, see Finucane, *The Rescue of the Innocents*, 59; Kuuliala, *Childhood Disability*, 115-16; Kuuliala, 'Love and Duty in the Time of Family Crisis'; on facial disfigurement and the society, see Skinner, *Living with Disfigurement in Early Medieval Europe*.

36 PC Nicholas of Tolentino, 236: 'Redite ad eam et dicatis ei ex parte mea quod si possem venire ad eam libenter venire; sed bene scit ipsa quod ego non possum ambulare, ita sum infirmus: veniat ipsa ad me et portet dictam Ceccham filiam suam, et non faciat eam tangi cum ferro'. See also PC Nicholas of Tolentino, 126: 'Redite ad eam et dicatis ex parte mea: quod si possem venire ad eam, libenter venirem, sed bene scit ipsa quod ego non possum ambulare ita sum infirmus, veniat ipsa ad me et portet dictam Ceccham filiam suam et non faciat eam tangi cum ferro aliquo.'

37 Saints who specialized in curing specific illnesses sometimes appear in canonization documents. St. Blasius (or St. Blaise) was, for example, popular in the area. Katajala-Peltomaa, *Gender, Miracles, and Daily Life*, 125. As another example, many of the people with ailing feet and legs evidently cured by the merits of St. Louis IX of France first sought help from St. Eloy, a known healer of legs. Guillaume de Saint-Pathus, *Les miracles de saint Louis*, 47, 100, 138, 143, 174. The belief in the powers of St. Eloy in such maladies was so great that Henri de Mondeville, the French surgeon, lamented it; Macdougall, 'The Surgeon and the Saints'. However, as pointed out by Bartlett, *Why Can the Dead Do Such Great Things?*, 353, although such examples are frequently recorded in modern dictionaries and encyclopedias, it 'was by no means a general or defining feature of the cult of the saints'.

38 PC Nicholas of Tolentino, 13; for the case of the stillborn child, see 128. The miracle also relates to Nicholas's triumph over the devil, since he had a vision in which the devil tried to steal the child. A parallel case concerning a saint's prophetic abilities in a case of an infirm devotee is recorded in Dauphine of Puimichel's process, in which *dominus* Raymundus de Agouto was suffering from the infirmity, which finally killed him. Although there was no certainty about his approaching death, Dauphine reportedly foresaw it. See PC Dauphine of Puimichel, 58-69, 253-54.

ill. Thus the state of his health was well-known to the family, with whom he was in frequent interaction, and as the family was also reported to have been of a high social standing and among those who spread Nicholas's *fama*, their knowledge was presumably shared by the other members of the community. The saint himself appears to have put some emphasis on his own infirmity here, with certain expectations of how his devotees should react to it. This is the only case where he reportedly recognized his situation as preventing him from doing something.

Similarly, Nicholas's infirmity at the time of a miracle was recorded in the depositions of Philippa and Ceccha Ugolini. They said that about a year before Nicholas's death, their father Hugolinus had been severely *infirmus*, apparently suffering from some form of paralysis as he could not use the left side of his body or open his left eye. After hearing about Nicholas's *fama*, Hugolinus sent his family and servants to fetch Nicholas to visit him. The two daughters testified that Nicholas himself was so infirm that he could not walk without a cane and without the help of his companions, who, in this case, enabled his acting as a living saint.[39] Despite his own infirmity, Nicholas arrived with the help of his companions, made the sign of the cross on Hugolinus and blessed him – after which he was healed.[40]

The records state that Philippa Ugolini was more than 26 and Ceccha Ugolini 26 years old when giving their witness accounts, which would make them between 5 and 7 years old at the time of the miracle. Both stated that they were present when their father sent for Nicholas, and also when he arrived and the miracle occurred.[41] The similarity of the Ugolini girls' narrations shows how reminiscing about the events within the family had shaped their views.[42] Nicholas's own ill health and walking problems were an important part of this memory. Among all the things that were significant for the two families in their interaction with the saint, repeated in the later recollections, his infirmity was one of the features whose memory they kept alive, merging it with his other saintly features, in this case especially his willingness to help his devotees and his miraculous powers.

39 The same can be said about the reports of St. Yves of Tréguier's final days and his companions helping him still celebrate the Mass. See note 58 (p. 151) below.

40 PC Nicholas of Tolentino, 272-74.

41 See Katajala-Peltomaa, *Gender, Miracles, and Daily Life*, 125, for the similarities between the testimonies to these miracles. According to her, any copying is highly improbable due to the regulations of canon law. On the importance of similarities in the depositions for proving a case, see also Goodich, *Miracles and Wonders*, 81-82; Goodich, 'Miseries of Dulcia and Cristina', 107.

42 On reminiscing about miraculous events within a family, see Katajala-Peltomaa, *Gender, Miracles, and Daily Life*, 262-67, 271-74.

There are, however, differences in how big a role Nicholas's infirmity played in the witnesses' minds when reporting the miracles *in vita* during his last years. There are instances when the testimony gives no information about whether the saint had any infirmity; such a case is the miraculous cure of Berardus Appillaterre himself from a recurring fever by Nicholas's touch. Berardus did not remember the exact time of the cure, but it must have been some time before Nicholas's death because the saint was still able to come to visit him.[43] Pucius Iohannis, on the other hand, testified about his tertian fever, of which he was cured about a year before Nicholas's death. He went to see the holy man with his father, and they found him in his cell, where he lay 'gravely infirm' ('fortiter infirmus').[44] Here the saint's infirmity was a way of reconstructing the time frame and the location. *Frater* Iohannucius de Tholentino also reported the miraculous cure of Dunzella, the wife of *magister* Iohannis Salvastie, who had *fluxum sanguinis*. Dunzella begged Iohannucius to take her to Nicholas, which he did, and, as usual, Nicholas's touch and benedictions cured her. In this testimony Nicholas's own infirmity only comes up when the commissioners asked Iohannucius about the time and place of the miracle. He said it occurred ten to twelve days before Nicholas died, in the *cella* where the friar lay infirm.[45] Unfortunately, we do not have Dunzella's own testimony about the matter, so we have no idea whether she put more emphasis on the saint's illness. Possibly this aspect of the miracle was not important for Iohannucius because it was not *his* miraculous cure, and since he was Nicholas's *infirmarius* the saint's infirmity must have been something he was used to at that point.[46] The saint's declining health during his last years is emphasized in the miracle testimonies primarily because a majority of the investigated miracles *in vita* occurred towards the end of his life. His activities despite the increasing infirmity helped to reinforce his *fama*.

As for the other saints known to have been infirm for a long period, their bodily ailments do not, rather surprisingly, come across in the witness accounts about their miracles *in vita*. For example, Dauphine of Puimichel's process includes a significant number of miracles done during her life.[47]

43 PC Nicholas of Tolentino, 122-23.

44 PC Nicholas of Tolentino, 228.

45 PC Nicholas of Tolentino, 486.

46 See PC Nicholas of Tolentino, 478, 481.

47 This was an important part of her *fama*, as testified, for example, by Philippe de Cabassole, the bishop of Cavaillon, who could provide an impressive list of names of those who had spread it, starting from King Robert of Naples and his wife Sancha. The bishop testified that God enacted many miracles through Dauphine's prayers, and after her death through her merits. After he

However, if we compare Dauphine's activities in her community, and how her infirmity is treated in the testimonies, with the process of Nicholas of Tolentino, the difference is striking. While in Nicholas's case several witnesses emphasized his infirmity and mentioned it when talking about his appearance among them and his humility, in Dauphine's hearing this aspect is much more subdued, although it was often investigated under the articles about her *vita*. This is an intriguing difference especially considering the tendency to highlight female saints' physical suffering. It is of course possible that her infirmity was less visible, at least at times, than Nicholas of Tolentino's, and it apparently started to incapacitate her seriously only during her last years. However, there are miracles *in vita* occurring around the same time as the settling of the quarrel in 1348, when Dauphine was reportedly too incapacitated to walk any distance or ride a horse.[48] Even in these cases the saint's own infirmity is not referred to, although she was occasionally reported to have visited the sick in person.[49]

That the only activity of Dauphine's where her bodily infirmity had specific importance for the witnesses was the settling of the quarrel is curious, especially because the witnesses saw her walking around asking for alms. This must have made her a very visible figure in the community, but in their testimonies they did not connect it with her infirmity,[50] except for the reference to the beggars complaining about her begging and big stomach mentioned earlier.[51] Otherwise the witnesses referring to her begging and self-humbling only reported the ridicule she faced when people called her

listed where this was being said, the commissioners inquired when he heard it. He replied that he had heard it being said for nearly fifty years that God had done many miracles in her lifetime. He similarly stated that he heard that God performed many miracles after Dauphine's death for her merits. PC Dauphine of Puimichel, 531-32.

48 See p. 78 above.

49 See e.g. PC Dauphine of Puimichel, 281-82, 510-12, for cures of people ill with the plague or otherwise ill at that time. For an analysis of these cures, see Archambeau, 'Healing Options during the Plague', 545-47. See also PC Dauphine of Puimichel, 294, for the testimony of Aycardus Boti, a cleric, who was cured of fever in 1347 by Dauphine's visit. He had not made a vow, but stated that the cure had occurred because of the joy and consolation of the saint's visit. Similarly, *nobilis et egregius vir* Guillelmus Henrici reported his own conversations with Dauphine and how the saint baptized his long-wished-for son in 1350, again with no references to the saint's old age or infirmity, and Dauphine's former vassal Bartholomea Marcella's cure of leprosy in 1357. PC Dauphine of Puimichel, 72-73, 309, 366-67, 453-54, 455-46. See also Archambeau, 'God Helps Those Who Help Themselves', 19-21, for an analysis of Bartholomea Marcella's case.

50 PC Dauphine of Puimichel, 432, 533, 537. As a point of comparison, one of the witnesses in Nicholas's hearing specified that he did not go begging often because he was so gravely infirm. PC Nicholas of Tolentino, 265.

51 PC Dauphine of Puimichel, 438. See also pp. 83-84 above.

a beguine or a *bizoca*.[52] This was related to the general mockery this type of religious woman faced, in northern Europe as beguines and in Italy as *pinzochere*.[53] Although the criticism penitent women faced makes this a gendered phenomenon,[54] in the hagiographic context a similar kind of ridicule could be used to construct male sanctity.[55] In Dauphine's case it was a more powerful tool to reconstruct her humility than her infirmities would have been.

The lack of references to infirmity is one facet of the testimonies about Dauphine's begging which suggests that infirmity did not have value to sainthood per se but only in certain contexts. For those ridiculing Dauphine's begging activities who came from the higher end of the social hierarchy, her swollenness (known by many to be caused by dropsy) or other infirmities did not serve a purpose, as the reason for their scorn was precisely her situation as a beggar. However, the beggars, whose voice is only heard through the testimony of Alasacia de Mesellano, a draper's widow from Apt, obviously saw the situation in a different light. Throughout the medieval period there was an ongoing discussion of voluntary and involuntary begging, as well as on the entitlement to beg.[56] For some beggars of the area Dauphine must have been a competitor, perhaps seen as using her status as a way to get a bigger

52 PC Dauphine of Puimichel, 223, 326-28, 395.

53 Such derision reflects the tensions in society about living a religious life within the community instead of inside the closed walls of a monastery. Furthermore, religious women choosing such a lifestyle took over many activities previously reserved for men, such as cloth-making or teaching, thus becoming their competitors. Miller, *The Beguines of Medieval Paris*, 21-22, 80-86, 126. For the situation in the south, see Lehmijoki-Gardner, 'Laywomen, Religious', 462-64, who also writes that the criticism and suspicion towards religious women in Italy is probably one reason why only one of them, St. Catherine of Siena, ended up being canonized. On the satirical literature about beguines and other religious women, see Deichmann, *Wayward Nuns in Medieval Literature*. The Council of Vienne (1311-12) famously forbade the beguine lifestyle, although it was not intended to forbid women from living a life of penance serving God. Simons, *Cities of Ladies*, 133.

54 This kind of attitude was also reported in the case of St. Elizabeth of Hungary. One of her handmaids testified that other people called her 'insane' (*insana*) after her decision to give away her possessions and start her religious life. Appropriately, she tolerated this with patience. PC Elizabeth of Hungary, 125.

55 Guillaume de Saint-Pathus's *Vie de saint Louis*, 118, for example, records a case where a woman called it a great shame that someone like Louis, dressed in his humble garments, was a king. As befitting his saintly nature, Louis was thankful for the criticism and derision. As pointed out by Miller, *Beguines of Medieval Paris*, 32-33, although the narration of Louis's piety is constructed with a hagiographic approach, it is clear that he had a reputation as a man who strongly expressed his piety already in his lifetime. Louis also supported the beguinage movement.

56 Scholarship on this topic is immense. See e.g. Farmer, *Surviving Poverty*, 44-50, 60-70; Geremek, *The Margins of Society*, 31-35; Metzler, *A Social History of Disability*, 154-98; Rubin, *Charity and Community*, 54-65.

share of the alms.[57] Since they appear to have lacked information about her health, they read the bodily signs as evidence of wealth instead of illness.

Although this book's focus is not on the death of a saint, the role of community members in defining a holy person's illness as fatal is a visible aspect of interaction and infirmity as well, especially since a saint's death was an essential part of their *fama publica*. The records of St. Yves of Tréguier's canonization hearing from the summer of 1330 include lengthy testimonies about his life, but they mainly focus on his ascetic habits and benevolence towards the poor. As mentioned above, references to any bodily ailments are mostly missing, except when recording the last days of his life.[58] The reports of the saintly priest's last days illustrate well the problem in reconstructing community members' interpretations from a later narrative. Guillelmus Petri, the perpetual vicar of the church of Tréguier, reported Yves's habit of using a hair shirt. The commissioners asked how Guillelmus knew about this; to which he replied that a certain lord of the witness, an *officialis* named Yvo Casini, visited Yves once when he had a 'certain infirmity' ('in quadam infirmitate') in his manor in Kermartin. Yvo Casini placed his hand on Yves's breast, 'as is the habit to touch the infirm', and then the witness saw the hair shirt.[59] Yvo Casini's and Guillelmus Petri's situation as clerics of high rank obviously had an impact on their touching the saint,[60] but other community members visited him at that time too. A man called Darianus de Bouaysalio testified that he visited Yves on the Friday before his death, which occurred on the following Sunday. Darianus reported seeing Yves's modest bed and 'cheap, black, and miserable mattress', and that he said to the holy man: 'Lord, will you not be healed, as your people say?' Yves responded: 'God knows.'[61]

While Guillelmus Petri's statement was intended to prove Yves's humility and abstinence, Darianus de Bouaysalio was asked if he was present at

57 See Geremek, *The Margins of Society*, 193, 206-7, on possible rules among beggars and their mobility.

58 One servant of Yves testified that he celebrated Mass every day unless debilitated by infirmity or impediment, but he may as well have referred to the saint's final days. The same servant testified that in the week when Yves died, he celebrated Mass with great devotion despite his great infirmity. PC Yves of Tréguier, 39-40.

59 PC Yves of Tréguier, 53: 'et tunc idem dominus officialis posuit manum supra pectus dicti domini Yvonis, sicut moris est palpare infirmos; et tunc dictus testis vidit per capsiliam dictum cilicium quod deferebat juxta carnem idem dominus Yvo.'

60 On *officialis*, see Smith, 'The *Officialis* of the Bishop in Twelfth- and Thirteenth-Century England'.

61 PC Yves of Tréguier, 110: 'et cum ipse qui loquitur dixisset sibi: "Domine, vos non estis curatus, sicut dicebant gentes vestre?" Tunc ipse respondit: "Deus scit et novit."'

Yves's death, which is why he recounted his last encounter with the saint during his fatal illness, although his testimony underlined his penitentiary lifestyle as well. The third witness who mentioned an encounter with the ailing saint was Sibilla de Gressilh. She was pregnant with twins when she heard that Yves, her confessor, was ill, and decided to walk to Kermartin to make a confession.[62] She found him in his chapel, celebrating the Mass, and so infirm that he could hardly stand on his own feet, being supported by two other men.[63] When Yves was taking off his sacerdotal clothes, he asked Sibilla what she wanted. She responded: 'Lord, I hear that you are infirm, and I want to confess to you.' Yves then sat down, heard her confession, and on the next Sunday he died.[64]

Saints' acceptance of their death and/or the ability to foresee it is a known hagiographic trope.[65] Though the testimonies refer to Yves's illness only when reporting his death or his approaching death, it is unclear whether the devotees themselves were aware of the fatality of the condition. In some cases the testimonies about the saint's final illness also show how the fatality of a condition, even in the case of holy men and women, was communally negotiated, and that physicians often played an important role in this process.[66] The fatal illness also looms large in the case of St. Louis of Toulouse (1274-97), the cadet of the royal house of Anjou who was made

62 Although the Fourth Lateran Council of 1215 ordered that laypeople had to confess once a year, pregnant women commonly sought confession more often. Due to the dangers of childbirth, they were also encouraged to take the Eucharist. Barr, *The Pastoral Care of Women*, 81-83; Taylor, *The Culture of Confession*, 57-58.

63 Yves celebrating Mass with the help of his associates was also reported by two other female witnesses, a mother and a daughter; paupers who had resided in Yves's household for eleven years. PC Yves of Tréguier, 98, 101.

64 PC Yves of Tréguier, 121-22: 'et erat adeo debilis et infirmus, quod vix se poterat sustinere; ymo abbas Belli Portus et dominus Alanus Le Bruec, archidiaconus Trecorensis, sustinebant eum. Et quando dictus dominus Yvo fuit exutus dixit testi loquenti: "Domina, quid vultis?" Et ipsa sibi repondens, dixit: "Domine, audivi dici quod eratis infirmus, et voleam confiteri vobis." Et tunc predictus dominus Yvo assedit se, et audivit confessionem ipsius testis; et die dominica sequenti bene mane, decessit, ut audivit dici.'

65 See Goodich, 'The Death of a Saint', 229, 233. For earlier examples, see Crislip, *Thorns in the Flesh*, esp. 129-30. For signs of death in miracles, see Nissi, 'Quomodo Scit Quod Mortuus Erat?'

66 This was not always the case, however. Thomas Aquinas's sanctity was primarily constructed by other means than corporality or suffering, but many of the witnesses in the Naples hearing reported his final days. Already ill, when residing at his sister's castle in Maenza, he told the fellow brothers that he should be transferred to a religious house. They took him to Fossanova, where he lay ill for some time (according to one witness for a month, according to another one for several days) before dying on 7 March 1274. No physicians are mentioned in the witness accounts. Thomas had a strong reputation as a saint among the other monks, which may explain this. PC Thomas Aquinas, 276-77, 378-79. See also Räsänen, *Thomas Aquinas's Relics*, esp. 30-34, on the

a bishop at a young age. The testimonies about Louis's *vita* included in the canonization inquest, conducted in the church of Notre Dame de Marseille in 1308, appropriately record his patience during his fatal fever, which lasted for two weeks.[67] The article and the corresponding witness statements record that he was in the care of physicians who believed that they had managed to cure him, but Louis himself foretold that they had not.[68] Similar situations were mentioned in the articles and witness depositions in other inquests as well. The articles in Clare of Montefalco's process record that during her final illness, a physician told her brother Franciscus that she was cured, and she also appeared like 'another healthy woman' to the brethren and nuns who were present. Clare herself, however, confessed her sins, stated that she was going to God, and died without any pain or other symptoms typical of dying.[69] Franciscus testified how Clare had told him to go back to his own monastery, and how on the following day, he had encountered the physician, who said that she was completely 'freed' ('liberata'), except from her raptures. Franciscus's testimony is exceptionally descriptive when it comes to his own emotions, as he refers to his own sorrow and tears several times.[70] This gives us a rare glimpse into the witness's own emotions in the narratives concerned with saints' infirmities and their personal significance to those close to them.

As they did in these saints' everyday lives, the various household and community members also paid close attention to their bodily symptoms and reactions just before their death. Especially the lack of pain when dying was a concept that had existed since the time of martyrs and their violent, gruesome deaths, and it was kept alive by medieval hagiographers.[71]

importance of Thomas's wish to stay in Fossanova forever and for the later disputes concerning the ownership of his relics.

67 For Louis's canonization process and cult, see Goodich, *Miracles and Wonders*, 52-54, and Toynbee, *S. Louis of Toulouse and the Process of Canonisation*, 146-232.

68 PC Louis of Toulouse, 49, 58, 70, 105.

69 PC Clare of Montefalco, 24-25. The statement about her apparent good health is clear: 'et stabat ipsa sancta Clara sedendo recta et pulcro colore et cum bona dispositione membrorum et loquebatur firma voce sicut aliqua mulier sana posset stare et loqui, et videbatur quod nullam infirmitatem haberet'. The description of Clare's death in Bérenger's *vita* is very similar to that in the articles; *Vita sanctae Clarae de Cruce*, ed. Semenza, 55-58.

70 PC Clare of Montefalco, 291-93. According to Sister Iohanna, it was Franciscus who declared to all bystanders that Clare was freed from her illness. PC Clare of Montefalco, 83.

71 Pincikowski, *Bodies of Pain*, 15; he also points out that this idea conflicted with that of *imitatio Christi*, and how with its rise the notion of impassability of pain had to fade, coming to only pertain to saints in heaven. In canonization testimonies, the saints are indeed portrayed as suffering, but the moment of death was one occasion in which the pain that might normally be suffered was absent.

The idea was clearly internalized by witnesses to canonization inquests, who reported not just lack of pain but lack of any symptoms. There are depositions regarding St. Elizabeth of Hungary and St. Yves of Tréguier stating that they did not appear to have any infirmity at the time of death,[72] and Catherine of Vadestena testified that just before she died St. Birgitta instructed her son Birger, her confessors, and Catherine 'as if she was not infirm' ('quasi non esset infirma').[73] Due to the importance of the lack of symptoms for a saintly death, the topic interested the commissioners of Clare of Montefalco's hearing. They asked Sister Marina how she knew there were no symptoms, to which she replied that Clare did not lament nor were there any other signs.[74] As written by Esther Cohen, 'norms of behaviour dictated not only the actions of people in pain but also how those actions were interpreted in subsequent recording'.[75] Marina – and probably the other bystanders – thus interpreted Clare's lack of lamenting as well as the other signs through the lens of a saintly death. It is possible that there was some disagreement regarding the completeness of Clare's cure among the witnesses to her final days, as Sister Francescha said that a couple of days before her death she saw her looking 'a lot better' ('multumullioratam'),[76] rather than stating explicitly that she was healthy. Then again, it is probably unsafe to make any judgement on the basis of nuances in verbal expression as recorded by a notary.

Although many community members encountered saints in their final illness, physicians were the ones whose verdicts gave scientific grounds for the lack of pain and for the acceptance of death. This is also interlinked with the treatments they provided. In St. Peter of Luxembourg's hearing, the seventy-ninth article and some corresponding depositions state that when he was infirm, he was taken, as the physicians had instructed, from Avignon to Villeneuve-lès-Avignon to get better air.[77] The seventy-ninth article, describing the moment of his death, states that it made the physicians desperate, especially 'an Italian one' who had promised to cure him.[78] This physician was, apparently, Blasius de Fortino, who testified in the hearing.

72 PC Elizabeth of Hungary, 139; PC Yves of Tréguier, 53.

73 See Catherine's testimony, PC Birgitta of Sweden, 319.

74 PC Clare of Montefalco, 149.

75 Cohen, *The Modulated Scream*, 114.

76 PC Clare of Montefalco, 338.

77 'Processus de vita & miraculis b. Petri de Luxemburgo', *AASS*, Iul. I, 557, 560.

78 'Processus de vita & miraculis b. Petri de Luxemburgo', *AASS*, Iul. I, 557: 'medicis tunc desperantibus de ipsius vita, & maxime medico Italico, qui ante speraverat, imo promiserat ipsum curare.'

In his own statement he claimed that he had not promised to cure Peter.[79] Joseph Ziegler reasonably points out that he must have known the basic rule of a doctor-patient relationship, namely that the physician must not promise too much.[80] The repeated narratives of physicians promising a cure to a fatally ill holy person appear in a rather singular light from this perspective. Healing depended on many factors, and a physician's failure to cure a patient did not mean a lack of expertise. Above all, God's will, the surroundings and the patients' behaviour determined whether a physician's treatment was a success or not.[81] For saints, death was a beginning of a new life, which gives one explanation for this apparent contradiction.

A physician's attendance at the holy person's deathbed allowed the saint to demonstrate his or her prophetic abilities. The problem, however, in analysing the narratives about saints' final illnesses from the viewpoint of communal 'diagnosis' is that a saint's death was such an important and well-established *topos*. Even if there was great uncertainty about the fatal nature of these conditions, they were necessarily interpreted as such retrospectively. Nevertheless, these depositions show the community's concern for the well-being of the holy person and how information about their infirmities was spread among the devotees, in monastic and lay communities. Furthermore, especially Sibylla de Gressilh's deposition demonstrates how this information influenced the devotees and their own spiritual and even corporeal well-being.

The Saint as a Medical Practitioner

Saints' charity towards those in need, including the infirm, was one of the most important factors in their lives, and their visits to the *infirmi* were related over and over again in *vitae* and canonization testimonies. The origin of such charitable acts lies in the biblical acts of mercy, and in Christ's vision of the Last Judgement, where obligation to visit the sick was among the good works required to receive salvation.[82] Furthermore, the

79 'Processus de vita & miraculis b. Petri de Luxemburgo', *AASS*, Iul. I, 561-62.

80 Ziegler, 'Practitioners and Saints', 217. See Pomata, *Contracting a Cure*, for the doctor-patient relationship in late medieval and Renaissance Italy.

81 See e.g. Siraisi, *Medieval and Early Renaissance Medicine*, 42.

82 Matthew 25:36: 'Infirmus fui et visitatis me' ('I was sick and you visited me'). This paragraph also became a guideline for medieval monastic rules, in which visiting the infirm and taking care of them in the name of Christ was an essential aspect of monastic life. See Vogüé, *La règle de Saint Benoît VI*, 1080-81.

developments of the early thirteenth century and the rise of Franciscan ideals placed charitable actions at the core of sanctity, and both clerical or monastic and lay saints performed their sanctity by taking care of the sick.[83] As pointed out by André Vauchez, especially the canonizations of St. Elizabeth of Hungary and her aunt St. Hedwig of Silesia (1231 and 1267, respectively) show that such acts were approved by the Roman Church.[84] Narrations about saints' encounters with the infirm reiterate their humility and patience and their lack of abhorrence towards even the most hideous physical conditions.[85] Witness depositions related to these topics only rarely touch upon the saint's own infirmities or corporality, but they are essential to the current discussion, both because they depict one of the ways in which suffering and the body functioned as a means for the manifestation of the holy and because the testimonies occasionally parallel the infirm body of a saint with those of their patients. In the narrations about saints taking care of the sick and infirm, the divine and the medical intermingle, providing one window onto the medical pluralism of the period.[86] Reports of saints' attitudes towards earthly medicine tend to follow a pattern – that is, they were keener on administering medicine to others than themselves, and many canonization testimonies portray living saints medicating their infirm community members.

Regarding the ways that infirm bodies were portrayed in the hearings, there is a striking difference in the emphasis witnesses gave to them. St. Elizabeth of Hungary is one of the most famous saints whose holiness was largely constructed by caring for others.[87] After the death of her husband, she used her whole fortune to found a leper house in Marburg, and even before this, her handmaids' statements underline her charitable activity

83 The ideals of the Mendicant Orders also had more far-reaching effects on the concepts of charity as well as voluntary and involuntary poverty. For this discussion, see Buhrer, 'From *Caritas* to Charity'; Farmer, *Surviving Poverty*, 60-70; Geremek, *The Margins of Society*, 32, 192-201; Mollat, *The Poor in the Middle Ages*; Rubin, *Charity and Community*, 54-65.

84 Vauchez, *Sainthood*, 376.

85 See Goodich, *Vita perfecta*, 186-205; Rawcliffe, *Leprosy in Medieval England*, 131-43; Vauchez, 'Lay People's Sanctity', 21-32.

86 The concept 'medical pluralism' includes the idea that there was no clear dichotomy between 'orthodox' and 'unorthodox' healing methods. Rather, a patient could choose from a wide array of healing options including mundane and religious/spiritual healing. See Gentilcore, *Healers and Healing*, for this concept in early modern Italy. Medical pluralism has been extensively analysed in Jütte (ed.), *Medical Pluralism*.

87 Such narrations are closely connected with her later *fama sanctitas*; she is portrayed as the carer for of lepers, and a majority of the miracles recorded in her canonization process concern cures of children. Wolf, ed. and trans., *The Life and Afterlife of St. Elizabeth*, 48; Demaitre, *Leprosy in Premodern Medicine*, 247; Klaniczay, 'Proving Sanctity', 134.

and how she took care of her patients at home. While their depositions regarding Elizabeth's infirmities are very brief, their statements are most detailed and even graphic in their descriptions of the bodies of her patients. Ysentrudis, for example, reported her visit to a hospital whose patients were abhorred by other people, but where Elizabeth happily cleaned their faces of the spittle and filth from their mouths and nostrils with her veil.[88] Similar emphasis on the gruesome details of infirmity appears in the hearing of St. Margaret of Hungary, who in her nunnery cleaned latrines and removed vomit, even catching it in her bare hands,[89] as well as in the hearing of St. Clare of Montefalco. Although she was largely associated with her own *imitatio Christi*, Clare's bodily symptoms were, as discussed above, described only in vague terms, whereas in the same testimonies the infirmities of the sick nuns she cared for are described far more explicitly. Sister Marina, for example, testified that a certain *domina* Vannola residing in their monastery had a horrid infirmity, a fever that caused her to emit foam from her mouth, but Clare treated her with compassion and humility.[90]

Despite the tropelike nature of these descriptions, they form an illuminating contrast to the descriptions of the saints' own corporality and even to the conditions they miraculously cured, which were very rarely described as causing repellence.[91] Leprosy, as an illness with very particular cultural connotations, is the most common infirmity connected with saints' charity towards the sick. However, other infirmities – or 'infirmity' in general – served the same purpose. The tendency to highlight the symptoms of the recipients of these saints' charity is a universal hagiographic phenomenon; although the level of emphasis varies,[92] the repugnant character of the

88 PC Elizabeth of Hungary, 119-21. Another servant, Elizabeth, reported that the holy woman took, among others, a one-eyed boy with *scabies* to her house, taking him to her bed; PC Elizabeth of Hungary, 128.

89 PC Margaret of Hungary, 144-45, 236-37. Undertaking such filthy tasks can also be read as Margaret's way of consciously counteracting the hedonistic court culture of her time. At the same time, it gave her special power as someone to imitate and to receive God's love. Klaniczay, *The Uses of Supernatural Power*, 104-5. The contradiction appears in some of the testimonies. One of the sisters testified that Margaret's family 'loved her very much', and Margaret herself wished she were the daughter of a poor man so that she could better serve God. PC Margaret of Hungary, 400-1.

90 PC Clare of Montefalco, 110.

91 Kuuliala, *Childhood Disability*, 71-81, 175-83.

92 Although St. Birgitta's process includes reports her taking care of the sick with her own hands, their symptoms are not highlighted in a manner similar to the hearings of Saints Elizabeth, Margaret, or Clare of Montefalco. See e.g. PC Birgitta of Sweden, 316. This accords with the subdued role corporality and infirmity have in the testimonies about her life.

patients' illnesses made the holiness of the saints shine all the more brightly.[93] The witnesses reporting these instances thus used sentiments, or expected sentiments, to highlight a very crucial aspect of sainthood. St. Elizabeth is exceptional among mendicant female saints in that although her *vita* shares a strong focus on tending the sick, which is largely in accordance with the ideas of Franciscan spirituality, it does not place the same importance on self-mortification and other types of infirmities.[94] In the depositions of Elizabeth's handmaids the suffering and even revolting bodies of others epitomized her patience, but not her own physical suffering.[95]

The same goes for Margaret of Hungary, in whose case the witnesses portrayed charity as the most extreme manifestation of humility, austerity, and penitence. This is highlighted in her confessor Marcellus's attempt to limit her charity. Marcellus testified that 'the more serious and contagious their ailments were, the more attentively she served them', which highlights her martyrlike attitude towards the task. He also referred to his fear that she would herself become ill.[96] Two of the nuns testified about the level of Margaret's self-sacrifice by mentioning her wish to carry on her tasks even when she herself was infirm; this is one of the few places where any long-term ailment of the saint was recorded in the process.[97] The testimonies in St. Clare of Montefalco's inquest do the same by emphasizing her own suffering

93 Rawcliffe, *Leprosy in Medieval England*, 133. See also Goodich, *Vita perfecta*, 186-205; Peyroux, 'The Leper's Kiss'; Touati, *Maladie et société*, 203-5; Vauchez, 'Lay People's Sanctity', 21-32.

94 See Vauchez, *Sainthood*, 340, 342, 350.

95 PC Elizabeth of Hungary, 119-21.

96 PC Margaret of Hungary, 440-43: 'Cum magna humilitate et devotione serviebat sororibus infirmis, et quanto graviores erat infirmitates et magis contagiose, tanto diligentius serviebat eis'. Similar fears were recorded in Catherine of Vadstena's and Bishop Alphonsus's depositions in St. Birgitta's canonization inquiry. According to them, Birgitta took Catherine to take care of the infirm so that both could console and tend their wounds with their own hands. Some people told her that she should not do such a thing to a young girl. Birgitta replied that because they were serving God, there would be no danger of infection. PC Birgitta of Sweden, 315, 374. Catherine's own canonization process also records her visiting the infirm and the poor and not being repelled by their condition. PC Catherine of Vadstena, 28, 43.

97 One of the nuns reported an incident where Margaret had been infirm for forty days, and fearing that the prioress would send her to the infirmary if she found out about it, did not tell her about the illness. The witness was asked how she knew about this, and replied that she was the only one in whom Margaret had confided. Interestingly, here the commissioners inquired after the type of the infirmity, perhaps searching for more credibility in the testimony. The witness told them that the infirmity was *fluxus ventri*. PC Margaret of Hungary, 354-55. Sister Candida testified how Margaret took care of other sick nuns even though she was not well herself; PC Margaret of Hungary, 392-95. The above incident also found its way into Margaret's *vita* based on the canonization documents by Garin de Guy-l'Evêque, written in 1340; 'Vita, Margarita Hungarica, virgo ordinis praedicat (b.)', *AASS*, Ian. II, 902. The *vita* similarly records her fasting

as a consequence of helping the infirm sisters in her monastery. The twenty-third article and the corresponding depositions report that she suffered from their infirmities more than the infirm sisters themselves, comparing her caring with her *imitatio Christi*. This creates a curious sickroom dynamic, in which suffering appears to have an agency of its own, moving from one victim to another but giving their experiences entirely different meanings.[98]

In many *vitae* women saints are associated with distributing food from their family's possessions, motivated at least in part by a desire to obtain some self-control.[99] In her survey of gender, charity, and sainthood in the later Middle Ages, P. H. Cullum has noted that men who followed the conventional model of male charity by being responsible and balancing the needs of their lineage and household with those of charity were more likely to receive official canonization than those who attempted to achieve a 'more heroically charitable' sainthood, like Charles of Blois. Women, on the other hand, were expected to provide charity under the direction of their male guardians, but in some cases their charity became femininely excessive. By being 'irresponsible' in this way, they could upset the power balance within a household or a community. In some cases, however, like that of St. Elizabeth, this could lead to obtaining papal canonization, and on the whole these women fared better than overcharitable men whose benevolence was considered excessive or 'feminine'.[100]

When it comes to treating the sick, the depositions discussed above can similarly be read as examples of excessively charitable behaviour, especially when expressions of charity were penitential. The importance of this behaviour for female saints derives partially from the nurturing role of women.[101] However, such gendered tendencies did not necessarily have much significance in the individual community to which a saint belonged, even if the depictions of female saints' nursing activities portray their patients' bodies in a more graphic way.[102] Nicholas of Tolentino's frequent acts of mercy are highlighted

and other self-disciplining practices, and how she abstained from eating meat for her entire life, except when gravely ill. See 'Preface to the Texts' in PC Margaret of Hungary, 33.

98 PC Clare of Montefalco, 4, 183.

99 Bynum, *Holy Feast and Holy Fast*, 222-27.

100 Cullum, 'Gendering Charity', esp. 148.

101 For this view and miracle testimonies in canonization inquests, see Katajala-Peltomaa, *Gender, Miracles, and Daily Life*, 114-22. There were, however, geographical differences; in northern material, men, especially fathers, had a more visibly nurturing role; Katajala-Peltomaa, 'Fatherhood, Masculinity and Lived Religion in Late Medieval Sweden'. On caring for an infirm spouse, see Kuuliala, 'Love and Duty in the Time of Family Crisis'.

102 In the case of leprosy, there appears to have been an idea that close proximity to lepers could help a female saint overcome the flaws of her sex. Rawcliffe, *Leprosy in Medieval England*, 149.

throughout the hearing, and occasionally his own infirmity adds to the significance of this habit and to the ties he had with his devotees. A witness called Raynalducius Andree, for instance, mentioned that Nicholas visited the infirm during daytime but also at night if they needed him, and on top of that he 'went visiting the infirm and had his companions helping him, because he could not walk by himself, and he did this because the people of Tolentino had great devotion to him, so that the infirm and others asked for him a lot.'[103]

Besides mentioning administering food and spiritual guidance and consolation, the witnesses in St. Nicholas's hearing did not describe the holy man's deeds when visiting the *infirmi*. Nevertheless, there are testimonies of male saints tending the sick, even if the descriptions are often – although not invariably – less detailed than in the case of female saints. St. Louis of Toulouse's hearing includes a textbook example of an encounter with a leper. Louis's brother, the duke of Calabria, was horrified by the sight of a severely deformed leper, and feared contagion. Louis, however, washed the leper's feet and kissed him in memory of Christ who was tortured and appeared *quasi leprosus*. The witness, who had heard about the incident from the duke, made a point of the leper's appearance by describing the maculae, swollen lips, and ulcers.[104] It is probably no coincidence that the witness was a Franciscan brother, given the fame of the legend of St. Francis kissing a leper.[105] Guillaume de Saint-Pathus's text shows that some witness(es) reported how St. Louis IX, who fed the sick on many occasions and in whose case the horridness of their conditions plays a major role, communicated with the sisters of a Maison Dieu to ask what malady a sick person had, what kind of food should be given to them, and then gave them precisely the food that was required.[106] Yves of Tréguier's charitable deeds were mostly described as giving paupers food, visiting the infirm and talking with them, but he even reportedly washed and buried the corpse of a pauper, a task that others could not stomach because of the stench.[107]

103 PC Nicholas of Tolentino, 209: 'et etiam tempore infirmitatis ibat visitando infirmos et faciebat se iuvare a socio suo, quia ipse per se non poterat ambulare, et hoc ideo faciebat quia homines de Tholentino habebant maximam devotionem in eo ita quod infirmi et alii multum requirebant eum.'

104 PC Louis of Toulouse, 94-96. For *Christus quasi leprosus*, see Rawcliffe, *Leprosy in Medieval England*, 135-43.

105 For the motif of kissing the lepers and its connection with St. Francis, see, Peyroux, 'The Leper's Kiss'.

106 Guillaume de Saint-Pathus, *Vie de saint Louis*, 96-97, also describes how horrified were people accompanying the king to the hospices.

107 PC Yves of Tréguier, 55, 60, 72-73, 100. Piety towards paupers was an essential element of Yves's sainthood, to a point that once he punished a Spanish man for failing to give alms to a

The connection between the infirm body, sainthood, and medicine becomes more nuanced in the depictions of saints administering medicine to the sick with their own hands. As was typical for the first generation of Mendicants, the Franciscan friar St. Ambrose of Massa's (d. 1240) mid-thirteenth-century inquest reports him as eagerly giving medical care not only to other brothers but also poor laypeople.[108] Similarly, Hugo, the barber of St. Thomas Cantilupe, testified that when someone in the bishop's *familia* was infirm, he not only visited them but also had medicine prepared for them, as was expected of a bishop. Hugo himself had received such assistance.[109] As a charitable action this form of help had an economic aspect as well as alleviating physical suffering. Using the help of educated physicians was expensive, and only the well-off were able to pay for their services, even though medical men were expected to treat the poor free of charge.[110] For this reason enabling institutionalized or educated medical assistance as an act of charity by rulers was common, as demonstrated by the large institutions founded by St. Louis IX, which he often visited.[111] Georgius de Lesnen testified that Charles of Blois visited the infirm and gave them medicine, but he also had Georgius and his other physicians do the same.[112] As noted by P. H. Cullum, Charles's charity reached a point where it became a problem to his peers,[113] but for his devotees these activities were undoubtedly of crucial importance.

pauper asking for them in God's and the saint's name. PC Yves of Tréguier, 185-88. Some of the infirm *paupers* that had received Yves's help also testified in the hearing. A man called Guillelmus Ballech had been *contractus* in one tibia, and at that time received a lodging and money from Yves. Years later, after the saint's death, he pondered this, made a vow to him, and was cured. PC Yves of Tréguier, 216-17. For a similar case, see PC Vincent Ferrer, 283-84.

108 'Processus canonizacionis b. Ambrosii Massani', *AASS*, Nov. IV, 574-75; Vauchez, *Sainthood*, 342.

109 BAV, MS Vat. lat. 4015, fols. 24v-25r. It is no wonder that when, years later, Hugo himself acquired a blinding condition, he turned to his now deceased master for help and miraculously received his eyesight back. BAV, MS Vat. lat. 4015, fols. 27r-28r. For the charity of holy bishops, see Cullum, 'Gendering Charity', 139-40.

110 Lett, '*Judicium Medicine* and *Judicium Sanctitatis*', 159. On the other hand, Carole Rawcliffe has pointed out that '[o]ne of the most striking features of medieval healing is the wide range of treatment [...] available at a price to suit almost every pocket'. Rawcliffe, 'Curing Bodies and Healing Souls', 113. Charity of physicians is rarely reported in canonization processes. The only direct mention of a medical professional treating someone 'out of charity' I have found is recorded in Thomas Cantilupe's hearing, in which *magister* Gilbertus treated the leg of a beggar girl 'for the love of God'; BAV, MS Vat. lat. 4015, fol. 66v.

111 See Guillaume de Saint-Pathus, *Vie de saint Louis*, 92-99; Farmer, *Surviving Poverty*, 89-90; O'Tool, 'Caring for the Blind', esp. 103-10; Wheatley, *Stumbling Blocks before the Blind*, 49-59.

112 BAV, MS Vat. lat. 4025, fol. 12 r-v; PC Charles of Blois, 29: 'ipsis medicinas et species et alia necessaria ministrari faciebat'.

113 Cullum, 'Gendering Charity', 147-48.

Mostly the canonization hearings do not make a connection between the ailing bodies of saints and those of their devotees that the saints gave medical assistance. An illuminating exception is the 1451 inquest of St. Frances of Rome. Of the late medieval saints, she was perhaps the one who most clearly lived among people who were, or who would become, her devotees.[114] The twenty-ninth article discusses the severity of her infirmities and her kindness towards other infirm people, paralleling these two. According to the article, despite her wealth, while infirm Frances never used their help or any medicine but lived in the same manner as she had when in good health. However, the article further states that she did not act in a similar manner towards other infirm people, but provided them with all possible help, including any medical help that was necessary for their bodily health.[115] This was a part of her role as a well-known benefactor who transformed the family's palazzo into a hospital.[116] Some witnesses specified that Frances's reason for refusing to use medicine was that she did not wish to provide pleasure to her body and that she kept eating vegetables as she did when she was healthy, so choosing not to alleviate her infirmity was a part of her penitence;[117] Agnes Pauli Lelli specified that at the time of infirmity, when she refused medicine, she said: 'Lord Jesus Christ, thy will be done'.[118] According to Frances's nephew Iohannes Antonius, the son of Iacobus magistri Laurentii, who had been a recipient of Frances's charitable actions, she gave infirm people medicines and remedies suitable for their specific infirmities. *Domna* Vannozia, another member of Frances's congregation, stated that she consulted physicians about these medicines.[119] The way the article and the testimonies are recorded does not tell us whether

114 See Esch, 'Santa Francesca Romana', 14; as Esch points out, the other contemporary female saints living in Rome, St. Birgitta of Sweden and St. Catherine of Siena, mostly moved in the most elite circles of the society. Although the Ponziani family was an elite one too, Frances's social circles and connections were far more diverse. Esch, 'I processi medioevali', 43, has demonstrated that her cult was propagated within families. In the first inquest, the witnesses mostly come from the same generation of Frances, whereas in the last one it is their children and grandchildren testifying. At the same time, many witnesses testified in one of the earlier hearings as well.

115 PC Frances of Rome, 242: 'Erga vero alios infirmos non ita faciebat, sed cum omni caritate et sollicitudine omnibus providebat et tam medicorum iuvamina, que ad salutem corporis necessaria erant, ministrabat.'

116 Another example of this was Frances distributing grain from the Ponziani granary as well as wine, during a terrible famine. Boanas and Roper, 'Feminine Piety in Fifteenth-Century Rome', 181-82; Parigi, *The Rationalization of Miracles*, 51.

117 See Elliott, *Proving Woman*, 81-82, for other examples.

118 PC Frances of Rome, 243: 'quod b. F^e^ tempore infirmitatis sue medicinalia recipere noluit, sed temper [*sic*] dixit: "Domine Iesu Christe, fiat voluntas tua".'

119 PC Frances of Rome, 242-43.

Frances openly expressed that she did not expect other people to follow her example by not using medicine or medical expertise, or whether it was something that was simply understood from her use of these same aids on behalf of others. Bodily ailments were treated very differently in canonization inquests depending on whether the body was that of a saint or that of a devotee. The ailing bodies of others provided vehicles for the saintly figure to demonstrate not only her miraculous powers but her charity and solicitude.

Frances's willingness to treat those in her community is reflected in testimonies about her *miracula in vita*. In these narrations, her thaumaturgic powers function in concert with the medical assistance she provides. Other saints were reported to have given petitioners ointments and other medical substances,[120] but the frequency of such reports is exceptionally high especially in Frances's 1451 inquest.[121] Unlike, for example, Dauphine of Puimichel, Frances was not portrayed as unwilling to perform miracles – or at least to help her devotees. Many of the testimonies portray Frances as being called to visit an infirm person, usually a woman from her circle, living in Campitelli or Trastevere,[122] and giving some ointment or other medicine, but the witness remaining convinced that the cure had a miraculous origin. The reason for this conviction, often inquired about by the commissioners, could be the lack of power in the medicine or its simplicity, or the speed of the cure, which might have appeared miraculous.[123] In two instances Frances even carried out operations: she performed a cauterization for her spiritual daughter Rita Covelli,[124] and stitched a festering wound of a pauper.[125] In these testimonies Frances's ability to administer medicine and her holiness are complementary aspects of her cures. Some witnesses even testified that they had specifically asked for medicine, or for medicine and divine intervention.[126] These remarks can also be read as the witnesses

120 For Nordic examples, see Krötzl, 'Saints, Healing and Communities', esp. 259-61.

121 See also Siraisi, *Medieval and Early Renaissance Medicine*, 44, 46, for Frances's healing activities.

122 Frances healed men too, but her cult appears to have been primarily female. Esposito, 'St. Francesca and the Female Religious Communities', 198.

123 PC Frances of Rome, 261, 264, 265-66, 268. Once Frances forbade the witness from trusting in a medical professional. This is the only instance in which such a dichotomy is visible. The medical man in question was a Jew, which may explain the statement. PC Frances of Rome, 272.

124 PC Frances of Rome, 180, 267. Cauterization with burning oil, known as one of the most painful medical treatments of the time, was a standard treatment for poisoned wounds. Siraisi, *Medieval and Early Renaissance Medicine*, 170-71, 176.

125 PC Frances of Rome, 170-71.

126 PC Frances of Rome, 263-64, 282.

formulating their experience into a proper miracle account after the events, in which traces of Frances's role as a lay healer are still visible.

Frances's hearing is only one, albeit rather exceptional, example of the overlapping nature of different healing methods. The witnesses to many of her healing miracles *in vita* appear to have regarded her as both a living saint and a semiprofessional healer. The gendered aspects of her cult may have played some role in all this, but her medical assistance was needed in a tumultuous period when there was a shortage of physicians in the city.[127] Her clientele were primarily female too, and her role as a 'mother figure' brought women and children into her care. In the rhetoric of the miraculous, male saints have, since late antiquity, been paralleled more directly with doctors.[128] The best-known examples of this connection are perhaps the early Christian martyrs and alleged physicians, Sts. Cosmas and Damian.[129] In our sources, such a comparison was made by St. Nicholas of Tolentino himself, when he told Margarita Appillaterre to take her daughter Ceccha to St. Blaise, since he was a better doctor than all the others. Furthermore, in some vows referred to in Nicholas's hearing the petitioner promised to bring the same sum of money to his grave as they would have paid to the doctors.[130] Although hagiographic texts, regardless of their type, generally portray 'divine medicine' as superior to the mundane one, in everyday life religious healing did not compete with medicine. The texts portraying saints as healers finely illustrate the role of a living saint in the medical pluralism of the time, in which religion, educated medicine, and various 'folk healing' practices were supplementary characteristics of medieval health care.[131]

Cure and the Benefits of Infirmity

As the discussion above has demonstrated, saints were by no means immune to pain, suffering, or bodily infirmity in general. Their endurance when

127 Morelli, 'Malattie e medicina a Roma nel XV secolo', 90-91.

128 For examples, see Bartlett, *Why Can the Dead Do Such Great Things?*, 349. To my knowledge, no large-scale comparison of saints and doctors has been done, but it appears that it was indeed more common in the case of male saints, unsurprisingly given that official doctors and surgeons were male. Giselle de Nie notes that an isolated reference to St. Radegund (compared with the numerous such references in the case of the contemporary St. Germanus of Paris) is reminiscent of the Roman tradition of female physicians. Nie, 'Fatherly and Motherly Curing', 62.

129 On these two saintly figures, see Duffin, *Medical Saints*.

130 Lett, '*Judicium Medicine* and *Judicium Sanctitatis*', 163.

131 For the relationship of medicine and religion, see Dinzelbacher, *Mystik und Natur*, 66; Wilson, 'Conceptions of the Miraculous'; Ziegler, 'Practitioners and Saints'; and pp. 127-28 above.

facing such experiences was a crucial factor in the definitions of sanctity, and physical infirmity played a major role in the negotiations concerning penitence and asceticism. When endured by saints, infirmity and pain was glorified and could be read as a mark of God's special grace given to the holy, who often thanked him for this gift. As a phenomenon belonging to the sphere of lived religion, suffering was not something to get rid of, but medieval texts depict ways of making physical pain, loss, defeat, or helpless contemplation of others' agony, something bearable.[132] Saints were the scapegoats (in the biblical sense of suffering on behalf of others) of the whole of Christendom in their infirmities, and they could be that for a smaller community as well. At the same time, they were, in their extraordinariness, model figures, even 'superhumans', whose *vitae* were widely read.[133] To what extent they were actually role models for those not aspiring to live a holy life is of course open to question, but their virtuousness was widely esteemed and learned theologians considered them an example of penance and virtue for the laity to follow.[134] In the final pages of this chapter, we will take a look at the way saints' infirmities were recorded as exemplary and as something to take one's cue from, and how all this intermingles with notions of cure and medicine.

There have been conflicting views on whether a person should seek secular medical treatment for infirmities since late antiquity. The ascetics in Egyptian and Cappadocian monasteries addressed the question, often condemning medical treatment, and this prompted St. Basil to write in the fourth century a lengthy chapter in favour of Galenic/Hippocratic treatment. According to Basil, medicine itself was a gift from God, given to humankind to ease the pain of infirmities caused by the fall. The ambiguity regarding medical treatment continued into the medieval period, for example within the Franciscan Order where Francis himself was more critical towards the assistance of physicians than later leaders. Mostly these discussions are visible in hagiographic texts and the monastic setting, and did not necessarily concern 'ordinary' people. For instance, the Fourth Lateran Council of 1215 was the first to address the usage of medical help, which implies that from the point of view of the church, it was expected that individuals would seek medical help when necessary.[135]

132 Clifford Geertz 1973, cited in Kleinberg, *Prophets*, 104.

133 Lewis, 'Male Saints and Devotional Masculinity in Late Medieval England', 116.

134 Goodich, *Miracles and Wonders*, 19, 45, 69.

135 Crislip, *From Monastery to Hospital*, 26-28; Trembinski, 'Illness and Authority', 115-16, 119-20. Chapter 22 of the Council states that because infirmity is sometimes caused by sin, the physician should take care that patients make confession before starting the treatment.

The relationship between saints and different attempts to cure is therefore an intriguing feature of the valorization of physical suffering and shows again how an aspect related to 'holy infirmity' could be given varying emphases and meanings in the course of a canonization hearing. Despite her attitude towards infirmities, Dauphine of Puimichel had her physician near her most of her life, and she also consulted him at times when she suffered from them.[136] Similarly, although Clare of Montefalco refused to ask for God's help and acknowledged the benefits of infirmity for the human soul, the canonization records include no examples of her refusing medicine or medical treatment. Her submission to physicians' continuous treatment was used to highlight her chastity.[137] Some of the witnesses whose depositions have been preserved confirmed this.[138] At the same time, as discussed above, Frances of Rome, who actively and wilfully gave medical care to other people and respected medical expertise, refused to be given any medical treatment, submitting herself to God's will.[139] The indications of her collaboration with physicians show her willingness to invest in caring for the infirm, and thereby emphasize the significance of her own abstinence from any medicine. Furthermore, she did adjust her ascetic behaviour to satisfy the requirements of health, but, as we have seen, according to the canonization process this moderation was imposed by her confessor rather than the physicians. Following the order of a confessor was a virtue in itself, and did not invalidate her choice of a life of penitence, which included refusal of medicine.

It is likely that in the case of these three women, both their gender and their situation in life played a role in how their own wishes regarding

Sacrorum conciliorum nova et amplissima collectio, ed. Mansi, XXII, col. 1010. The chapter does not emphasize the sinfulness of an infirm person, although it recognizes the possible connection between sin and illness. Instead, it concerns the worry that if a physician recommends confession, as he should, a patient might give up all hope. See McVaugh, *Medicine before the Plague*, 170-71; Metzler, *Disability in Medieval Europe*, 67. Medical professionals also wrote about medicine being a creation of God, as is visible in the report of Paris medical faculty in 1348 (quoted in Horrox, *The Black Death*, 163), stating that '[w]e must not overlook that the pestilence proceeds from the divine will, and our advice can therefore only be to return humbly to God. But this does not mean forsaking doctors. For the Most High created earthly medicine, and although God alone cures the sick, he does so through the medicine which in his generosity he has provided'.

136 See pp. 43-44 above.

137 PC Clare of Montefalco, 10: 'et si medicus intrabat ad eam visitandam in infirmitatibus, ipsa sancta Clara cohoperiebat se totam cum mantelo et faciem etiam cum velo, et declinabat occulos in terram, et vitabat respicere homines.' See also pp. 133-34 above.

138 PC Claire of Montefalco, 98, 330.

139 Two witnesses specified in their depositions that when refusing it, she simply cited Lord's Prayer, saying: 'let your will be done' ('fiat voluntas tua'). PC Frances of Rome, 243.

medical treatment were adjusted and how this aspect was later retold and investigated. Especially before she became an abbess, Clare of Montefalco is unlikely to have had a say in how her own infirmity should be treated, and for the investigation into her sanctity, her acquiescence was beneficial. This view is emphasized in her brother Franciscus's statement that she did not care for her body or the medical treatment.[140] As pointed out by Nancy Siraisi, Franciscus is probably not saying that there was anything wrong in the use of medical help as such, but stating that it was not compatible with Clare's ascetic lifestyle.[141] Dauphine of Puimichel was a noblewoman, and especially in her youth the situation may have been quite similar, although partly for different reasons. The incident concerning her and Elzéar's claimed infertility discussed above[142] shows what an important role the lay authorities of one's life could play in situations related to health, for male as well as female holy figures. Like illness and impairment, cure was also something communally negotiated, and in the texts discussed here, these negotiations were modelled to fit into the hagiographic framework.[143] The need for medical intervention appears often to have pertained to the ability to function in a social role, as was the case with Elzéar and other such lay figures; after all, it has been proposed that in late medieval and early modern Europe, it was precisely the ability to fulfil one's social role that defined 'health'.[144] Charles of Blois was even reported as having treated the wounds caused by his use of a hair shirt with an ointment. Although this incident was reported by his *barbitonsor* and *cubicularius* as proofs of the habit, it also shows the saintly duke's constant need to balance his saintly corporality with his official duties.[145] However, Frances of Rome

140 PC Clare of Montefalco, 270.

141 Siraisi, *Medieval and Early Renaissance Medicine*, 39.

142 See pp. 102-3 above.

143 There are accounts in early modern German family books, which portray the fact that laity could also face pressure from their peers for medical treatment. Frohne and Horn, 'On the Fluidity of "Disability"', 37-38; presumably the situation could be similar in earlier centuries as well. At the same time, hagiographic sources include examples where no attempts to cure appear to have been used in the case of congenital or otherwise chronic conditions. For examples, see Kuuliala, *Childhood Disability*, 192-20. For conceptions of incurability, see Metzler, *Disability in Medieval Europe*, 71; Metzler, *A Social History of Disability*, 6.

144 Gentilcore, *Healers and Healing*, 163, 185-86.

145 BAV, MS Vat. lat. 4025, fol. 67r; PC Charles of Blois, 163: 'Dicens iste quod per asperitate dicte corde qua cinctus erat, et cilicii quo induebatur, plures lesiones seu incisiones habebat et paciebatur in corpore circumquaque, quas aliquociens ungebat dictus D. C. quodam unguento vocato alborasis. 'Alborasis' – or 'albo Rasis' – refers to what is known as the white ointment of Rhazes, which includes olive oli, ceruse, beeswax, egg yolks, and camphor. See Norri, *Dictionary of Medical Vocabulary*, 1143.

appears to have managed to regulate the treatments of her own infirmities throughout her life – or at least this was how the witnesses interpreted the situation. Gender alone does not, therefore, explain the variety in the tone of the canonization processes when describing a saintly figure's exemplary suffering and medicine; their personal situation, age, and social environment played an important part.

The question of gender, medical help, and suffering, as well as of asking for divine help, gets more nuance in the case of St. Nicholas of Tolentino. As already discussed, he was the saint who seems to have rejected medical professionals more than any other, and his community members attempted to intervene. André Vauchez's study implies that this might have something to do with Nicholas being an eremitic saint;[146] this may be true, but it does not mean that other types of saints did not follow similar ideals, as the case of St. Frances shows. According to the articles, Nicholas was 'repelled by physicians' advice' ('repulsis consiliis medicorum') to eat more at the time of his bodily infirmities,[147] which Didier Lett reads as an example of 'the inferiority of human acts when compared to divine work' mode of thought.[148] When testifying about Nicholas's patience, Mancinus Fortis de Castro Sancti Angeli, who also reported his *gutta salsa* and *plaga magna*, stated that he told the saint to take baths and to follow physicians' advice. Nicholas responded that he did not want to do that, but that God, who gave him the wound, would cure it when it pleased Him, as He was the physician.[149] Brother Nucius testified that he had once asked why Nicholas did not have the wound on his thigh treated, to which the saint replied that God would be allowed to cure it.[150] *Magister* Thomas Bartolucii further testified that the more Nicholas suffered the more he praised God,[151] and Nicholas's *infirmarius* Iohannucius de Tholentino said that during his infirmities, the saint sweetly called for the Virgin Mary's

146 See Vauchez, *Sainthood*, 332. The same may explain why in Celestine V's inquest a brother of his Order explicitly states that he followed his ascetic regime in health as well as in infirmity. PC Celestine V, II, 300-1.

147 PC Nicholas of Tolentino, 19.

148 Lett, '*Judicium medicine* and *judicium sanctitatis*', 160.

149 PC Nicholas of Tolentino, 257: 'Et ipse frater Nicholaus respondit: Nolo ire ad balneum, frater, non, nec ad medicos propter istam causam; sed ille Deus, qui dedit michi istam plagam, auferet quando placebit sibi: et ipse erit medicus.'

150 PC Nicholas of Tolentino, 550: 'dum extrageret sibi calzarium, quia calzarius multum tragebat et dilatabat illud vulnus: O quare non facis tibi sanari istud vulnus? Respondit dictus fratre Nicolaus cum magna patientia: Permittas, fili, permittas quia Deus sanabit.'

151 PC Nicholas of Tolentino, 553: 'quanto magis afficiebatur, tunc magis laudabat Deum, dicendo: Te Deum laudamus, te Deum laudamus.'

help.[152] Nicholas's reluctance to receive medical assistance, as well as his succumbing to the help and mercy of God and the Virgin Mary, were a part of his *fama publica*, also recorded in his fourteenth-century *vita* by Petrus de Monte Rubiano.[153]

For several reasons, when thinking about saints' attitudes towards medical help, whether it was ministered for them or by them for their devotees, making comparisons between different saints and their communities is tricky. First, in only a few cases was this attitude specified and of fundamental importance for the hearing. St. Nicholas of Tolentino and St. Frances of Rome are the only ones whose refusal to accept any medicine is mentioned in an article. Furthermore, several witnesses to John Buoni's sanctity mentioned that he refused the help of medicine or physicians, saying that God was his physician in a manner similar to St. Nicholas.[154] These are probably references to Book 10 of Augustine's *Confessions*, but the same idea is also inherent in Matthew 8:17 ('ut adimpleretur quod dictum est per Isaiam prophetam, dicentem: Ipse infirmitates nostras accepit: et aegrotationes nostras portavit').[155] Physicians' presence is also crucial in the hearing of St. Clare of Montefalco, not only in relation to the relics found inside her body after her death, but also during her lifetime. It is quite possible that these saints simply had this kind of *fama*, being known to have been ill for a long time. Nicholas and Frances were well-known figures among the laity already during their lifetime, but it is also plausible that the executors of their hearings decided to make a point of the medical aspects.

It is also likely that the geographic location and the dating of these hearings had an influence, as has been suggested regarding the investigation into the marks of the passion in Clare of Montefalco's heart.[156] Compared with many other areas of Europe, late medieval Italy was a much more medicalized society, so the importance of medical expertise shows in the miracle testimonies of Italian and some other southern European processes but far less frequently in those from northern Europe.[157] Therefore, the presence

152 PC Nicholas of Tolentino, 481: 'et quod dulciter vocabat dictus frater Nicolaus in infirmitatibus suis dicendo: Beata Maria, adiuva me.'

153 'Vita, Nicolaus Tolentinas, ord. eremitarum s. Augustini', *AASS*, Sept. X, 649.

154 'Processus apostolici, de b. Joanne Buono', *AASS*, Oct. IX, 816, 818, 821, 831, 838.

155 The English translation (New King James Bible) reads: 'that it might be fulfilled which was spoken by Isaiah the prophet, saying: "He Himself took our infirmities, and bore our sicknesses."' In *Confessions*, bk. 10, ch. 28, sec. 39, Augustine writes: 'Woe is me! Lo, I hide not my wounds; Thou art the Physician, I the sick; Thou merciful, I miserable' (trans. Pilkington). For *Christus Medicus* see e.g. Henderson, *Renaissance Hospital*, 113-18; McAvoy, 'Bathing in the Blood'.

156 Park, 'Relics of a Fertile Heart'.

157 Finucane, *The Rescue of the Innocents*, 5, 95-96; Kuuliala, *Childhood Disability*, 205-9; Lett, '*Judicium Medicine* and *Judicium Sanctitatis*', 157-58.

of medicine and medical knowledge brought prestige to different kinds of testimonies concerning saints' lives, and perhaps the witnesses became accustomed to interpreting religious phenomena also from a more medical perspective. Geographical differences did not wholly exclude the possibility of defining sanctity, or at least saintly patience, by the holy person's attitude towards medicine,[158] but the issue was undoubtedly much more topical in areas where refusing medical treatment given by university-trained professionals was an actual statement.

Saints' refusal to accept medical help is rooted in the valorization of pain and suffering. The biblical passage 'Cum infirmor potens sum' already referred to above, was essential to the medieval conception of the beneficial nature of bodily weakness. Furthermore, in the later Middle Ages, regardless of its origins, pain was considered to have a purifying effect.[159] Consequently, expressing the benefits of infirmity for one's soul is a hagiographic trope,[160] frequently appearing in *vitae* and canonization testimonies as well. For instance, in Jacques de Vitry's *Life of St. Mary of Oignes* it is stated, 'she thanked Our Lord who chastises like children those whom He loves' with so much joy that the apostle's word was plainly fulfilled in her. Jacques went on to explain that Our Lord had thus tested Mary as his 'chosen child'.[161] Paul's passage was also referred to by canon Joannes Tennagotti in the diocesan hearing of Jeanne-Marie de Maille in 1414/15, where he testified about her long-lasting infirmities, and compared the state of her body and soul to that of Paul and others who excelled in their infirmities.[162]

158 See a Swedish example in PC Brynolf of Skara, 148, where he is reported to have scorned the remedies of physicians: 'adiecerunt, quod ipse beatus Brynolphus spreto remedio medicorum, diuine dispositione in huiusmodi infirmitate se commisit similiter dirigendum.'

159 Elliott, *Proving Woman*, esp. 83.

160 As an example, in St. Francis of Assisi's thinking, 'our sisters, the illnesses', are vital opportunities for salvation. Le Goff, *Saint Francis of Assisi*, 26, and Francis's early *vitae* show that Francis and the writers of those early biographies believed that his suffering and disability were beneficial for his spiritual growth; Trembinski, 'Illness and Authority', 113, 115. As another example, Julian of Norwich wrote that a sickness in youth was one of the three gifts desirable from God and it initiated her revelations. Julian of Norwich, *Revelations of Divine Love*, 25-26.

161 McNamer, 'Middle-English Version of Jacques de Vitry's *Life of St. Marie d'Oignies*', 726.

162 'Processus informativus pro canonizatione d. Mariae de Maillye', *AASS*, Mar. III, 752: 'Dicit vltra quod pluries vidit dictam Dominam varijs infirmitatibus laborantem [...]: adeo quod assistentes et superuenientes spiritu et corpore mirabiliter recreabat, secundum quod legitur de Apostolo et B. Laurentio et alijs, qui in suis infirmitatibus gloriabantur.' The allusion to St. Lawrence may refer to the *Passio Polychronii*, which was a popular text in the Middle Ages, and which provided the basis for the last days of the saint in the martyrologies. For these texts, see Ziolkowski's introduction to *Passio sancti Laurentii Martiris* in *The Passion of St. Lawrence: Epigrams and Marginal Poems*.

It has been proposed that the valorization of suffering was a female phenomenon.[163] Based on their statistical analysis, Donald Weinstein and Rudolph M. Bell write that suffering an illness is 'the one category of activity in which women were not merely statistically overrepresented but constituted an absolute majority'.[164] However, as with many other aspects related to holy infirmity, although quantitative analysis shows that infirmity was more of a requirement for female sanctity, our sources show that similar views were associated with both male and female saints. When we look at the saints for whom we have a canonization process, it turns out that there is no similar, statistical difference – *if* such an observation can be made based on these sources in the first place. Most male saints for whom a canonization process exists, St. Louis of Toulouse, St. Yves of Tréguier, and St. Thomas Aquinas excluded,[165] reportedly had some kind of chronic infirmity. As an example, *frater* Bonusvisus, who took care of St. Dominic at the time of his infirmity, reported that the saint rejoiced in his infirmity, as he did of all tribulations.[166] The valorization of an infirm, holy body was very much a reality for the devotees of these (male) saints, as well as for the official sanctity. Conversely, as discussed already, a female saint did not *have* to have any reported sufferings or ecstatic states.[167]

The topic of glorious suffering was, nevertheless, more often elaborated on in the processes of especially fourteenth- and fifteenth-century female saints, which is one of the few temporal changes regarding saints' infirmities visible in the canonization processes. When testifying about Dorothea of Montau's wounds, Johannes Marienwerder's explanation for them was that God chastises those He loves. He was asked for proofs of this, and among other things specified that God took Dorothea as his spouse in several

163 See Bynum, *Fragmentation and Redemption*, 188; Bynum, *Holy Feast and Holy Fast*, 189; Metzler, *Disability in Medieval Europe*, 47-48.

164 Weinstein and Bell, *Saints and Society*, 234-35.

165 St. Ambrose of Massa could be added to the list. Then again, the testimonies to his life are very short and summarized, and the duration of the infirmity in which he reportedly was a patient is not recorded. One of the friars, for example, testified that he saw him being patient in his infirmities and bringing his life to perfection in his penitence and good deeds ('Vidit etiam in suis infirmitatibus patientem et sic in penitentia et bonis operibus vite sue cursum in Domino consummavit') which may also relate to his final illness. 'Processus canonizacionis b. Ambrosii Massani', *AASS*, Nov. IV, 574.

166 PC Dominic of Caleruega, 140-41.

167 An example is St. Isabel of Aragon. See McCleery, 'Isabel of Aragon (d. 1336): Model Queen or Model Saint?', 679. Of our female saints, St. Birgitta can also be used as an example of a female saint whose physical suffering was not emphasized, although she was known for her raptures and revelations.

revelations, as well as endowing her with various virtues.[168] Sister Marina, for her part, testified that St. Clare of Montafalco was pleased with her various infirmities and tribulations and grateful to God because of them.[169] Another witness, Sister Thomassa, testified that during her infirmities and especially her stomach pains, some sisters said to Clare that she was doing penance, to which she replied that she did that penance happily and freely, although the penance was not sufficient to atone for her sins. Thomassa also said that once the other sisters told Clare that she should ask God to free her from the infirmity. She replied that she would never do so, but that she prayed God would rather increase her pains and infirmities, and if it pleased Him, she would happily have these infirmities all her life.[170]

The idea that infirmity was created to halt sin had been stated a thousand years before by St. Basil,[171] but Thomassa's testimony provides a revealing counterpart to the endless narrations in healing-miracle accounts about the communally negotiated invocations of a saint. In these stories, the person proposing a vow to the saint or the one making a successful vow is usually portrayed as the hero of the events.[172] Here the role of the other sisters' suggestion was merely to prove Clare's willingness to preserve her infirmities and provide glory to the divine indirectly. As mentioned in the Introduction, throughout the medieval period, the terminology of infirmity, dis/ability, or illness was notably inexact. Given that descriptions of the symptoms of our saints' non-self-inflicted infirmities were also vague, the modern reader is faced with an interesting methodological problem. It is well known that in the hagiographic and religious context, pain and suffering were valorized, but although this can be read in the canonization testimonies, it is not emphasized. Even the terms *dolor* or *poena* appear relatively rarely in the depositions concerning infirm saints, if you exclude descriptions of Clare of Montefalco's and Thomas Cantilupe's stomach pains, and some references to *imitatio Christi*.[173] Since the symptoms were

168 PC Dorothea of Montau, 260-61.

169 PC Clare of Montefalco, 109.

170 PC Clare of Montefalco, 181.

171 Crislip, *Thorns in the Flesh*, 90.

172 Smoller, 'Miracle, Memory, and Meaning', 435. See also Andrić, *The Miracles of St. John Capistran*, 323, for the various roles of people in miracle narratives. On negotiations concerning asking for saints' help as well as the common rumours as a source of information, see also Finucane, *Miracles and Pilgrims*, 156; Krötzl, 'Fama volat'; Krötzl, 'How to Choose a Saint?'; Kuuliala, *Childhood Disability*, 228-42.

173 This kind of reference is much more common in the Processo Castellano of Catherine of Siena, however, and especially so in Tommaso Caffarini's own testimony. See *Il processo Castellano*, ed. Laurent, 136, 190-93, 273, 338.

usually not elaborated on, we cannot detect details of suffering in them in the same way that we often can in miracle testimonies emphasizing painful symptoms or severely disabling consequences of a somatic condition. I am inclined, however, given all that we know about the medieval understanding of *infirmitas* and its implications, to think that the concept in the case of these saints already included all its connotations, such as pain, discomfort, and incapacity, even if we cannot apportion respective importance to them. In the context of canonization, it was not of crucial importance to highlight or specify physical pain as such, as it was inbuilt in the patience they showed during infirmities.

Esther Cohen has pointed out the variations in the gendered descriptions of pain behaviour, and the tendency in medieval texts to describe what ought to happen. Pain behaviour – or the expected pain behaviour – differed between genders, but there were also other norms and codes that influenced the way the subject's acts were recorded. As Cohen puts it, 'the sort of vocalization that was permissible to or demanded of parturient women in the twelfth century might have been shameful for a male knight at the time but proper for a contemporary abbot with mystical inclinations'.[174] This perspective is vital to the discourse on gender, holiness, and infirmity. Because sanctity itself, and consequently the meanings of saints' infirmities, were negotiated within a community, the ways holy men and holy women performed their infirmity or its symptoms such as pain or discomfort were of crucial importance.[175] Following a train of thought similar to Cohen's, Sharon Farmer has written extensively of the fluidity of medieval gender categories. There were not just 'men' and 'women' in later medieval society, as intersectionality played a major role. Different characteristics and expectations were attributed to wealthy and poor men and women.[176] Although in the sources living saints are primarily living saints, they were not just that, nor were they just men or women. They were nuns, friars, hermits, abbots, abbesses, bishops, rulers, mothers, and wives, and therefore they, and their expressions of infirmities, cannot be interpreted only according to their gender.

Despite the shared theological background of holy suffering, our saintly figures were reported as expressing their corporality and infirmity in varying

174 Cohen, *The Modulated Scream*, 114.
175 Within the hagiographic genre, this idea does not pertain only to saints. When asking for their help, their devotees, in certain situations, also benefitted from their performance of pain or disability. It could also help beggars with various infirmities to gain their bread. See Craig, *Wandering Women*, 100-1; Kuuliala, *Childhood Disability*, 288-94; Kuuliala, 'Unlikely Heroes'.
176 Farmer, *Surviving Poverty*, 30-32, 39-49, 78, 118-19.

manners, and sometimes the witnesses just referred to 'pain behaviour' without specifying it. This was done in Clare of Montefalco's hearing, when the witnesses stated that she demonstrated the sufferings of Christ that she felt.[177] Overall, descriptions of evident expressions of pain or discomfort are rare among testimonies to a saint's life, because the concept of *patientia* implied lack of wailing and complaining. Nonetheless, Bertrandus Iusberti testified that due to her fever and 'several other pains', he heard Dauphine of Puimichel wailing 'as if she was giving birth'. Bertrandus was giving testimony to the article about Dauphine's patience in infirmity, and apparently the commissioners inquired as to what words she used when crying or wailing, for had she been complaining, her patience would have been severely compromised. Bertrandus said, appropriately, that she thanked God for the pains.[178] In Bertrandus's testimony, the verb *dolere* is revealing regarding the multifaceted nature of pain and the vocabulary concerning it. The word combines the sensation of pain with the action as an expression, that is, crying. Furthermore, it highlights the idea of pain as an emotion, grief.[179] The depositions to this article are, however, somewhat inconsistent. Durandus Andree's testimony also mentions Dauphine thanking God, but does not refer to any precise expressions of pain from her, and, interestingly for the gendered approach to pain, crying and wailing were not mentioned by the two female witnesses, Bertranda Bartholomea or Catherina de Podio.[180] It is true that the 'gendered' aspect of canonization testimonies is complicated because, as Catherine Mooney puts it, 'women's testimony, whatever it may have been when orally delivered, would then be recorded, abbreviated, or omitted entirely according to the judgment of the supervising males'.[181] However, as already pointed out, the commissioners' duty was to record the statements truthfully, and there is no need to assume that they would have deliberately expunged cries of pain from their record of the female

177 PC Clare of Montefalco, 120, 193.

178 PC Dauphine of Puimichel, 229: 'dixit quod vidit eciam quod paciebatur febres et dolores multos alios in corpore suo, et specialiter quando mingebat, audivit eam clamantem et dolentem ac si parturiret. Interrogatus que verba pacinedo illos dolores clamabat, dixit quod regraciabatur Deo de dictis doloribus in generali, tamen non recordatur in speciali.' For pain and childbirth, see Cohen, *The Modulated Scream*, 131-33; for the pains of childbirth in miracles, see Craig, *Wandering Women*, 101-5, 113-14.

179 On pain as an emotion in late medieval discourse, see Cohen-Hanegbi, 'Pain as Emotion'. For the medieval vocabulary of pain, especially in the context of medicine and law, see Cohen, *The Modulated Scream*, 147-67, and on pain as an emotion in the modern world, see the article compilation, Boddice (ed.), *Pain and Emotion in Modern History*.

180 PC Dauphine of Puimichel, 264, 333, 399.

181 Mooney, 'Voice, Gender, and the Portrayal of Sanctity', 8.

companions' testimonies when they did record it in the deposition of a male witness.

A specific expression of pain was also recorded in Guillaume de Saint-Pathus's *Vie* of St. Louis IX. We have seen above how the holy king reportedly had a long-term infirmity unrelated to crusading, and how that interlinked with his patience towards an elderly servant. According to the narrative, during bouts of this *maladie*, the king had trouble hearing or understanding as well as eating and sleeping, and he lamented and wailed ('compleignoit et gemissaint').[182] As usual with this text, we have no way of knowing what the original depositions about Louis's malady had said about his behaviour, but there is no reason to suspect that no one of them would have reported this wailing. As portrayed, this behaviour in response to pain seems neither saintly, knightly, nor manly; after all, elite men were supposed to be able to stand pain and not to show physical weakness,[183] and therefore his behaviour appears rather feminine. In this case, however, Louis's sanctity provides a different framework for his expression of pain; crying and wailing underlined the severity of his malady and consequently highlighted the message of the passage, which was his good nature.[184]

Otherwise canonization documents are mostly silent about saints' pain behaviour or any expressions of discomfort caused by infirmities. This was presumably because of the existing concept of patience, but as Bertrandus Iusberti's testimony shows, distinct 'pain behaviour' did not exclude *patientia* – the saint's words and intention were the key. From this viewpoint the testimonies of St. Nicholas of Tolentino's 'sweet cries of help' directed to the Virgin can be interpreted as one of the ways the witnesses reshaped the actions of a saint in pain or discomfort to fit the established pattern of sanctity, and the same can be said of St. Vincent Ferrer's calls for Jesus.[185] Even in the case of saints such as Clare of Montefalco, who is portrayed as a very traditional suffering female saint, the testimonies concerning her infirmities remain silent about the exact manifestations of her pain. Unlike in the case of raptures, which were observable to witnesses by their corporeal signs, the infirm saints did not emphasize – or perhaps even *need* to emphasize – their pain. Perhaps infirmity was a self-evident aspect of being human, which included pain and/or discomfort, and which fits the pattern of sanctity as a

182 Guillaume de Saint-Pathus, *Vie de saint Louis*, 116. See pp. 65-67 above for this text.
183 Pincikowski, *Bodies of Pain*, 5-6, 23.
184 Not being able to sleep because of pain is a trope appearing every now and then in miracle narratives as a way of showing the severity of the condition to be cured. See Kuuliala, *Childhood Disability*, 267-68.
185 PC Vincent Ferrer, 21. See note 152 (p. 169) above for the quotation concerning St. Nicholas.

relatively simple concept. Therefore, it was enough to reconstruct holy suffering within the framework of patient tranquillity.[186] These depositions are in accordance with the *vitae* of many suffering saints who emphasized their physical suffering very little unless it was religiously charged or self-inflicted. Even in the latter case they often remained relatively silent.[187]

It is worth noting that in the pleas of the infirm saints or in reports of the lack of them, the divine agent most often discussed is God, and occasionally Christ or the Virgin. Other saints were mostly referred to in the depositions as models whose lives the saints under investigation took as an example, or in the visions leading to celibacy, not as potential helpers at times of infirmity; only in St. Frances of Rome's process does St. Alexis appear as both a model and a saintly helper.[188] God decided when a physical cure was necessary for the saintly path.[189] As an example of this, Johannes Marienwerder's *Vita Lindanea* of St. Dorothea of Montau tells us that she made a pilgrimage to Rome in 1390, and ended up severely infirm and spending eight weeks in a hospital until the 'great physician, who cures all our infirmities' ('medicus magnus, qui sanat omnes infirmitates nostras') revived her. Onlookers considered this a wondrous event. She was then able to walk with the help of another person and with the support of a cane, and thinking that she would have to 'crawl' for the rest of her life, decided to beg at the steps of St. Peter's until she died. Johannes's narration is related to Dorothea's *patientia*, since when God finally cured her, He 'revealed' that he had tested her patience and faith.[190] As is usual in Dorothea's case, the canonization inquest gives far less attention to her bodily tribulations. Her pilgrimage to Rome is included in the articles without further details, and the infirmity is reported only sporadically by the witnesses.[191] A Gdansk woman Metza

186 There is a parallel with miracle accounts in here as well. Although the *miraculées* were occasionally reported as having suffered from excessive pain and being liberated of precisely that by saints, canonization depositions in particular tend to be taciturn about pain as a symptom or an illness, using other symptoms to prove a condition genuine. Didactic miracle collections recorded at shrines emphasize pain more frequently. See Frohne and Kuuliala, 'The Trauma of Pain in Later Medieval Miracle Accounts'; Cohen, *The Modulated Scream*, 134-35; Craig, *Wandering Women*, 100-1.

187 See Cohen, *The Modulated Scream*, 120-21.

188 See pp. 46-47 above.

189 St. Margaret of Città di Castello is an exception, as her parents took her on a futile pilgrimage to the shrine of James of Castello. Since a miraculous healing always happens by God's will, the same principle holds here.

190 'Vita b. Dorotheae Lindana', *AASS*, Oct. XIII, 529. See also Stargardt, 'Dorothy of Montau', 476-77.

191 Johannes's *Libellus de vita* includes the event, making a point that this infirmity was also God-sent. PC Dorothea of Montau, 310: 'Fuit denique dictus languor plus ex amore quam dolore

Hugische testified to having seen Dorothea gravely infirm in Rome, but her deposition does not give any more details of this.[192] Another woman from the city said she had heard about Dorothea's infirmity,[193] so there appears to have been some kind of common *fama* about it.

In addition to God, the Virgin often appeared in visions related to the saints' infirmities, an example of a distinguishing characteristic of her cult,[194] showing the special grace she gave them. In their exploration of their inner selves and in their attempts to avoid sin, the late medieval religious had Mary as their companion, and she was increasingly invoked in nuns and monks' prayers. She was considered to have 'unique powers to mentor and assist'.[195] In the case of female saints, the Virgin Mary, and also Mary Magdalene, who were at the top of the hierarchy of saints, became models to conform to.[196] The significance of the Virgin for our saints and those testifying about their lives shows in the pleas of St. Nicholas discussed above, which act as a counterpoint to the suggestions of using medical help, as well as in the visions of saints in their infirmities. Clare of Montefalco's hearing reports an instance where she had a revelation that cured her of an unspecified *infirmitas*, during which it was revealed that she would live for a further fifteen days, after which she would join the glory of saints. Fifteen days turned out to be fifteen years, but the symbolism held.[197] Similarly, the *Miracoli* of Catherine of Siena reports an occasion where she was severely ill and had a vision of the Virgin, who explained that Christ still wanted her to remain on earth to guide more people, after which Catherine decided not to die yet.[198] Another healing vision was recorded in the diocesan hearing of

seu ex corporis egritudine.' ('In the end, the said feebleness was more because of love than because of pain or bodily illness.')

192 PC Dorothea of Montau, 108.

193 PC Dorothea of Montau, 116.

194 Visions of the Virgin appearing together with another saint, common in late medieval hagiographic material, could also enhance a saint's cult. See Adams, *Visions in Late Medieval England*, 70-74.

195 Rubin, *Emotion and Devotion*, 84.

196 Jansen, *The Making of the Magdalen*, 286-306.

197 PC Clare of Montefalco, 11. For Clare's visions, see Paoli, 'Le visioni di Chiara da Montefalco'

198 'The *Miracoli* of Catherine of Siena', ed. and trans. Lehmijoki-Gardner, 102. Tommaso da Siena, in his *libellus* of St. Catherine, also writes that because of the violence Catherine inflicted upon herself, she suffered from bleeding from her sides, but because she was drawn in such a way to God, she could not bear it and suffered from severe *infirmitas*. Christ and Mary Magdalene appeared to her and their touch cured her. Thomas of Siena, 'The *Libellus* concerning Catherine of Siena', ed. and trans. Lehmijoki-Gardner, 188-89. See also n. 45 on p. 292 of the same volume concerning the problems in defining this particular *infirmitas*. I think the infirmity in Catherine's sides may refer to her habit of wearing a hair shirt and an iron chain, since the author of 'The

Jeanne-Marie de Maille in 1414/15. Petrus des Aubuys, a presbyter, explained that in 1389, when she was 58 years old, Jeanne-Marie had been cured of a severe infirmity by a vision in which Christ had anointed her. This happened after she had dragged herself to her window to hear the vespers. Later, when she took part in a procession, she had a vision of the Virgin presenting her Son at the temple, and subsequently received the infant Jesus in her arms.[199]

In male and female saints' *vitae*, visions were frequently used to highlight key points in their lives, those where they were comforted for their torment or imprisonment being particularly common. In general, visions tied the saintly candidates to the divine. Many of them also received miraculous help. Belief in miraculous intervention in dreams or visions permeated the whole culture, and visions were also used for pedagogical and propagandist purposes, exposure to these stories being spread through various media.[200] In the cases discussed here, infirmity is an element emphasizing the connection the saint had with the divine. In Clare's case, the miraculous healing highlighted her status as one among the holy; in Catherine's case, her role as an instructor; and in Jeanne-Marie's, her devotion to the Virgin. Dorothea's infirmity and cure were both meant to underscore her patience and willingness to suffer. The episode is not a vision in any traditional sense, but in recording God's words, Johannes Marienwerder brought it towards such narratives. In none of these examples did the cure happen just to alleviate the suffering of the saint, but for a more noble purpose.[201] The cases discussed here are relatively few, concern only female saints,[202] and even fewer were recorded in a canonization inquest, but they nevertheless provide an interesting parallel to those leading to the path of sainthood, discussed in the first chapter of this book. It turns out that the idea of a saint asking to be cured by God's will or wanting to be miraculously

Miracoli of Catherine of Siena', 94-95, mentions it causing her pain in her sides. On the other hand, a seemingly non-self-inflicted pain in her sides was also reported in Francesco Malavolti's testimony, see *Il processo Castellano*, ed. Laurent, 338.

199 'Processus informativus pro canonizatione d. Mariae de Maillye', *AASS*, Mar. III, 757. Visions including lactation, and the veneration of the baby Jesus in general, are common in later medieval hagiography. See e.g. Klapisch-Zuber, *Women, Family, and Ritual in Renaissance Italy*, 324-27; Bynum, *Holy Feast and Holy Fast*.

200 Adams, *Visions in Late Medieval England*, 83; Goodich, *Miracles and Wonders*, 100-16.

201 The cures of saints' devotees could have spiritual associations as well. Miracles were meant to educate and enlighten, as well as to fight heresies. Occasionally they are also reported as enhancing the community's devotion. Goodich, *Miracles and Wonders*, 8-10; Goodich, 'The Politics of Canonization', 182; Katajala-Peltomaa, *Gender, Miracles, and Daily Life*, 169-70.

202 However, in saints' *vitae* male saints were also recorded as having such visions. See Adams, *Visions in Late Medieval England*, 83.

cured without asking for it was acceptable if it could later be ascribed to a life-changing moment enhancing holiness and did not reduce the *fama* of patience and *imitatio Christi*.

The importance of St. Paul's statement about strength in infirmity pertained not only to saints, but had great significance for the consolation of the suffering.[203] Furthermore, it was used in the crusading context when preachers explained the usefulness of suffering for God. For them, infirmity enabled humility. Like saints, crusaders who put themselves in danger suffered for Christ.[204] Our sources are very reticent about the matter, but it seems that sometimes the saintly figures could also make use of the benefits of infirmities when encountering their devotees. The depositions reporting St. Nicholas of Tolentino telling people to look for help from a saint instead of physicians can be read as one example of this.[205] They portray the living saint as a community member actively taking part in the negotiations regarding healthcare, in which his own, saintlike views of the superiority of divine healing predominate. They are also one example of how hierarchies of a given community were intervowen into these negotiations.[206]

That being said, reports given in canonization processes of saints pronouncing the spiritual benefits of infirmity to their devotees are sparse. St. Frances of Rome's hearing includes the case of *domna* Andrea (or Andreotzia) Petri Cecchi Pauli, who suffered from excessive pain to the point that she was unable to get up from her bed, and whom Frances medicated with herbs and clay. *Domna* Ceccha, who was present when Frances arrived, testified that she comforted Andrea, saying that she should put her hope in God and endure her infirmity with *patientia*.[207] Andrea herself did not mention these words, and the testimonies are generally curt. St. Frances's words are especially interesting when compared with the article stating that she did not expect other people to have a similar attitude to infirmity and medicine to her own. In this context, the words appear to have been consolatory.[208]

A more straightforward case of a saint expressing her attitude when encountering an infirm devotee was recorded in the process of Dauphine

203 See e.g. McClure, *Sorrow and Consolation in Italian Humanism*, 9-11. For consoling the suffering, see esp. Rittgers, *The Reformation of Suffering*.

204 Tamminen, 'The Crusaders' *Stigmata*', 110-11; see also Pincikowski, *Bodies of Pain*, 13.

205 See p. 146 above.

206 For communal strategies concerning invocation of saints, see Katajala-Peltomaa, 'Devotional Strategies in Everyday Life'.

207 PC Frances of Rome, 282.

208 As another example of Frances's consoling role, she comforted a woman whose daughter died of 'pestis', telling her that her daughter was in heaven. PC Frances of Rome, 277.

of Puimichel, who reportedly spoke very openly about the beneficial side of enduring infirmity. The thirty-third article, which records Dauphine's patience, states that she thought that if people considered how infirmities benefitted the soul by separating it from worldly things, they would go and buy the infirmities from a market if that were possible.[209] The testimonies also give hints that her attitude towards infirmities had some influence on her dealings with her devotees. As noted already, Dauphine was a very 'reluctant' saint, especially as a performer of miracles *in vita*. This was to some extent expected of her, being also typical of her form of sanctity.[210] Dauphine was not portrayed as a great visitor of the sick like many other saints discussed here, regardless of the social standing of the parties involved, although witnesses mentioned that she did occasionally do this, the most famous instance being her journey to console Sancia of Majorca during her illness.[211] A witness called *dominus* Petrus Audenqui, a canon and a precentor, testified about the cure of his own recurring fever, which left him so weak that he could only walk if assisted by others. A presbyter named Raymunus Raynaudi gave him cordial as a medicine, but he could not swallow it. Seeing his suffering, Raymundus asked Dauphine to visit Petrus, which she agreed to do. Among other good words, she repeated those of Paul to him, that one is stronger when one is weak. She explained that furthermore, if Petrus, like other Christians, knew how much good bodily infirmities did for the sufferer, especially if endured with patience, they would allow them to take their course. Dauphine then promised to cure Petrus but added that he should make his life better through God.[212]

In her discussion of Petrus's cure, Nicole Archambeau suggests that it was precisely the unsuccessful medical care, as well as the priest's request to act in the spirit of mercy, that made Dauphine consider interceding for him. Otherwise Dauphine's attitudes to physical suffering and her own infirmities presumably added to her reluctance to perform miracles *in vita*.[213] The report that she made her views about the benefits of infirmity so explicit to a

209 PC Dauphine of Puimichel, 33: 'ac eciam dicebat, et dicere consuevit, quod si gentes huius mundi considerarent quantum corporales infirmitates sunt utiles et quantum separant animum ab amore terrenorum, ipsas infirmitates corporeas, si esset possibile, in foro emerent sicut emunt res alias necessarias ad vivendum.'

210 For the varying ways in which devotees obtained the holy woman's help despite this, see Archambeau, 'God Helps Those Who Help Themselves', esp. 15-16. For saints' humility to perform cures as a counterpoint to the 'cunning folk', see Rider, *Magic and Religion*, 66-67.

211 See e.g. Philippe de Cabassole's testimony in PC Dauphine of Puimichel, 541.

212 PC Dauphine of Puimichel, 415-16.

213 Archambeau, 'God Helps Those Who Help Themselves', 14-16, 17, 23.

supplicant is indeed exceptional. In most canonization processes that portray the saintly candidate's own physical infirmity, it is discussed separately from the suffering of the devotees.[214] So, were the attitudes to physical infirmity of saints interlinked with those of others? Does hagiographic material in general tell us anything about the meaning of the benefits of infirmity in everyday life?

Pierre-André Sigal has calculated that in the miracle collections from eleventh- and twelfth-century France, women and girls are clearly under-represented as beneficiaries of a miraculous cure. He explains this by the attitudes of the time, which valued male children more than female, by the greater difficulty in getting to the shrine for women, and how their cures were a lesser preoccupation of their milieu.[215] Ronald C. Finucane has come to similar conclusions, writing that among children far more boys were beneficiaries of miracles than girls because 'in a profoundly male-dominated society, male children were valued more highly than female offspring. The greater care of boys could be seen as a passive, indirect, or attenuated form of female infanticide, or "selective neglect".'[216] Based on Sigal's calculations and reasoning, as well as those of Donald Weinstein and Rudolph M. Bell,[217] Caroline Walker Bynum concluded in an essay first published in 1989 that statistics show that medieval society perceived illnesses and impairments as something to be endured when the sufferer was a woman and as something that needed to be cured when the patient was a man.[218] She has returned to the topic more recently, this time based on a quantitative analysis of female saints' *vitae*.[219] Irina Metzler has written that there is a strong gendered difference in whether illness was to be endured or healed, but that physical conditions were seen as positive only in the case of certain (holy) women, who were considered different from the ordinary members of their communities.[220] In another study she asks what medieval people thought

214 The benefits of infirmity appear in a different context in the documents concerning St. Louis IX. In the letters addressed to his eldest son and daughter Philip and Isabella, the king broaches the question of infirmity. He writes that in the case of illness or any other adversity sent by Our Lord, the children should 'suffer it graciously and thank him and be grateful for it, because you should believe that he did it for your good'. The reason for the benefits of illness were, according to Louis, his son's possible errors, especially his failure to serve and love God sufficiently. Ashley, 'French *Enseignemenz*', 8, 19.

215 Sigal, *L'Homme et le miracle*, 259-61.

216 Finucane, *The Rescue of the Innocents*, 161.

217 Weinstein and Bell, *Saints and Society*, 234-35, calculate that of women saints, 1 in 6 suffered from a debilitating illness while the corresponding number for men was 22 of 713.

218 Bynum, *Fragmentation and Redemption*, 188-89.

219 Bynum, *Holy Feast and Holy Fast*, 189.

220 Metzler, *Disability in Medieval Europe*, 48.

about women who did seek cures, and contrasts their suffering with that of mystics such as Julian of Norwich, for whom sickness and impairment were not disabilities but facilitators towards achieving a spiritual goal.[221]

In some of these analyses, there is a source-critical problem in that miracles recorded at shrines or in canonization inquests are not statistically representative of the lived reality. While it is impossible to prove that there was no favouring of boys or men in the invocation of saints, quantitative analysis of miracle collections does not provide firm proof that there was, or, even if this were the case, that such a situation would hold true for every community and every cult. First, there is a significant variation in the sex ratios of the various collections of miracles, and in some of them, the proportion of female beneficiaries is in fact higher than that of males.[222] This is an example of the problems of using quantitative analysis in hagiographic research, if the analysis does not take into account the practicalities and preferences of individual cults and those recording and investigating the miracles. Second, certain types of miracles were favoured universally, and certain types in each process.[223] In the course of time, cures of accidents and resuscitations came to be favoured more than cures of chronic infirmities. The latter were showy and dramatic proofs of the saint's power, as well as easier to establish. Their prevalence has also been explained by the changes in the rituals. When making a *votum* or using portable relics became a common way of imploring saints in the late Middle Ages, there were more means available to invoke them in an acute situation.[224] Among the *miraculées* cured of injuries or resuscitated,

221 Metzler, 'Indiscriminate Healing Miracles', 162.

222 For example, while in St. Yves of Tréguier's process men were beneficiaries of his miraculous powers twice as often as women (this is partly due to the high number of miracles helping seafarers), Guillaume de Saint-Pathus's *Les miracles de saint Louis*, based on the lost canonization protocols, includes thirty-three male and thirty-four female beneficiaries. St. Clare of Assisi's hearing, which largely contains nuns as witnesses and reports miracles done in the monastic setting, only includes four miracles performed for boys or men, and around 60 per cent of the miracles in St. Frances of Rome's hearings were performed for girls and women.

223 As an example of this, St. Elizabeth of Hungary was venerated especially as a helper of children and, consequently, about two-thirds of the cures recorded in her inquest were done for children under the age of 15. Klaniczay, 'Proving Sanctity', 134. St. Birgitta of Sweden's canonization protocols, on the other hand, include an exceptionally high number of miraclous cures of demonic possession. For these cases, see Katajala-Peltomaa, 'Demonic Possession as Physical and Mental Disturbance'. The miracles of St. Peter Martyr include an unusually high number of punishment miracles, which the cult promoters saw as an effective tool in fighting heresy and disbelief. Prudlo, *The Martyred Inquisitor*, 147.

224 Andrić, *The Miracles of St. John Capistran*, 310; Krötzl, 'Miracles au tombeau – miracles à distance', 561-66; Vauchez, *Sainthood*, 468. See also Gentilcore, *Healers and Healing*, 194-95,

men and boys are more common, while women were more often reported to have been cured of chronic or prolonged conditions.[225] This most likely reflects the real-life situation. Men's lifestyles made them more prone to suffer various injuries,[226] and the greater tendency of male children to get hurt in accidents is recognized in modern society, and is found also in, for example, medieval coroners' rolls.[227]

Furthermore, whose miracle ended up being recorded was tightly interlinked with questions of trustworthiness. Women and girls may be statistically under-represented as *miraculées*, but so are poor people, which does not mean that they were not cured by saints as often as the wealthy, but that they were considered less trustworthy, so that their miracles required more witnesses and were considered harder to prove.[228] Men were favoured over women as witnesses for the same reason, although there are differences between various canonization processes and women were considered important witnesses in miracles done to children.[229] Therefore, the statistical analyses are most likely a reflection of the more frequent recording, and perhaps reporting, of male petitioners' cures than those of women and girls, because cures of males were valued more as proofs of saintly power. The question becomes one of emphasis in the sources, comparable to the highlighting of holy women's suffering by male hagiographers, rather than lived reality. It is very doubtful that the statistics gleaned from our sources tell us much about everyday gendered attitudes towards illness and impairment. And, at the risk of repeating myself, it is important to emphasize here that physical infirmity could be and often was a way to enable one's spiritual goal for male saints as well as female.

who writes that in the early modern Italian collections, cures of sudden conditions are more common than others in the collections with more clerical influence, while the division is much less significant in collections with less clerical influence. This is one demonstration of the impact of those selecting miracles to be recorded, as contrasted with the lived religion of the laity.

225 Craig, *Wandering Women*, 94-95; Finucane, *Miracles and Pilgrims*, 148.

226 Craig, *Wandering Women*, 94-95.

227 Finucane, *The Rescue of the Innocents*, 141-42; Hanawalt, *The Ties that Bound*, 145. In my own analysis of children's cures of prolonged physical impairments in later medieval canonization processes, the sex ratio is much more even than in all miracles done to children. Presumably it is precisely the selection of cases to be studied that has an influence here. See Kuuliala, *Childhood Disability*, 17.

228 Farmer, *Surviving Poverty*, 50-56; Goodich, *Miracles and Wonders*, 82; Krötzl, 'Prokuratoren, Notare und Dolmetscher', 122-23.

229 Golinelli, 'Social Aspects in Some Italian Canonization Trials', 170-71; Goodich, 'The Politics of Canonization', 177; Katajala-Peltomaa, *Gender, Miracles, and Daily Life*, 29, 36; Kuuliala, *Childhood Disability*, 29-30; Lett, *L'Enfant des miracles*, 32. See also p. 29 in the Introduction.

In her discussion of female saints gladly welcoming or even looking for illness and pain, Irina Metzler also writes that 'one can on no account surmise that such attitudes extended to the "everyday" illnesses, including impairments, of ordinary kinds of people, of whichever gender'.[230] This is a reasonable assumption, considering that despite all the theological messages about the benefits of pain, which most likely reached the masses, alleviating pain was preferable for the laity.[231] The physicians and writers of recipe collections also recognized the dangers of physical pain, but pain relief was usually recommended only when the pain was so severe that it threatened the patient's life.[232] At the same time, especially given the limited means of alleviating pain and treating many prolonged or chronic physical conditions, coping with pain or bodily discomfort suffered by oneself and/or by a family or community member was a profoundly human experience. It could not be marginalized or institutionalized as is often the situation in modern, western society, but it was visible to everyone and an ever-present threat to those who did not already experience it. 'Health' in premodern societies largely meant the ability to fulfil one's social role and a full cure was not necessarily the main expectation of an infirm person.[233] The concept of 'health' included a wide range of abilities, sentiments, and conditions on a line from 'excruciating pain' to 'no pain at all'. Therefore, hagiographic concepts and understanding of valorized infirmity as recorded in the case of holy men and women did not necessarily run counter to the search for the alleviation of the symptoms of illness and impairment.

It has been concluded that miracle narratives provided a means for people to make sense of traumatic experiences.[234] As a part of the hagiographic tradition and culturally internalized ideas about sainthood and suffering, that was one purpose of saints' lives as well. In consoling their infirm devotees,

230 Metzler, *Disability in Medieval Europe*, 48. See also Metzler, 'Indiscriminate Healing Miracles', 164.

231 In addition to hagiographic texts, pain and suffering were valorized by many preachers, and in the *Ars moriendi*. Cohen, *The Modulated Scream*, 32-35, 50.

232 Cohen, 'If You Prick Us, Do We Not Bleed?', 30; Cohen, *The Modulated Scream*, 87-103; Siraisi, *Medieval and Early Renaissance Medicine*, 171-72.

233 See Gentilcore, *Healers and Healing*, 186; Kuuliala, 'Heavenly Healing or Failure of Faith?'; R. Scott, *Miracle Cures*, 11-12. See also Pomata, *Contracting a Cure*, esp. 27-28, where she analyses legal contracts between a physician and his patient. The contracts state that the physician would receive a payment only when the patient was again able to perform his or her daily tasks. (In one of the cases, a full payment would be given only when the patient felt fully cured.)

234 See Gentilcore, *Healers and Healing*, 196-98; Klaniczay, 'Speaking about Miracles', 369; Smoller, 'Miracle, Memory, and Meaning', 433.

living holy men and women had a therapeutic value to their community,[235] which also holds true for the stories told about their patience and *imitatio Christi*. Although all this did not necessarily lead people to hope for an illness or infirmity,[236] saints were role models, and their lives gave people a way to explain and understand, perhaps even tolerate pain, discomfort, disability, and the threat of their occurrence.

235 The role of the saint as a mental counsellor has been examined in the case of Dauphine of Puimichel in Archambeau, 'Tempted to Kill'.

236 Examples of literary channelling of saints' attitudes towards their bodies and infirmities are sparse and rather extreme. As an example, it is known that Dorothea of Montau's mysticism and extreme asceticism influenced other people prone to similar views and behaviour, including the famous English mystic Margery Kempe. Ute Stargardt, 'The Influence of Dorothea von Montau on the Mysticism of Margery Kempe', PhD diss., University of Tennessee, Knoxville, 1981, cited in Classen, 'Wounding the Body and Freeing the Spirit', 426.

Conclusions

Infirmity, Community, and Canonization

In this book I have analysed the varying ways physical infirmity was used to delineate and prove sanctity in canonization trials by those conducting the inquests and those testifying in them. Because the corporality of late medieval sanctity and the cultural importance of *imitatio Christi* emerged and developed simultaneously with the canonization procedure itself, these concepts have been at the core of my investigations into saintly candidates' lives. Physical infirmity – be it illness or impairment causing pain, discomfort, functional restrictions, or threat of dying – was a prevalent aspect of the everyday experience of all medieval communities, but the cultural attitudes towards it were not uniform. In the testimonies of canonization inquests the veneration of saints, which was one of the key elements of late medieval lived religion, is especially entangled with cultural ideas of the beneficial sides of infirmity.

Canonization processes are juridical sources but behind them lies a lived, religious experience, which the commissioners, the cult promoters, and the witnesses interpreted in varying ways, depending on culturally internalized models, their personal preferences, and the communal memories and ways of narrating them. Temporal changes in the inquests also played some role. The first ones in the early and middle of the thirteenth century were less organized and full than the later ones, which obviously influenced the amount of detail that was recorded. Those testifying about a saint's life in detail were a specific set of people who usually belonged to the clerical or secular elite or a monastic community, and who had known the holy man or woman personally. Often they also knew each other. Therefore, their communal practices and their lived religious reality played a crucial role in the formation of the saint's *fama*, even if their narrations were remodelled and reshaped by the notaries of the inquest. Each of the inquests also had their own practicalities, which shaped the way sainthood was constructed. Partly these derived from geographical differences, especially in a sense that the holiness of Italian saints was usually investigated in more corporeal terms

Kuuliala, Jenni, *Saints, Infirmity, and Community in the Late Middle Ages.*
Taylor & Francis Group 2020
DOI: 10.5117/9789462983373_CONCL

than elsewhere. Gender played a part to some extent as well, but its role was not as crucial for individual communities of devotees as sometimes proposed by modern scholars. The suffering of especially Italian female saints has been highlighted in studies concerning late medieval hagiography. Canonization process records, however, show that the corporality of gender was varying and fluid. Although patient suffering may have become a prerequisite for female sainthood, for individual witnesses the suffering of male saints – even outside Italy – could be of crucial importance. And, at the same time, the holiness of suffering female saints had other important characteristics as well. Saints' devotees interpreted the bodily manifestations of holiness in terms of their own memories and experiences, but they are unlikely to have thought that their holy person's gender should influence what they saw or sensed, or how they interpreted it. Furthermore, it is worth emphasizing that although extreme imitation of Christ's passion was primarily a female phenomenon, as such it was a positive characteristic of the feminine.

Infirmity had several functions in the investigation and proof of a person's holiness. The start of a putative saint's 'career' was a key point when it could be presented as playing an important role. Although conversion prompted by infirmity is a hagiographic trope up to a point, it does not come up in the *inquisitiones in partibus* analysed in this study. This is in accordance with the lessening importance of such narratives for official sanctity. Instead, infirmity could induce another type of action which led to the path that later defined a person's sainthood; St. Louis IX of France taking the cross when lying ill is a textbook example. For some of the married female saints, infirmity played a major role in their attempts to secure a celibate marriage or as a proof of their reluctance to have any sexual encounter. They and their devotees could interpret a bout of ill health as a God-sent event that justified and explained their position as married women.

Almost all later medieval canonization inquiries specifically investigated the holy person's *patientia*, and infirmity was usually among the tribulations saints reportedly faced. There are nevertheless big differences in the emphases and definitions these infirmities were given in the articles and by different witnesses. Here different aspects of sanctity and the canonization inquest came into play. Cult promoters and procurators selected the aspects of the holy person's life to be specifically investigated, and their choices guided the witnesses as well. The saint's gender and especially the type of sainthood and situation in life played a big part. Typically, the sanctity of male hermits and religious women was constructed in the most corporeal terms, but even here the categorizations are not watertight. A male saint's holiness could be highlighted and reminisced in terms of his physical suffering, of which St. Louis IX is the most illuminating example, while those conducting the hearing of a cloistered nun, such as St. Margaret of Hungary, did not necessarily investigate their long-term infirmities, even if they were among the memories the witnesses reported.[1]

Furthermore, cult promoters, commissioners, and witnesses occasionally had differing views of the meanings of infirmity, and the commissioners were most keen to categorize the infirmity in question when it was necessary to discern its spiritual origins. This is clearly visible in the inquest of St. Nicholas of Tolentino, where those conducting the process were much keener than the witnesses to investigate his suffering in relation to his battles with the devil. For the devotees, his infirmity was a visible aspect of their interaction with the holy man, and one they primarily used to highlight his humility and willingness to attend the Mass. The other instances where such definitions were of crucial importance were raptures and other mystic experiences – in the sources of this study experienced by female saints. Their devotees primarily interpreted them by corporeal marks that were part of a religious experience, but when asked to do so by the inquisitors, they were also able to interpret them in medical terms and to separate them from somatic conditions. Although these doubts primarily appear as a phenomenon attached to holy women, St. Elzéar of Sabran's example, albeit from a *vita* and not a canonization inquest, shows that such negotiations also occurred in cases of male saints.

Other types of infirmities that the saints endured were very rarely subject to any diagnosis; even if a specific medical term was given, it was not emphasized. This is one example of the way the medicalization of society worked in the late Middle Ages. In the inquiries into saints' lives, medical terminology and precision was used when it served a clear inquisitorial purpose, but corporeal forms of religious experience and sainthood were not subordinate to it. The witnesses usually simply stated that the saint had an *infirmitas*, and for them and for the commissioners it was crucial to find out what her or his reactions towards it were. Even the symptoms were only sporadically recorded. Pain was mentioned as a specifically defined symptom surprisingly rarely, and the witnesses mention a saint as having problems in walking only occasionally. It is possible that there was no need for further specification, because the consequences and symptoms were inbuilt in holy *infirmitas*. Infirmity thus served mainly as a tool for proving

1 There even emerged reports of her alleged stigmatization in the mid- and late fourteenth century The fame of these *stigmata* was, however, short-lived. The topic is covered in Klaniczay, 'On the Stigmatization of Saint Margaret of Hungary'.

and reconstructing *patientia* and every now and then other key elements of a holy person's *fama sanctitatis*.

Gender and the saint's social position intermingle with the witnesses' lived experience in the testimonies about holy infirmities. Especially in the case of the military leaders Louis IX of France and Charles of Blois, the defeats during which the future saints became ill or were injured must have been long-term, striking memories for the witnesses who took part in these campaigns. For them, reminiscing about the holy men's suffering may have provided a way to make sense of a military fiasco, especially as these men's injuries were easily interpreted as Christlike sacrifices for the sake of their community or Christendom. At the same time, infirmity suffered as a crusader was easier to incorporate into the official *fama*. A shared corporeal religious experience in which a saint's infirm body and *patientia* played a role is detectable in the communities of religious women. They observed 'their' saint's *imitatio Christi*, raptures, and patience from close proximity, often quite literally participating in these activities. This holds true also for the male saints who belonged to monastic orders and/or were known hermits. The members of their Orders and others observing their asceticism and corporal endurance were included in their devotional sphere, where they could become part of their religious practice or at least be moved to admire and wonder at it. The suffering saints can thus be interpreted as intermediators between the passion of Christ and the devotees, providing a tool for taking part in affective veneration.

Patientia was also associated with the suffering of a saint's family – this, obviously, mainly pertaining to lay saints, and usually to women. Although these kinds of topics were rarely investigated in canonization inquests, when they were, they were among those that place the actions of the saintly figure most clearly within their communities. Despite – or perhaps because – of her uniqueness as a societally active saintly laywoman,[2] Frances of Rome's *patientia* in taking care of her infirm husband at the time when the city of Rome was going through a tumultuous period in its history is particularly telling. A person with a holy reputation could be a role model and a source of comfort in coping with a situation that could occur anywhere: the infirmity of a family member.

Infirmity played a key role in the inquests regarding a putative saint's pentitential practices. Asceticism, austerity, and to an extent devotion,

2 See Esch, 'I processi medioevali', 48-51, who attributes the failure of Frances of Rome's canonization to her nonconformity as a saint. This nonconformity was, however, mostly related to her active role as a laywoman.

were acts that were crucial for a *fama sanctitatis* on the one hand and easily considered imprudent on the other. While virtually every saint had to be shown to have lived an ascetic life, *discretio* was valued and lack of it considered harmful for the cause. As saints always performed and put their holiness into practice in relation to a community, the community also had its say in their ascetic practices. In all these activities, infirmity served as a border or a tool that delineated harmful self-discipline. Saints might be reported as having tormented their bodies with fasting, harsh sleeping conditions, and the use of a hair shirt, but the witnesses were aware that it was not proper to do this to such an extent that it caused permanent or excessive infirmity. Herein also lies a contradiction, since it was precisely the ability to endure rigorous asceticism and penitence without obtaining infirmity that made saints' bodies extraordinary and different from those of their devotees. This contradiction demonstrates the fluidity of conceptions of austerity and infirmity; they had to be renegotiated under each individual saint, most likely over and over again, and this need for renegotiation continued into the canonization inquest.

Quite a large array of elite community members or servants could partake in the negotiations concerning a holy person's austerity and self-discipline, and the reminiscing about their role later was undoubtedly also a way for these people to enhance their own social position. However, actual regulation was mainly reserved for confessors, (religious) superiors, and physicians, and the witnesses used these persons' actions to prove both the holy person's firmness in their asceticism and their discretion. The role of confessors was especially emphasized in the lives of female saints, but there are references to their regulatory role in the documents concerning some male saints' lives as well. Other religious superiors – abbesses, priors, or even the pope – could also regulate austerity out of fear of the infirmity it might cause. In the case of prelates, one of the pronounced reasons for these fears was the effect of austerity on the holy person's ability to function in their office, which shows that the concern had practical implications as well, and only became a problem when it caused an impediment, or even a disability. Often these leading figures teamed up with physicians, whose role in the inquiries was not just to testify about putative saints' lives but to give scientific, medical background to their lifestyles and their corporeal manifestations and consequences. Even a ruler like Charles of Blois, the duke of Brittany, could not escape the physician's orders, especially when he acted in concert with his confessor.

Self-discipline, particularly fasting, is one of the aspects of saints' corporality that earlier researchers have interpreted as the most gender-specific. Most of the depositions that heavily emphasize a holy person's austerity and its bodily consequences concern female saints' lives. However, in comparison with many of those (female) saints and mystics in whose *vitae* extreme austerity and painful experiences play a significant role, the picture given in canonization inquests and in the *vitae* of many female saints for whom a canonization inquest was opened was usually more conventional. It must be noted, however, that there are male saints in whose cases these experiences are highlighted, eremitical saints being the most obvious examples, as their sainthood was more corporeal than that of other male saints. Compared with royal and clerical male saints, they were usually from a relatively low-status background, which may also have made them more corporeal in the eyes of their devotees and hagiographers. At the same time, there are female saints in whose processes the witnesses and clearly also the commissioners primarily focused on other things, even in the course of reporting severe austerity and self-discipline. Therefore, even though asceticism and especially fasting to the point of self-torture was generally associated with female saints, when we look at an individual saint's community and an individual process, the role of gender was not carved in stone, but the type of sanctity had influence as well. Furthermore, the general trend of emphasizing female saints' austerity – or the tendency of female saints to practise it for religio-cultural reasons – did not need to have a big impact on the ways devotees of an individual saint interpreted their corporality.

The witnesses in a majority of the testimonies in canonization inquests referred to a holy person's infirmity precisely when asked to testify about their patience and penitence. There are, however, other types of testimonies here and there in the dossiers which demonstrate that the role of infirmity in performing and reconstructing sanctity could acquire meanings outside those parameters. When a saint performed their public role as a benefactor, as a devoted ruler, as a healer, or as a religious role model and counsellor, their infirmity could underline the significance of these actions. A saint who was hardly able to walk and still came to meet his or her sick devotees, perhaps to settle their quarrels, or who performed a religious act such as attending a Mass or making a pilgrimage with great physical difficulty was seen – and perhaps also consciously emphasized – as an example of the willingness to suffer for their community. This held true for male and female saints alike. In a similar way, visiting the *infirmi* could also have been considered dangerous to a saint, especially given the risk of contagion; in respect of the hazards involved, these visits resembled the practices of austerity, but here the extravagant charity – or the generosity shown to repugnant *infirmi* – was primarily reserved for female saints. Saintly figures were suffering for the benefit of whole Christendom. The devotees who witnessed these situations also discussed saintly figures' bodily states, at least whether they were considered fatal or not, and these negotiations could, in turn, be used in the inquest to highlight the holy men and women's prophetic abilities and acceptance of their suffering.

In the canonization documents, the bodies of the saints and the bodies of the infirm are usually treated separately, as two completely different aspects of sainthood. Here the hearing of St. Frances of Rome makes an exception. The articles specifically state that she refused medicine for herself but gave it to infirm community members, not expecting the same from them as she gave to them. Medicine itself was generally considered a gift from God and not bad per se, and at least in St. Frances's case the refusal to take it was primarily connected with her unwillingness to indulge in any comforts. At the same time, refusal to accept physicians' assistance and succumbing to God's will were frequently reported as a sign of a saint's austerity as well as of their trust in God. As shown by the testimony of the notary Berardus Appillaterre in Nicholas of Tolentino's hearing, even here the (elite) community members could have a delineating role, aiming at control over the saint's body. All in all, the witnesses referred to physicians to prove varying points – in the case of female saints, it could be proof of virginity and chastity. Geography played a role here as well, just as in miracle depositions. The varying meanings given to secular medicine appear much more frequently in the southern European inquests, for the obvious reason that it was more regularly used in the areas where educated physicians were commonly available.

A more complicated question is that of the relationship between the valourization and significance of saints' infirmities and those of other community members not considered 'holy'. Of our saints, Dauphine of Puimichel reportedly stated that if people knew how beneficial infirmities were for one's soul, they would buy them from a marketplace if possible, and medieval literature is full of examples of praise for the benefits of infirmity and pain. Some holy figures even prayed to suffer from them. Even an infirmity considered to have a mundane origin could be used as a way of penance and *imitatio Christi*. Laypeople, on the other hand, most certainly sought to alleviate pain by the available means, whether spiritual or mundane. There have been some attempts in earlier research, mainly based on hagiographic sources, to show that in medieval society pain and discomfort were considered something that women should endure whereas men could more readily seek help. My own reading of these sources does not support this view, however, especially given the source-critical issues that arise in quantitative analysis. Whether the ailing layperson was a man or a woman, a boy or a girl, the knowledge of saintly characters' ailments and their positive connotations most likely had a therapeutic function. Although this knowledge may not have enabled laypeople to accept pain willingly or persuaded them to stop treating it, it gave a meaning and explanation for physical suffering, which was unavoidable in the lives of the great majority of medieval people.

In the introduction to this book I wrote that of the various proposed disability theories, my study is mostly applicable to the 'cultural history of dis/ability'. But can we find 'disability' in the depositions about saints' infirmities? The many different ways in which *infirmitas* was used to reconstruct patience clearly demonstrate the fluidity of medieval categorizations of 'illness' and 'impairment'. Their uses and roles in the investigations into saints' lives illustrate this variability in meaning well. With a caveat, perhaps, and if we think of the term in the spectrum from ability to disability. At least in hagiographic sources, the infirmity, or some kind of bodily 'condition' of laypeople, became a disability that needed a cure when it prevented the person from fulfilling their social role, and/or caused unbearable discomfort and distress. In the case of saints, infirmity was reported, investigated, and highlighted when it enhanced the fulfilling of their role as saints and occasionally in other religious roles like that of bishop as well. Often their infirmities were not very different from those of other humans, and they could occasionally render the holy person unable to take care of their earthly duties, but their behaviour while suffering gave specific meaning to the condition itself.

The mechanisms and negotiations that determined the kinds of meanings given to saints' infirmities depended to varying degrees on the saint's position in society, including their status and gender and up to a point their geographic origin, as well as the preferences of their communities and those conducting the canonization inquest. A saint's *fama* was formed, reminisced about, and negotiated within a community of devotees, which can also be seen as an emotional community, where emotions and sentiments played an important role in formulating a saintly reputation. This community was not, however, comprehensive, as only a fraction of an individual saint's following of devotees was given the chance to express their views in front of the inquisitorial committee, and voices of doubt were very rarely recorded. General views of what constituted a holy life were internalized, but these ideas were put into practice in varying manners, formulated in the interaction between the witnesses and the conductors of the inquest. Most of those who testified in detail about a saint's life had lived in their monastery or household, and for them the matter held clear personal significance. In their narrations, infirmity and suffering, which were a profound part of human experience and crucial in late medieval religion, were a tool for the saints and their communities to regulate and demonstrate holiness, just as it was often a way for the divine to manifest itself on earth.

Bibliography

Manuscripts

Vatican City, Archivio Apostolico Vaticano

MS Archivum Arcis, Arm. 1, XVIII, 3328: *Processus canonizationis b. Laurentii Sublacensis, eum copia eiusdem et reliquis ut in inventaris.*

Vatican City, Biblioteca Apostolica Vaticana

MS Vat. lat. 4015: *Inquisitio de fide, vita et moribus et fama et miraculis recolende memorie domine Thome de Cantilupo quondam episcope dicte ecclesie Herefordensis.*

MS Vat. lat. 4019: *Testes super uita et conuersatione Philippi quondam Bituricensis archiepiscopo.*

MS Vat. lat. 4020: *Rubrica examinis canonizationis Philippi archiepiscopi Bituricensis.*

MS Vat. lat. 4025: *Liber canonizationis dominis Karoli ducis Bretanie.*

MS Vat. lat. 4027: *Rubrice examinationis et recollectionis sumpte de processu inquisitione miraculis et arcestati omnibus habitis et receptis super vita conversatione et miraculis recolende memorie Nicholai de Tolentino ordinis heremitarum sancti Augustiniani Cameriensis diocese et relatio super hiis et relatio processus.*

Paris, Bibliothèque nationale de France

MS Fr. 2829: *Le livre des faiz monseigneur saint Loys, composé à la requête du cardinal de Bourbon et de la duchesse de Bourbonnois.*

Printed Sources

Acta et processus canonizacionis beate Birgitte, ed. Isaac Collijn (Uppsala: Samlingar utgivna av Svenska Fornskrift, 1924-30).

Acta sanctorum quotquot toto orbe coluntur vel a catholicis scribtoribus celebrantur, ed. Société des Bollandistes, vols. 1-68 (Brussels/Antwerp: Société des Bollandistes, 1863-87), citations from Acta Sanctorum Database, Chadwyck-Healey, Cambridge, 2000.

'Acta Francisca Romana vidua, Fundatrix Oblatarum Turris-speculorum Romae (s.)', *AASS*, Mar. II, pp. 92-176.

'Processus apostolici, de b. Joanne Buono', *AASS*, Oct. IX, pp. 771-886.

'Processus canonizacionis b. Ambrosii Massani', *AASS*, Nov. IV, pp. 571-886.

'Processus de vita & miraculis b. Petri de Luxemburgo, duobus annis cum dimidio a beati obitu formatum', *AASS*, Iul. I, pp. 527-607.

'Processus informativus pro canonizatione d. Mariae de Maillye', *AASS*, Mar. III, pp. 747-65.

'Proemium ad processus in causa canonizationis b. Joannis Boni confectos', *AASS*, Oct. IX, pp. 768-71.

'Vita, Aemiliana seu Humiliana, vidua Florentie tertii ordinis s. Francisci (b.)', *AASS*, Maii IV, pp. 386-401.

'Vita, auctore Ambrosio Calepino, ordinis eremitarum s. Augustini', *AASS*, Oct. IX, pp. 748-67

'Vita b. Augustini novelli ord. erem.', *AASS*, Maii IV, pp. 616-26.

'Vita b. Dorotheae Lindana', *AASS*, Oct. XIII, pp. 499-560.

'Vita, Catharina Suedica, filia s. Brigittae, Vastenae in Suecia (s.)', *AASS*, Mar. III, pp. 505-19.

'Vita, Elisabetha regina Portugalliae (s.)', *AASS*, Jul. II, pp. 173-97.

'Vita gallice scripta per Agnetem de Harcourt abbatissam de Longi-Campi, et Latine reddita interprete J.S.', *AASS*, Aug. VI, pp. 798-808.

'Vita, Guilielmus archiepiscopus Bituricensis, in Gallia (s.)', *AASS*, Ian. I, pp. 628-36.

'Vita, Hugo episcopus Gratianopolitanus, in Gallia (s.)', *AASS*, Apr. I, pp. 37-46.

'Vita, Ludovicus Francorum rex, prope Tunetum in Africa (s.)', *AASS*, Aug. V, pp. 541-58.

'Vita, Margarita Hungarica, virgo ordinis praedicat (b.)', *AASS*, Jan. II, 900-6.

'Vita, Nicolaus Tolentinas, ord. eremitarum s. Augustini Tolentini in Piceno (s.)', *AASS*, Sept. X, pp. 644-64.

'Vita, Petrus de Luxemburgo S.R.E. cardinalis, episcopus metensis, Avenione in Gallia (b)', *AASS*, Iul. I, pp. 509-16.

'Vita s. Elzearii de Sabrano, conf.', *AASS*, Sept. VII, pp. 576-94.

'Vita s. Vincenti Ferrerii', *AASS*, Apr. I, pp. 484-512.

Benedict XIV [Prospero Lambertini], *De servorum Dei beatificatione et beatorum canonizatione*, in *Opera omnia*, III, app. 4 (Prato, 1840), pp. 662-93.

Chronique de Richard Lescot: religieux de Saint-Denis (1328-1344) suivie de la continuation de cette chronique (1344-1364), ed. Jean Lemoine (Paris: Librairie Renouard, 1896).

The Confessions of St. Augustine, trans. J. G. Pilkington (Altenmünster: Jazzybee, 2012).

Conrad of Marburg, *Summa vitae*, in *The Life and Afterlife of St. Elizabeth of Hungary: Testimony from her Canonization Hearings*, ed. and trans. Kenneth Baxter Wolf (Oxford: Oxford University Press, 2010), pp. 91-96.

Déposition de Charles d'Anjou pour la canonisation de saint Louis, ed. M. le comte Riant, in *Notices et documents publiés pour la Société de l'histoire de France à l'occasion du cinquantième anniversaire de sa foundation*, ed. Ch. Jourdain (Paris: Renouard, 1884), pp. 155-76.

Dicta quatuor ancillarum, in *The Life and Afterlife of St. Elizabeth of Hungary: Testimony from her Canonization Hearings*, ed. and trans. Kenneth Baxter Wolf (Oxford: Oxford University Press, 2010), pp. 193-216.

Die Akten des Kanonisationsprozess Dorotheas von Montau, ed. Richard Stachnik, with Anneliese Triller and Hans Westpfal (Vienna/Cologne: Böhlau, 1978).

Die Akten des Kanonisationsprozess in dem Codex zu Sulmona, in *Monumenta Coelestiniana: Quellen zur Geschichte des Papstes Coelestin V*, ed. Franz Xaver Seppelt, Quellen und Forschungen aus dem Gebiete der Geschichte 19 (Paderborn: F. Schöningh, 1921), pp. 211-331.

Die ältesten Viten Papst Cölestins V. (Peters vom Morrone), ed. Peter Herde, Monumenta Germaniae Historica: Scriptores rerum Germanicarum, n.s., 23 (Hannover: Monumenta Germaniae Historica, 2009), pp. 101-222.

Enquête pour le procès de canonisation de Dauphine de Puimichel Comtesse d'Ariano, Apt et Avignon, 14 mai-30 octobre 1363: édition critique, ed. Jacques Cambell (Turin: Bottega d'Erasmo, 1978).

Fragments de l'enquête faite à Saint-Denis en 1282 en vue de la canonisation de Saint Louis, ed. H.-F. Delaborde, *Mémoires de la Société de l'histoire de Paris de l'Ile-de-France*, 23 (1896): 1-71.

'Geoffrey of Beaulieu's *Life and Saintly Comportment of Louis, Former King of Franks, of Pious Memory*', in *The Sanctity of Louis*, IX: *Early Lives of Saint Louis by Geoffrey of Beaulieu and William of Chartres*, trans. Larry F. Field, ed. M. Cecilia Gaposchkin and Sean L. Field (Ithaca/London: Cornell University Press, 2013), pp. 69-128.

Gerson, Jean, *On Distinguishing True from False Revelations*, in *Jean Gerson: Early Works*, ed. and trans. Bernard McGinn (New York/Mahwah: Paulist Press, 1998), pp. 334-64.

Guillaume de Nangis, *Vie et vertus de Saint Louis*, ed. René de Lespinasse (Paris: Librairie de la société de bibliographique, 1877).

Guillaume de Saint-Pathus, *Les miracles de saint Louis*, ed. Percival B. Fay (Paris: Librairie Ancienne Honoré Champion, 1931).

—, *Vie de saint Louis*, ed. H.-F. Delaborde (Paris: Alphonse Picard et Fils, 1899).

I processi inediti per Francesca Bussa dei Ponziani (Santa Francesca Romana) 1440-1453, ed. Placido Tommaso Lugano, Studi e Testi 120 (Vatican City: Biblioteca Apostolica Vaticana, 1945).

Il processo Castellano con appendice di documenti sul culto e la canonizzazione di s. Caterina da Siena, ed. M.-H. Laurent (Milan: F.lli Bocca, 1942).

Il processo di canonizzazione di Bernardino da Siena (1445-1450), ed. Letizia Pellegrini, Analecta Franciscana, XVI, n.s., Documenta et Studia 4 (Grottaferrata: Frati editori di Quaracchi, 2009).

Il processo di canonizzazione di Celestino V, I-II, ed. Alessandra Bartolomei Romagnoli and Alfonso Marini (Florence: Sismel, 2015)

Il processo di canonizzazione di Chiara da Montefalco, ed. Enrico Menestò, Quaderni del Centro per il collegamento degli studi medievali e umanistici nell'Università di Perugia (Florence/Perugia: La Nuova Italia, 1984).

Il processo per la canonizzazione di s. Nicola da Tolentino, ed. Nicola Occhioni, Collection de l'Ecole française de Rome 74 (Rome: École française de Rome, 1984).

Jean de Joinville, *Histoire de saint Louis*, ed. Natalis de Vailly (Paris: Librairie de Firmin Didot Frères, Fils et Cie, 1874).

Johannes Matteotti, *Vita s. Francesca Romana*; *Tractatus de visionibus; Tractatus de conflictibus*, in *Santa Francesca Romana: edizione critica dei trattati latini di Giovanni Mattiotti*, ed. Alessandra Bartolomei Romagnoli (Vatican City: Libreria Editrice Vaticana, 1994), pp. 319-812.

Julian of Norwich, *Revelations of Divine Love*. Translated from British Library Additional MS 37790, ed. and trans. by Frances Beer (Cambridge: DS Brewer, 1998).

Legenda vetus: acta processus canonizationis et Miracula sanctae Margaritae de Hungaria/The Oldest Legend: Acts of the Canonization Process, and Miracles of Saint Margaret of Hungary, ed. Ildikó Csepregi, Gábor Klaniczay, and Bence Péterfi, trans. Ildikó Csepregi, Clifford Flanigan, and Louis Perraud (Budapest: Central European University Press, 2018).

Les grandes chroniques de France, ed. Jules Viard, 10 vols. (Paris: Libraire Ancienne Honoré Champion, 1920-53), IX (1937).

'Le sommaire de l'enquete pour la canonisation de s. Elzear de Sabran, TOF (d. 1323)', ed. Jacques Cambell, *Miscellanea Francescana*, 73 (1973): 438-73.

McNamer, Sarah, 'The Middle-English Version of Jacques de Vitry's *Life of St. Marie d'Oignies*', in *Medieval Hagiography: An Anthology*, ed. Thomas F. Head (New York/London: Routledge, 2000), pp. 709-28.

Matthew Paris, *Chronica Majora*, ed. Henry Richards Luard, 7 vols. (London: Longman & Co., 1872-83), V (1880).

Matthew Paris's English History, ed. and trans. J.A. Giles, 2 vols. (London: Henry G. Bohn, 1852-1853), II (1853).

Miracula sancti Stanislai, ed. Wojciech Kętrzyński, in *Monumenta Poloniae historica*, IV (Lviv: Nakł. Akademii Umiejętności, 1884), pp. 238-318.

'The *Miracoli* of Catherine of Siena', ed. and trans. Maiju Lehmijoki-Gardner, in *Dominican Penitent Women*, ed. Maiju Lehmijoki-Gardner, Classics of Western Spirituality: A Library of the Great Spiritual Masters (New York: Paulist Press, 2005), pp. 87-104.

Monuments du procès de canonisation du bienheureux Charles de Blois, duc de Bretagne, 1320-1364, ed. A. de Sérent (Saint-Brieuc: Imprimerie de Prud'homme, 1921).

The Passion of St. Lawrence: Epigrams and Marginal Poems, ed. Jan M. Ziolkowski (Leiden: Brill, 1994).

Patrologiae cursus completus: series latina, ed. Jacques-Paul Migne, 221 vols. (Paris: Migne, 1844-64).

Procès de la canonisation de saint Vincent Ferrier pour faire suite à l'histoire du même saint, ed. P.-H. Fages (Paris: A. Picard, 1904).

Processus canonizationis s. Dominici, ed. A. Waltz, *Monumenta Ordinis fratrum praedicatorum historica*, 16 (1935): 88-194.

Processus canonizationis s. Ludovici ep. Tolosani, in *Analecta Franciscana sive chronica aliaque varia documenta*, VII: *Processus canonizationis et legendae variae sancti Ludovici O.F.M. episcopi Tolosani*, ed. Collegio S. Bonaventura (Florence: Ad Claras Aquas, 1951), pp. 1-269.

Processus canonizationis s. Thomae, Neapoli, fasc. 4 of *Fontes vitae s. Thomae Aquinatis 1-4*, ed. M.-H. Laurent (Saint-Maximin: Revue Thomiste, 1911).

Processus de vita et miraculis sancti Yvonis, in *Monuments originaux de l'histoire de saint Yves*, ed. A. de La Borderie, J. Daniel, R. P. Perquis, and D. Tempier (Saint-Brieuc: Imprimerie L. Prud'homme, 1887), pp. 1-299.

Processus seu negocium canonizacionis b. Katerine de Vadstenis: efter Cod. Holm. A 93, ed. Isaak Collijn, *Samlingar utgivna av Svenska Fornskriftsäilskapet*, ser. 2, 3 (Uppsala, 1942-46).

Quellenstudien zur Geschichte der hl. Elisabeth: Landgräfin von Thüringen, ed. Albert Huyskens (Marburg: Elwert, 1908).

The Revelations of St. Birgitta of Sweden, ed. and trans. Denis Searby and Bridget Morris, 4 vols. (Oxford: Oxford University Press, 2006-2015), III, *Liber caelestis*, bks. 6-7 (2012).

Sacrorum conciliorum nova et amplissima collectio, ed. Johannes Dominicus Mansi, 53 vols. (Venice, 1692-1769), XXII (1778).

Santa Chiara di Assisi: i primi documenti ufficiali; lettera di annunzio della sua morte, processo e bolla di canonizzazione, ed. Giovanni Boccali (Santa Maria degli Angeli: Edizioni Porziuncola, 2002).

Thomas of Siena, 'The *Libellus* concerning Catherine of Siena (Part One)', ed. and trans. Maiju Lehmijoki-Gardner, in *Dominican Penitent Women*, Classics of Western Spirituality: A Library of the Great Spiritual Masters, ed. Maiju Lehmijoki-Gardner (New York: Paulist Press, 2005), pp. 177-91.

Tommaso di Celano, *Vita prima*, in *Analecta Franciscana*, X: *Legendae s. Francisci Assisiensis: saeculis XIII et XIV conscriptae*, ed. Collegio S. Bonaventura (Florence: Ad Claras Aquas, 1926).

Vie de s. Auzias, comte d'Ariano, in *Vies occitanes de saint Auzias e de sainte Dauphine, avec traduction française, introduction et notes*, ed. Jacques Cambell, Bibliotheca Pontificii Athenaei Antoniani 12 (Rome: Ponficium Athenaeum Antonianum, 1963), pp. 41-127.

Vie de Ste Dauphine, comtesse d'Ariano, in *Vies occitanes de saint Auzias e de sainte Dauphine avec traduction française, introduction et notes*, ed. Jacques Cambell, Bibliotheca Pontificii Athenaei Antoniani 12 (Rome: Ponficium Athenaeum Antonianum, 1963), pp. 129-246.

Vies occitanes de saint Auzias e de sainte Dauphine avec traduction française, introduction et notes, ed. Jacques Cambell, Bibliotheca Pontificii Athenaei Antoniani 12 (Rome: Ponficium Athenaeum Antonianum, 1963).
Vita beatae Margaritae virginis de Civitate Castelli, ed. A. Poncelet, *Analecta Bollandiana*, 19 (1900): 23-36.
Vita Margaritae de Città de Castello, in *La plus ancienne légend de la b. Marguerite de Città di Castello*, ed. M.-H. Laurent, special issue of *Archivum Fratrum Praedicatorum*, 10 (1940): 109-41.
Vita s. Brynolphi episc. Scarensis, com processu euis canonizationis, ed. C. Annerstedt, *Scriptores rerum svecicarum medii aevi*, III (Uppsala, 1876).
Vita s. Philippi archiepiscopi Bituricensis, in *Thesaurus novus anecdotorum*, III: *Complectens chronica varia aliaque cùm ecclesiastica tùm civilia omnium pene nationum monumenta historica*, ed. Edmond Martene and Ursin Durand (Lutetiae Parisiorum, 1717), cols. 1927-46.
Vita sanctae Clarae de Cruce, ordinis eremitarum s. Augustini: ex Codice Montefalconensi saeculi XIV desumpta, ed. P. Alfonsus Semenza (Vatican City: Typis Polyglottis Vaticanis, 1944).
The Writings of Agnes of Harcourt: The Life of Isabelle of France and the Letter of Louis IX and Longchamp, ed. and trans. Sean L. Field (Notre Dame, IN: University of Notre Dame Press, 2003).

Literature

Adams, Gwenfair Walters, *Visions in Late Medieval England: Lay Spirituality and Sacred Glimpses of the Hidden Worlds of Faith* (Leiden: Brill, 2007).
Adams, Jonathan, *The Revelations of St. Birgitta: A Study and Edition of the Birgittine-Norwegian Texts, Swedish National Archives, E 8902* (Leiden: Brill, 2015).
Allmand, Christopher, *The Hundred Years War: England and France at War c.1300-c.1450* (Cambridge: Cambridge University Press, 1989).
Andenna, Cristina, 'Women at the Angevin Court between Naples and Provence: Sancia of Majorca, Delphine of Puimichel, and the "Struggle" for a Female Franciscan Life', in *Queens, Princesses and Mendicants: Close Relations in a European Perspective*, ed. Nikolas Jaspert (Münster: LIT, 2019), pp. 29-52.
Andrić, Stanko, *The Miracles of St. John Capistran* (Budapest: Central European University Press, 2000),
Archambeau, Nicole, 'God Helps Those Who Help Themselves: Negotiating a Miracle in Fourteenth Century Provence', *Anuario de Estudios Medievales*, 43 (2013): 7-25
—, 'Healing Options during the Plague: Survivor Stories from a Fourteenth-Century Canonization Inquest', *Bulletin of the History of Medicine*, 85 (2011): 531-59.

—, 'Remembering Countess Delphine's Books: Reading as a Means to Shape a Holy Woman's Sanctity', in *Writing Medieval Women's Lives*, ed. C. Goldy and A. Livingstone (New York: Palgrave Macmillan, 2012), pp. 33-49.

—, 'Tempted to Kill: Miraculous Consolation for a Mother after the Death of her Infant Daughter', in *Emotions and Health, 1200-1700*, ed. Elena Carrera (Leiden: Brill, 2013), pp. 47-66.

Armstrong, Regis J., ed. and trans., *The Lady: Clare of Assisi; Early Documents* (New York: New City Press, 2006).

Arnold, John H., *Belief and Unbelief in Medieval Europe* (London: Hodder Education, 2005).

—, 'Histories and Historiographies of Medieval Christianity', in *The Oxford Handbook of Medieval Christianity*, ed. John H. Arnold (Oxford: Oxford University Press, 2014), pp. 23-41.

Ashley, Kathleen, 'The French *Enseignemenz a Phelippe* and *Enseignement a Ysabel* of Saint Louis', in *Medieval Conduct Literature: An anthology of Vernacular Guides to Behaviour for Youths, with English Translations*, ed. Kathleen M. Ashley and Mark David Johnston (Toronto: University of Toronto Press, 2009), pp. 3-22.

Atkinson, Clarissa W., *The Oldest Vocation: Christian Motherhood in the Middle Ages* (Ithaca/London: Cornell University Press, 1994).

Barone, Giulia, 'Il processo di canonizzazione di Chiara da Montefalco', in *Santa Chiara da Montefalco monaca agostiniana (1268-1308) nel contesto socio-religioso femminile dei secoli XIII-XIV*, ed. Enrico Menestò (Spoleto: Fondazione Centro italiano di studi sull'alto medioevo, 2009), pp. 181-92.

Barr, Beth Allison, *The Pastoral Care of Women in Medieval England* (Woodbridge: Boydell Press, 2008).

Bartlett, Robert, *The Hanged Man: A Story of Miracle, Memory, and Colonialism in the Middle Ages* (Princeton: Princeton University Press, 2006 [2004]).

—, *Why Can the Dead Do Such Great Things?: Saints and Worshippers from the Martyrs to the Reformation* (Princeton: Princeton University Press, 2013).

Bartolomei Romagnoli, Alessandra, 'Vita di santa Francesca Romana', in *Santa Francesca Romana: edizione critica dei trattati latini di Giovanni Mattiotti*, ed. Alessandra Bartolomei Romagnoli (Vatican City: Libreria Editrice Vaticana, 1994), pp. 59-138.

—, ed., *Francesca Romana: la santa, il monastero e la città alla fine del Medioevo* (Florence: Tavernuzze, 2009).

—, and Giorgio Picasso, eds., *La canonizzazione di santa Francesca Romana: santità, cultura e istituzioni a Roma tra medioevo ed età moderna* (Florence: Edizione del Galluzzo per la fondazione Ezio Franceschini, 2013).

Bejczy, István P., 'The *sacra infantia* in Medieval Hagiography', *in The Church and Childhood: Papers Read at the 1993 Summer Meeting and the 1994 Winter Meeting of the Ecclesiastical History Society*, ed. Diana Wood (Oxford: Ecclesiastical History Society, 1994), pp. 143-51.

Bell, Rudolf M., *Holy Anorexia* (Chicago/London: University of Chicago Press, 1987 [1985]).

Black, Rhonda and Lori Pretes, 'Victims and Victors: Representation of Physical Disability on the Silver Screen', *Research and Practice for Persons with Severe Disabilities*, 32 (2007): 66-83.

Blumenfeld-Kosinski, Renate, *Poets, Saints, and Visionaries of the Great Schism, 1378-1417* (Philadelphia: Penn State Press, 2010).

—, and Timea Szell, eds., *Images of Sainthood in Medieval Europe* (Ithaca/London: Cornell University Press, 1991).

Boanas, Guy and Lyndal Roper, 'Feminine Piety in Fifteenth-Century Rome: Santa Francesca Romana', in *Disciplines of Faith: Studies in Religion, Politics and Patriarchy*, ed. James Obelkevich and Lyndal Roper (London/New York: Routledge, 2006 [1987]), pp. 177-93.

Bodawré, Katrinette, 'Abbesses', in *Women and Gender in Medieval Europe: An Encyclopedia*, ed. Margaret Schaus (London/New York: Routledge, 2006), pp. 1-4.

Boddice, Rob, ed., *Pain and Emotion in Modern History* (Basingstoke: Palgrave Macmillan, 2014).

Bolton, Brenda M., '*Vita ascetica:* A Papal Quandary', in *Monks, Hermits and the Ascetic Tradition. Papers Read at the 1984 Summer Meeting and the 1985 Winter Meeting of the Ecclesiastical History Society*, ed. W. J. Sheils (Padstow: Basil Blackwell, 1985).

Boquet, Damien and Piroska Nagy, *Medieval Sensibilities: A History of Emotions in the Middle Ages*, trans. R. Shaw (Cambridge: Polity, 2018).

Bouchard, Constance Brittain, *Strong of Body, Brave and Noble: Chivalry and Society in Medieval France* (Ithaca/London: Cornell University Press, 1998).

Bouley, Bradford A., *Pious Postmortems: Anatomy, Sanctity, and the Catholic Church in Early Modern Europe* (Philadelphia: University of Pennsylvania Press, 2017).

Boureau, Alain, *Satan the Heretic: The Birth of Demonology in the Medieval West*, trans. Teresa Lavender Fagan (Chicago/London: University of Chicago Press, 2006).

Buhrer, Eliza, 'From Caritas to Charity: How Loving God Became Giving Alms', in *Poverty and Prosperity in the Middle Ages and Renaissance*, ed. A. Scott and C. Kosso, Arizona Studies in the Middle Ages and Renaissance 19 (Turnhout: Brepols 2012), pp. 113-28.

Burr, David, *Spiritual Franciscans: From Protest to Persecution in the Century after Saint Francis* (Philadelphia: Pennsylvania State University Press, 2003).

Burrow, J. A., *The Ages of Man: A Study in Medieval Writing and Thought* (Oxford: Clarendon Press, 1986).

Bynum, Caroline Walker, *Fragmentation and Redemption: Essays on Gender and the Human Body in Medieval Religion* (New York: Zone Books, 1992) pp. 181-238.
—, *Holy Feast and Holy Fast. The Religious Significance of Food to Medieval Women* (Los Angeles: University of California Press, 1988).

Caciola, Nancy, *Discerning Spirits: Divine and Demonic Possession in the Middle Ages*, Conjunctions of Religion and Power in the Medieval Past (New York: Cornell University Press, 2003).
Cadden, Joan, *The Meanings of Sex Difference in the Middle Ages: Medicine, Science, and Culture* (Cambridge: Cambridge University Press 1995).
Camille, Michael, *Gothic Art. Visions and Revelations of the Medieval World* (London: Everyman, 1996).
—, 'The Image and the Self: Unwriting Late Medieval Bodies', in *Framing Medieval Bodies*, ed. Sarah Kay and Miri Rubin (Manchester: Manchester University Press, 1996), pp. 62-99.
Cassard, Jean-Christophe, 'Les coulisses de la sainteté? Charles de Blois vu par son entourage', *Annales de Bretagne et des Pays de l'Ouest* [online resource], 116 (2009), http://abpo.revues.org/165 (accessed 2 October 2016).
—, 'Propagande partisane et miracles engagés dans la guerre de Succession de Bretagne', *Annales de Bretagne et des Pays de l'Ouest* [online resource], 102 (1995): 7-24, http://abpo.revues.org/165 (accessed 2 October 2016).
—, *Saint Yves de Tréguier: un saint du XIII*[e] *siècle* (Paris: Beauchesne, 1992).
Claassens, Geert H. M., 'Jacob van Maerlant on Muhammed and Islam', in *Medieval Christian Perceptions of Islam: A Book of Essays*, ed. John Victor Tolan (London/New York: Routledge, 2013), pp. 211-42.
Classen, Albrecht, 'Introduction: Friendship – The Quest for a Human Ideal and Value from Antiquity to the Early Modern Time', in *Friendship in the Middle Ages and Early Modern Age: Explorations of a Fundamental Ethical Discourse*, ed. Albrecht Classen and Marilyn Sandidge (Berlin: De Gruyter, 2010), pp. 1-184.
—, 'Wounding the Body and Freeing the Spirit: Dorothea von Montau's Bloody Quest for Christ: A Late-Medieval Phenomenon of the Extraordinary Kind', in *Wounds and Wound Repair in Medieval Culture*, ed. Larissa Tracy and Kelly DeVries (Leiden: Brill, 2015), pp. 417-47.
Coakley, John, 'Friars as Confidants of Holy Women in Medieval Dominican Hagiography', in *Images of Sainthood in Medieval Europe*, ed. Renate Blumenfeld-Kosinski and Timea Szell (Ithaca/London: Cornell University Press, 1991), pp. 222-46.
—, *Women, Men, and Spiritual Power. Female Saints and their Male Collaborators* (New York: Columbia University Press, 2006).

Cohen, Esther, 'If You Prick Us, Do We Not Bleed? Reflections on the Diminishing of Other's Pain', in *Knowledge and Pain*, ed. Esther Cohen, Leona Toker, Manuela Consonni, and Otniel E. Dror (Amsterdam/New York: Rodopi, 2012), pp. 25-41.

—, *The Modulated Scream: Pain in Late Medieval Culture* (Chicago/London: The University of Chicago Press, 2010).

Cohen-Hanegbi, Na'ama, 'Pain as Emotion: The Role of Emotional Pain in Fifteenth-Century Italian Medicine and Confession', in *Knowledge and Pain*, ed. Esther Cohen, Leona Toker, Manuela Consonni, and Otniel E. Dror (Amsterdam/New York: Rodopi, 2012), pp. 63-82.

Courtenay, William, 'Curers of Body and Soul: Medical Doctors as Theologians', in *Religion and Medicine in the Middle Ages*, ed. Peter Biller and Joseph Ziegler (York: York Medieval Press, 2001) pp. 69-76.

Craig, Leigh Ann, *Wandering Women and Holy Matrons: Women as Pilgrims in the Later Middle Ages*, Studies in Medieval and Reformation Traditions 138 (Leiden: Brill 2009).

Crislip, Andrew T., *From Monastery to Hospital: Christian Monasticism and the Transformation of Health Care in Late Antiquity* (Ann Arbor: University of Michigan Press: 2005).

—, *Thorns in the Flesh: Illness and Sanctity in Late Ancient Christianity*, Divinations: Rereading Late Ancient Religion (Philadelphia: University of Pennsylvania Press, 2013).

Cullum P. H., 'Feasting Not Fasting: Men's Devotion to the Eucharist in the Later Middle Ages', in *Religious Men and Masculine Identity in the Middle Ages*, ed. P. H. Cullum and Katherine J. Lewis (Woodbridge: Boydell Press, 2013), 184-200.

—, 'Gendering Charity in Medieval Hagiography', in *Gender and Holiness: Men, Women and Saints in Late Medieval Europe*, ed. Sam Riches and Sarah Salih (London/New York: Routledge, 2011 [2002]), pp. 135-51.

—, and Katherine J. Lewis, eds., *Holiness and Masculinity in Medieval Europe* (Toronto: University of Toronto Press, 2004).

—, and Katherine J. Lewis, eds., *Religious Men and Masculine Identity in the Middle Ages* (Woodbridge: Boydell Press, 2013).

Daileader, Philip, *Saint Vincent Ferrer, his World and Life: Religion and Society in Late Medieval Europe* (New York: Palgrave Macmillan, 2016).

Dalarun, Jacques, *L'Impossibile sainteté: la vie retrouvée du Robert d'Arbrissel (v. 1045-1116), fondateur de Fontevraud* (Paris 1985).

Debby, Nirit Ben-Aryeh, *The Cult of St. Clare of Assisi in Early Modern Italy* (Aldershot: Ashgate, 2014).

—, 'St. Clare Expelling the Saracens from Assisi: Religious Confrontation in Word and Image', *Sixteenth Century Journal* 43.3 (2012): 643-65.

Deichmann, Graciela, *Wayward Nuns in Medieval Literature* (Syracuse: Syracuse University Press, 1986).

Demaitre, Luke, *Leprosy in Premodern Medicine: A Malady of the Whole Body* (Baltimore: Johns Hopkins University Press, 2009).

—, *Medieval Medicine: The Art of Healing, from Head to Toe*, Praeger Series on the Middle Ages (Santa Barbara/Denver/Oxford: Praeger, 2013).

Devaney, Thomas C., 'Everyday Miracles in Seventeenth-Century Spain', in *Lived Religion and Everyday Life in Early Modern Hagiographic Material*, ed. Jenni Kuuliala, Rose-Marie Peake, and Päivi Räisänen-Schröder, Palgrave Studies in the History of Experiences (New York: Palgrave Macmillan, 2019), pp. 189-213.

DeVries, Kelly, *Infantry Warfare in the Early Fourteenth Century: Discipline, Tactics, and Technology* (Woodbridge: Boydell Press, 1996).

Diekstra, F. N. M., ed., *The Middle English 'Weye of Paradys' and the Middle French 'Voie de Paradis': A Parallel-Text Edition* (Leiden: Brill, 1991).

Dinzelbacher, Peter, 'Der Kampf der Heiligen mit den Dämonen', in *Santi e demoni nell'alto medioevo occidentale (secoli V-XI)*, Settimane di studio del centro italiano di studi sull'alto medioevo 36, II (Spoleto: Presso la Sede del Centro, 1989), pp. 647-95.

—, *Heilige oder Hexen? Schicksale auffälliger Frauen* (Düsseldorf: Patmos, 2004).

—, *Körper und Frömmigkeit in der mittelalterlichen Mentalitätsgeschichte* (Paderborn: Schöningh 2007).

—, *Mystik und Natur: zur Geschichte ihres Verhältnisses vom Altertum bis zur Gegenwart* (Berlin: De Gruyter, 2009).

Dubisch, Jill, *In a Different Place: Pilgrimage, Gender and Politics at a Greek Island Shrine* (Princeton: Princeton University Press, 1995).

Du Cange, C. et al., *Glossarium mediae et infimae latinitatis* (Niort: L. Favre, 1883-87).

Duffin, Jacalyn, *Medical Miracles: Doctors, Saints and Healing in the Modern World* (Oxford: Oxford University Press, 2009).

—, *Medical Saints: Cosmas and Damian in a Postmodern World* (Oxford: Oxford University Press, 2013).

Elliott, Dyan, 'Authorizing a Life: The Collaboration of Dorothea of Montau and John Marienwerder', in *Gendered Voices: Medieval Saints and their Interpreters*, ed. Catherine M. Mooney (Philadelphia: University of Pennsylvania Press, 1999), pp. 168-91.

—, *The Bride of Christ Goes to Hell: Metaphor and Embodiment in the Lives of Pious Women 200-1500* (Philadelphia: University of Pennsylvania Press, 2012).

—, *Fallen Bodies: Pollution, Sexuality, and Demonology in the Middle Ages* (Philadelphia: University of Pennsylvania Press, 1999).

—, 'Flesh and Spirit: Women and the Body', in *Medieval Holy Women in the Christian Tradition c. 1100-c. 1500* (Turnhout: Brepols, 2010), 13-46.

—, 'The Physiology of Rapture and Female Spirituality", in *Medieval Theology and the Natural Body*, ed. Peter Biller and Alastair J. Minnis (York: York Medieval Press, 1997), pp. 141-74.

—, *Proving Woman: Female spirituality and inquisitional culture in the later Middle Ages* (Princeton: Princeton University Press, 2004).

—, *Spiritual Marriage: Sexual Abstinence in Medieval Wedlock* (Princeton: Princeton University Press, 1995).

Enenkel, K. A. E., 'Vorwort zur Textausgabe', in *Francesco Petrarca: De vita solitaria*, bk. 1: *Kritische Textausgabe und ideengeschichtlicher Kommentar*, ed. K. A. E. Enenkel (Leiden: Brill, 1990), pp. 1-51.

Esch, Arnold, 'Die Zeugenaussagen im Heiligsprechungsverfahren für S. Francesca Romana als Quelle zur Sozialgeschichte Rom im frühen Quattrocento', *Quellen und Forschungen aus italienischen Archiven und Bibliotheken*, 53 (1973): 93-151

—, 'Francesca Bussa, santa', in *Dizionario Biografico degli Italiani*, XLIX (1997), Treccani – la cultura Italiana [portal], www.treccani.it/enciclopedia/santa-francesca-bussa_%28Dizionario-Biografico%29/ (Accessed 20 May 2018).

—, 'I processi medioevali per la canonizzazione di santa Francesca Romana (1440-1451)', in *La canonizzazione di santa Francesca Romana: santità, cultura e istituzioni a Roma tra medioevo ed età moderna*, ed. Alessandra Bartolomei Romagnoli and Giorgio Picasso (Florence: Edizione del Galluzzo per la fondazione Ezio Franceschini, 2013), pp. 39-52.

—, 'Santa Francesca Romana e la società romana del suo tempo', in *Francesca Romana: la santa, il monastero e la città alla fine del medioevo*, ed. Alessandra Bartolomei Romagnoli (Florence: Edizione del Galluzzo, 2009), pp. 3-21.

Esposito, Anna, 'St. Francesca and the Female Religious Communities of Fifteenth-Century Rome', in *Women and Religion in Medieval and Renaissance Italy*, ed. Daniel Bornstein and Roberto Rusconi, trans. Margery J. Schneider (Chicago/London: University of Chicago Press, 1996), pp. 197-218.

Eyler, Joshua R., 'Introduction', in *Disability in the Middle Ages: Reconsiderations and Reverberations*, ed. Joshua R. Eyler (Aldershot: Ashgate, 2010), pp. 1-15.

Fanous, Samuel, 'Becoming the Theotokos: Birgitta of Sweden and Fulfilment of Salvation History', in *Motherhood, Religion, and Society in Medieval Europe, 400-1400: Essays Presented to Henrietta Leyser*, ed. Conrad Leyser and Lesley Smith (Aldershot: Ashgate, 2011), pp. 251-80.

Farmer, Sharon, 'The Beggar's Body: Intersections of Gender and Social Status in High Medieval Paris', in *Monks and Nuns, Saints and Outcasts: Religion in Medieval Society; Essays in Honor of Lester K. Little*, ed. Sharon Farmer and Barbara H. Rosenwein (Ithaca/London: Cornell University Press, 2000), pp. 153-71.

—, 'Introduction', in *Gender and Difference in the Middle Ages*, ed. Sharon Farmer and Carol Braun Pasternack (Minneapolis: University of Minnesota Press, 2003), pp. ix-xxvii.

—, *Surviving Poverty in Medieval Paris: Gender, Ideology, and the Daily Lives of the Poor* (Ithaca/London: Cornell University Press, 2005).

—, 'Young, Male and Disabled', in *Le petit peuple dans l'Occident médiéval: terminologies, perceptions, réalités*, ed. Pierre Boglioni, Robert Delort, and Claude Gauvard (Paris: Publications de la Sorbonne, 2002), pp. 437-51.

Ferzoco, George, 'The Processo Castellano and the Canonization of Catherine of Siena', in *A Companion to Catherine of Siena*, ed. Carolyn Muessig, George Ferzoco, and Beverly Kienzle (Leiden: Brill, 2012), pp. 185-202.

Field, Sean L., *Isabelle of France: Capetian Sanctity and Franciscan Identity in the Thirteenth Century* (Notre Dame: University of Notre Dame Press, 2006).

Finucane, Ronald C., *Contested Canonizations: The Last Medieval Saints, 1482-1523* (Washington, DC: Catholic University of America Press, 2011).

—, *Miracles and Pilgrims: Popular Beliefs in Medieval England* (New York: St. Martin's Press, 1995 [1977]).

—, *The Rescue of the Innocents. Endangered Children in Medieval Miracles* (New York: St. Martin's Press, 2000).

Frohne, Bianca, 'The Cultural Model of Dis/ability', in *Dis/ability History der Vormoderne: ein Handbuch/Premodern Dis/ability History: A Companion*, ed. Cordula Nolte, Bianca Frohne, Uta Halle, and Sonja Kerth (Affalterbach: Didymos, 2017), pp. 61-63.

—, *Leben mit 'kranckhait': der gebrechliche Körper in der häuslichen Überlieferung des 15. und 16. Jahrhunderts; Überlegungen zu einer Disability History der Vormoderne* (Affalterbach: Didymos, 2014).

—, 'Moderne Begriffe und Definitionen – so unentbehrlich wie problematisch', in *Dis/ability History der Vormoderne: ein Handbuch/Premodern Dis/ability History: A Companion*, ed. Cordula Nolte, Bianca Frohne, Uta Halle, and Sonja Kerth (Affalterbach: Didymos, 2017), pp. 52-58.

—, and Klaus-Peter Horn, 'On the Fluidity of "Disability" in Medieval and Early Modern Societies: Opportunities and Strategies in a New Field of Research', in *The Imperfect Historian: Disability Histories in Europe*, ed. Sebastian Barsch, Anne Klein, and Pieter Verstraete (Frankfurt am Main: Peter Lang, 2013), pp. 17-40.

—, and Jenni Kuuliala, 'The Trauma of Pain in Later Medieval Miracle Accounts', in *Trauma in the Middle Ages*, ed. Christina Lee and Wendy J. Turner (Leiden: Brill, 2018), pp. 215-36.

Fröjmark, Anders, 'The Canonization Process of Brynolf Algotsson', in *Procès de canonisation au Moyen Âge: aspects juridiques et religieux*, ed. Gábor Klaniczay, Collection de l'École française de Rome 340 (Rome: Ecole française de Rome, 2004), pp. 87-100.

—, *Mirakler och helgonkult* (Uppsala: Almqvist och Wiksell, 1992).

Gaposchkin, M. Cecilia, 'Boniface VIII, Philip the Fair, and the Sanctity of Louis IX', *Journal of Medieval History*, 28 (2003): 1-26.

—, 'The Captivity of Louis IX', *Quaestiones Medii Aevi Novae*, 18 (2013), 85-114.

—, 'Louis IX and Liturgical Memory', in *Memory and Commemoration in Medieval Culture*, ed. Elma Brenner, Mary Franklin-Brown, and Meredith Cohen (Aldershot: Ashgate, 2013), pp. 261-76.

—, 'Louis IX, Crusade and the Promise of Joshua in the Holy Land', *Journal of Medieval History*, 34.3 (2008): 245-74.

—, *The Making of Saint Louis: Kingship, Sanctity, and Crusade in the Later Middle Ages* (Ithaca: Cornell University Press, 2006).

—, 'The Place of the Crusades in the Sanctification of Saint Louis', in *Crusades – Medieval Worlds in Conflict*, ed. Thomas F. Madden, James L. Naus, and Vincent Ryan (Aldershot: Ashgate, 2010), pp. 195-209.

—, 'Place, Status, and Experience in the Miracles of Saint Louis', *Cahiers de recherches médiévales et humanistes*, 19 (2010): 249-66.

—, and Sean L. Field, 'Introduction', in *The Sanctity of Louis IX: Early Lives of Saint Louis by Geoffrey of Beaulieu and William of Chartres*, trans. Larry F. Field, ed. M. Cecilia Gaposchkin and Sean L. Field (Ithaca/London: Cornell University Press, 2013), pp. 1-60.

Garber, Rebecca L. R., *Feminine Figurae: Representations of Gender in Religious Texts by Medieval German Women Writers 1100-1375* (New York/London: Routledge, 2003).

Gemi-Iordanou, Effie, Stephen Gordon, Robert Matthew, Ellen McInnes, and Rhiannon Pettitt, eds., *Medicine, Healing and Performance* (Oxford: Oxbow, 2014).

Gentilcore, David, *Healers and Healing in Early Modern Italy* (Manchester: Manchester University Press, 1998).

Geremek, Bronisław, *The Margins of Society in Late Medieval Paris*, trans. Jean Birrell (Cambridge: Cambridge University Press, 2006 [1987, 1991]).

Getz, Faye Marie, *Medicine in the English Middle Ages* (Princeton: Princeton University Press, 1998).

Gigon, André, 'Histoire de la canonisation de s. Thomas d'Aquin', *Revue Thomiste*, 28 (1923), 142-54.

Goetz, Hans-Werner, 'Vorstellungen von menschlicher Gebrechlichkeit in frühen Mittelalter', in *Homo debilis: Behinderte-Kranke-Versehrte in der Gesellschaft des Mittelalters*, ed. Cordula Nolte (Affalterbach: Didymos, 2009), pp. 21-55.

Goldy, C. and A. Livingstone, eds., *Writing Medieval Women's Lives* (New York: Palgrave Macmillan, 2012).

Golinelli, Paolo, 'Social Aspects in Some Italian Canonization Trials: The Choice of Witnesses', in *Procès de canonisation au Moyen Âge: aspects juridiques et religieux*, ed. Gábor Klaniczay, Collection de l'École française de Rome 340 (Rome: École française de Rome, 2004), pp. 165-80.

—, '*Velut alter Alexius*: The Saint Alexis Model in Medieval Hagiography', in *Church and Belief in the Middle Ages: Popes, Saints, and Crusaders*, ed. Sari Katajala-Peltomaa and Kirsi Salonen (Amsterdam: Amsterdam University Press, 2016), pp. 141-52.

Goodich, Michael, 'The Death of a Saint. A Hagiographical Topos', in *Hoping for Continuity: Childhood, Education and Death in Antiquity and the Middle Ages*, ed. Katariina Mustakallio, Jussi Hanska, Hanna-Leena Sainio, and Ville Vuolanto, Acta Instituti Romani Finlandiae 33 (Rome: Institutum Romanum Finlandiae, 2005), pp. 227-38.

—, '*Mirabilis Deus in sanctis suis*: Social History and Medieval Miracles', in *Signs, Wonders, Miracles. Representations of Divine Power in the Life of Church, Studies in Church History*, ed. Kate Cooper and Jeremy Gregory (Woodbridge: Boydell & Brewer, 2005), pp. 135-56.

—, *Miracles and Wonders: The Development of the Concept of Miracle, 1150-1350*, Church, Faith, and Culture in the Medieval West (Aldershot: Ashgate, 2007).

—, 'Miseries of Dulcia St. Chartier (1266) and Cristina of Wellington (1294)', in *Voices from the Bench: The Narratives of Lesser Folk in Medieval Trials*, ed. Michael Goodich (New York: Palgrave Macmillan, 2006), pp. 99-125.

—, 'The Politics of Canonization in the Thirteenth Century: Lay and Mendicant Saints', in *Saints and their Cults: Studies in Religious Sociology, Folklore and History*, ed. Stephen Wilson (Cambridge: Cambridge University Press, 1983), pp. 169-88.

—, *Violence and Miracle in the Fourteenth Century: Private Grief and Public Salvation* (Chicago: University of Chicago Press, 1995).

—, *Vita perfecta: The Ideal of Sainthood in the Thirteenth Century* (Stuttgart: Anton Hiersemann, 1982).

Gordon, Sarah, 'Representations of Aging and Disability in Early Sixteenth-Century France', in *Old Age in the Middle Ages and the Renaissance: Interdisciplinary Approaches to a Neglected Topic*, ed. Albrecht Classen, Fundamentals of Medieval and Early Modern Culture 2 (Berlin: De Gruyter, 2007), pp. 421-36.

Green, Monica H., *Making Women's Medicine Masculine: The Rise of Male Authority in Pre-modern Gynaecology* (Oxford: Oxford University Press, 2008).

Haas, Louis, *The Renaissance Man and his Children: Childbirth and Early Childhood in Florence, 1300-1600* (New York: Palgrave Macmillan, 1998).

Hanawalt, Barbara A., *'Of Good and Ill Repute': Gender and Social Control in Medieval England* (Oxford: Oxford University Press, 1998).

—, *The Ties that Bound: Peasant Families in Medieval England* (Oxford: Oxford University Press, 1986).

Hanska, Jussi, 'The Hanging of William Cragh: Anatomy of a Miracle', *Journal of Medieval History*, 27 (2001): 121-38.

Harlow, Mary and Ray Laurence, 'Age, Agency and Disability: Suetonius and the Emperors of the First Century CE', in *Infirmity in Antiquity and the Middle Ages: Social and Cultural Approaches to Health, Weakness and Care*, ed. Christian Krötzl, Katariina Mustakallio, and Jenni Kuuliala (Aldershot: Ashgate, 2015), pp. 15-27.

Hartmann, Sieglinde, 'Bridal Mysticism and the Politics of Anchorhold: Dorothy of Montau', in *Anchoritism in the Middle Ages: Texts and Traditions*, ed. Catherine Innes-Parker and Naoë Kukita Yoshikawa (Cardiff: University of Wales Press, 2013), pp. 101-16.

Heinonen, Meri, 'Henry Suso and the Divine Knighthood', in *Holiness and Masculinity in Medieval Europe*, ed. P. H. Cullum and Katherine J. Lewis (Toronto: University of Toronto Press, 2004), pp. 79-92.

Henderson, John, *The Renaissance Hospital: Healing the Body and Healing the Soul* (New Haven/London: Yale University Press, 2006).

Heng, Geraldine, *Empire of Magic: Medieval Romance and the Politics of Cultural Fantasy* (New York: Columbia University Press, 2003).

Héry, Laurent, 'Le culte de Charles de Blois: résistances et réticenses', *Annales de Bretagne et des Pays de l'Ouest* [online resource], 103 (1996): 39-56, http://abpo.revues.org/165 (accessed 2 October 2016).

Heβ, Cordelia, *Heilige machen im spätmittelalterlichen Ostseeraum: die Kanonisationsprozesse von Birgitta von Schweden, Nikolaus von Linköping und Dorothea von Montau* (Berlin: Akademie, 2008)

Hollywood, Amy, 'Inside Out: Beatrice of Nazareth and her Hagiographer', in *Gendered Voices: Medieval Saints and their Interpreters*, ed. Catherine M. Mooney (Philadelphia: University of Pennsylvania Press, 1999), pp. 78-98.

—, *The Soul as Virgin Wife: Mechtild of Magdeburg, Marguerite Porete, and Meister Eckhart* (Notre Dame: University of Notre Dame Press, 1995).

Horrox, Rosemary, trans. and ed., *The Black Death*, Manchester Medieval Sources (Manchester: Manchester University Press, 1994).

Houts, Elisabeth van, *Memory and Gender in Medieval Europe 900-1200* (Hampshire/London: Macmillan Press, 1999).

Hughes, B. and K. Paterson, 'The Social Model of Disability and the Disappearing Body: Towards a Sociology of Impairment', *Disability and Society*, 12.3 (1997): 325-40.

Hughes-Edwards, Mari, *Reading Medieval Anchoritism: Ideology and Spiritual Practices* (Chicago/New York: University of Chicago Press, 2012).

Ilardi, Vincent, *Renaissance Vision from Spectacles to Telescopes* (Philadelphia: American Philosophical Society, 2007).

Jackson, Peter, *The Seventh Crusade 1244-1254: Sources and Documents* (Aldershot: Ashgate, 2009).

Jacquart, Danielle, *Milieu médical en France du XIIe au XVe siècle: en annexe 2e supplément au 'Dictionnaire' d'Ernest Wickersheimer* (Genova: Droz, 1981).

Jannuccelli, Gregorio, *Memorie di Subiaco e sua badia* (Genova: Gio. Fassi-Como, 1856).

Jansen, Katherine Ludwig, *The Making of the Magdalen: Preaching and Popular Devotion in the Later Middle Ages* (Princeton: Princeton University Press, 1999).

Jones, Michael, 'Politics, Sanctity and the Breton State: The Case of the Blessed Charles de Blois, Duke of Brittany (d. 1364)', in *The Medieval State. Essays Presented to James Campbell*, ed. J. R. Maddicott and D. M. Palliser (London: Hambledon Press, 2000), pp. 215-32.

Jordan, William C., 'Anti-corruption Campaigns in Thirteenth-Century Europe', *Journal of Medieval History*, 35 (2009): 205-7.

—, *Louis IX and the Challenge of the Crusade: A Study in Rulership* (Princeton: Princeton University Press, 1979).

—, *Men at the Center: Redemptive Governance under Louis IX* (Budapest: Central European University Press, 2012).

Jotischky, Andrew, *A Hermit's Cookbook: Monks, Food and Fasting in the Middle Ages* (New York: Continuum, 2011).

Jütte, Robert, ed., *Medical Pluralism: Past – Present – Future* (Stuttgart: Franz Steiner Verlag, 2013).

Karras, Ruth Mazo, *From Boys to Men: Formations of Masculinity in Late Medieval Europe* (Philadelphia: University of Pennsylvania Press, 2003).

Katajala-Peltomaa, Sari, 'Bishops Fighting with Demons in Swedish Canonization Processes', in *Saintly Bishops and Bishops' Saints: Proceedings of the 3rd Hagiography Conference, organized by Croatian Hagiography Society 'Hagiotheca' and International Hagiography Society, Poreč, 27-30 May 2010*, ed. John S. Ott and Trpimir Vedris (Zagreb: Hagiotheca, 2012), pp. 217-33.

—, *Demonic Possession and Lived Religion in Later Medieval Europe* (Oxford: Oxford University Press, 2020).

—, 'Demonic Possession as Physical and Mental Disturbance', in *Mental (Dis)Order in Later Medieval Europe*, ed. Sari Katajala-Peltomaa and Susanna Niiranen (Leiden: Brill, 2014), pp. 108-26.

—, 'Devotional Strategies in Everyday Life: Laity's Interaction with Saints in the North in the Fourteenth and Fifteenth Centuries', in *Lived Religion and the Long Reformation in Northern Europe c. 1300-1700* (Leiden: Brill, 2016), pp. 21-45.

—, 'Fatherhood, Masculinity and Lived Religion in Late Medieval Sweden', *Scandinavian Journal of History*, 38 (2013): 223-44.

—, *Gender, Miracles, and Daily Life: The Evidence of Fourteenth-Century Canonization Processes* (Turnhout: Brepols, 2009).

—, 'Gender, Networks and Collaboration: Pilgrimages in Fourteenth-Century Canonization Processes', in *De Amicitia: Friendship and Social Networks in Antiquity and the Middle Ages*, ed. Katariina Mustakallio and Christian Krötzl (Rome: Institutum Romanum Finlandiae, 2011) pp. 231-43.

—, 'A Good Wife? Demonic Possession and Discourses of Gender in Late Medieval Culture', in *Gender in Late Medieval and Early Modern Europe*, ed. Marianna Muravyeva and Raisa Maria Toivo, Routledge Research in Gender and History (London/New York: Routledge, 2013), pp. 73-88.

—, 'Recent Trends in the Study of Medieval Canonizations', *History Compass*, 8/9 (2010), pp. 1083-92.

—, and Christian Krötzl, 'Approaching Twelfth-Fifteenth-Century Miracles', in *Miracles in Medieval Canonization Processes*, ed. Christian Krötzl and Sari Katajala-Peltomaa (Turnhout: Brepols, 2018), pp. 1-39.

—, and Raisa Maria Toivo, 'Religion as an Experience', in *Lived Religion and the Long Reformation in Northern Europe c. 1300-1700* (Leiden: Brill, 2016), pp. 1-19.

Kay, Sarah and Miri Rubin, 'Introduction', in *Framing Medieval Bodies*, ed. Sarah Kay and Miri Rubin (Manchester: Manchester University Press, 1996), pp. 1-15.

Kelly, Kathleen Coyne, *Performing Virginity and Testing Chastity in the Middle Ages* (London/New York: Routledge, 2000).

Kieckhefer, Richard, 'Holiness and the Culture of Devotion: Remarks on Some Late Medieval Male Saints', in *Images of Sainthood in Medieval Europe*, ed. Renate Blumenfeld-Kosinski and Timea Szell (Ithaca/London: Cornell University Press, 1991), pp. 288-305.

—, *Unquiet Souls: Fourteenth-Century Saints and their Religious Milieu* (Chicago/London: University of Chicago Press, 1987).

Kirkham, Anne and Cordelia Warr, 'Introduction', in *Wounds in the Middle Ages*, ed. Anne Kirkham and Cordelia Warr (London/New York: Routledge, 2014), pp. 1-16.

Klaniczay, Gábor, *Holy Rulers and Blessed Princesses: Dynastic Cults in Medieval Central Europe*, trans. Éva Pálmai (Cambridge: Cambridge University Press, 2002).

—, 'Illness, Self-inflicted Body Pain and Supernatural Stigmata: Three Ways of Identification with the Suffering Body of Christ', in *Infirmity in Antiquity and the Middle Ages: Social and Cultural Approaches to Health, Weakness and Care*, ed. Christian Krötzl, Katariina Mustakallio, and Jenni Kuuliala (Aldershot: Ashgate, 2015), pp. 119-36.

—, 'The Inquisition of Miracles in Medieval Canonization Processes', in *Miracles in Medieval Canonization Processes: Structures, Functions, and Methodologies*, ed. Christian Krötzl and Sari Katajala-Peltomaa (Turnhout: Brepols, 2019), pp. 43-73.

—, 'Miracoli di punizione e *maleficia*', in *Miracoli: dai segni alla storia*, ed. Sofia Boesch Gajano and Marilena Modica (Rome: Viella, 2000), pp. 109-36.

—, 'On the Stigmatization of Saint Margaret of Hungary', in *Medieval Christianity in Practice*, ed. Miri Rubin (Princeton: Princeton University Press, 2009), pp. 274-84.

—, 'The Power of the Saints and the Authority of the Popes: The History of Sainthood and Late Medieval Canonization Processes', in *Church and Belief in the Middle Ages: Popes, Saints, and Crusaders*, ed. Sari Katajala-Peltomaa and Kirsi Salonen (Amsterdam: Amsterdam University Press, 2016), pp. 117-40.

—, 'Proving Sanctity in the Canonization Processes (Saint Elizabeth and Saint Margaret of Hungary)', in *Procès de canonisation au Moyen Âge: aspects juridiques et religieux*, ed. Gábor Klaniczay, Collection de l'École française de Rome 340 (Rome: École française de Rome, 2004), pp. 117-48.

—, 'Saint Elizabeth: A European Saint', in *Schola Europaea: les valeurs de l'Europe – l'Europe des valeurs*, ed. Ladislaus Havas, Ladislaus Takács, and Emericus Tegyey, Classica-Mediaevalia-Neolatina 3 (Debrecen: Soc. Neolatina Hungarica, 2009), pp. 201-22.

—, 'Sainte Élisabeth comme modèle: l'image de la sainteté féminine dans le Libellus de dictis quattuor ancillarum', in *Le plaisir de l'art du Moyen Âge: commande, production et réception de l'oeuvre d'art; mélanges en hommage à Xavier Barral i Altet*, ed. Rosa Alcoy Pedrós and Dominique Allios (Paris: Picard, 2012), pp. 967-75.

—, 'Speaking about Miracles: Oral Testimony and Written Record in Medieval Canonization Trials', in *The Development of Literate Mentalities in East Central Europe*, ed. Anna Adamska and Marco Mostert, Utrecht Studies in Medieval Literacy 9 (Turnhout: Brepols, 2004), pp. 365-95.

—, *The Uses of Supernatural Power: The Transformations of Popular Religion in Medieval and Early Modern Europe*, trans. Susan Singerman (Princeton: Princeton University Press, 1990).

Klapisch-Zuber, Christiane, *Women, Family, and Ritual in Renaissance Italy*, trans. Lydia G. Cochrane (Chicago/London: University of Chicago Press, 1985).

Kleinberg, Aviad, 'Canonization without a Canon', in *Procès de canonisation au Moyen Âge: aspects juridiques et religieux*, ed. Gábor Klaniczay, Collection de l'École française de Rome 340 (Rome: Ecole française de Rome, 2004), pp. 7-18.

—, *Prophets in their Own Country: Living Saints and the Making of Sainthood in the Later Middle Ages* (Chicago/London: University of Chicago Press, 1992).

Knight, Kimberley-Joy, '*Si puose calcina a' propi occhi*: The Importance of the Gift of Tears for Thirteenth-Century Religious Women and their Hagiographers', in *Crying in the Middle Ages*, ed. Elina Gertsman (London/New York: Routledge, 2011), pp. 136-55.

Knox, Lezlie S., *Creating Clare of Assisi: Female Franciscan Identities in Later Medieval Italy* (Leiden: Brill, 2008).

Koopmans, Rachel, *Wonderful to Relate: Miracle Stories and Miracle Collecting in High Medieval England* (Philadelphia: University of Pennsylvania Press, 2011).

Krafft, Ortrfried, *Papsturkunde und Heiligsprechung: die päpstlichen Kanonisationen vom Mittelalter bis zur Reformation. Ein Handbuch* (Cologne/Weimar/Wien: Böhlau, 2005).

Kroll, Jerome and Bernard Bachrach, *The Mystic Mind: The Psychology of Medieval Mystics and Ascetics* (London/New York: Routledge, 2005).

Krötzl, Christian, '"Fama volat": On Propagation, Decision-Making and Influence in the Later Middle Ages', in *Changing Minds: Communication and Influence in the High and Later Middle Ages*, ed. Christian Krötzl and Miikka Tamminen (Rome: Institutum Romanum Finlandiae 2013), pp. 79-86.

—, 'How to Choose a Saint? On Propagation, Advice, and Decision-Making in Medieval Communities', in *Agiografia e culture popolari/Hagiography and Popular Cultures: in ricordo di Pietro Boglioni*, ed. Paolo Golinelli, Biblioteca di Storia Agraria Medievale 37 (Bologna: Clueb, 2012), pp. 371-416.

—, 'Miracles au tombeau – miracles à distance: approches typologiques', in *Miracle et Karama: hagiographies médiévales comparées*, ed. Denise Aigle, Bibliothèque de l'Ecole des Hautes Etudes, Sciences Religieuses 109 (Turnhout: Brepols, 2000), pp. 557-76.

—, *Pilger, Mirakel und Alltag: Formen des Verhaltens im skandinavischen Mittelalter (12.-15. Jahrhundert)*, Studia Historica 46 (Helsinki: Suomen Historiallinen Seura, 1994).

—, 'Prokuratoren, Notare und Dolmetscher: zu Gestaltung und Ablauf der Zeugeneinvernahmen bei spätmittelalterlichen Kanonisationsprozessen', *Hagiographica*, 5 (1998): 119-40.

—, 'Saints, Healing and Communities in the Later Middle Ages: On Roles and Perceptions', in *Infirmity in Antiquity and the Middle Ages: Social and Cultural Approaches to Health, Weakness and Care*, ed. Christian Krötzl, Katariina Mustakallio, and Jenni Kuuliala (Aldershot: Ashgate, 2015), pp. 255-64.

—, '*Sexaginta vel circa*: zur Wahrnehmung von Alter in hagiographischen Quellen des Spätmittelalters', in *Alterskulturen des Mittelalters und der frühen Neuzeit: Internationaler Kongress, Krems an der Donau, 16. bis 18. Oktober 2006*, ed. Elisabeth Vavra (Vienna: Verlag der Österreichischen Akademie der Wissenschaften, 2008), pp. 109-15.

Kuuliala, Jenni, *Childhood Disability and Social Integration in the Middle Ages: Constructions of Impairments in Thirteenth- and Fourteenth-Century Canonization Processes* (Turnhout: Brepols, 2016).

—, 'Disability and Religious Practices in Late Medieval Prussia: Infirmity and the Miraculous in the Canonization Process of St. Dorothea of Montau (1404-1406)', in *Lived Religion in the Baltic Sea Region during the Long Reformation*, ed. Sari Katajala-Peltomaa and Raisa Maria Toivo (Leiden: Brill, 2016), pp. 46-74.

—, 'Heavenly Healing or Failure of Faith? Partial Cures in Later Medieval Canonization Processes', in *Church and Belief in the Middle Ages: Popes, Saints, and Crusaders*, ed. Sari Katajala-Peltomaa and Kirsi Salonen (Amsterdam: Amsterdam University Press, 2016), pp. 171-99.

—, '*Infirmitas* in Monastic Rules', in *Disability in Antiquity*, ed. Christian Laes (London/New York: Routledge, 2017), pp. 342-56.

—, 'Love and Duty in the Time of Family Crisis: Physical Disability and Marriage in Later Medieval (*c.* 1200-1500) Miracle Testimonies', *Mirator*, 14.2 (2013): 111-22.

—, 'Nobility, Community and Physical Disability in Later Medieval Canonization Processes', in *Infirmity in Antiquity and the Middle Ages: Social and Cultural Approaches to Health, Weakness and Care*, ed. Christian Krötzl, Katariina Mustakallio, and Jenni Kuuliala (Aldershot: Ashgate, 2015), pp. 67-82.

—, 'Unlikely Heroes: A Study on Three Miracle Narratives of Disabled Beggar Children in LateThirteenth-Century Hagiographic Sources', *Agents and Objects – Children in Pre-modern Europe*, ed. Katariina Mustakallio and Jussi Hanska, Acta Instituti Romani Finlandiae 42 (Rome: Institutum Romanum Finlandiae, 2015), pp. 149-69.

—, Katariina Mustakallio, and Christian Krötzl, 'Introduction: *Infirmitas* in Antiquity and the Middle Ages', in *Infirmity in Antiquity and the Middle Ages: Social and Cultural Approaches to Health, Weakness and Care*, ed. Christian Krötzl, Katariina Mustakallio, and Jenni Kuuliala (Aldershot: Ashgate, 2015), pp. 1-13.

Lamberg, Marko, 'Anger as a Spiritual, Social and Mental Disorder in Late Medieval Swedish Exempla', in *Mental (Dis)order in Late Medieval Europe*, ed. Sari Katajala-Peltomaa and Susanna Niiranen (Leiden: Brill, 2014), pp. 70-90.

Langum, Virginia, *Medicine and the Seven Deadly Sins in Late Medieval Literature and Culture* (New York: Palgrave Macmillan, 2016).

—, 'Medicine, Female Mystics and Illness Experience', in *Revisiting Gender in European History, 1400-1800*, ed. Elise M. Dermineur, Åsa Karlsson Sjögren, and Virginia Langum (London/New York: Routledge 2018), pp. 100-20.

Lawrence, C. H., *The Friars: The Impact of Mendicant Orders on Medieval Society* (London/New York: I. B. Tauris, 1994).

—, *Medieval Monasticism: Forms of Religious Life in Western Europe in the Middle Ages* (Essex: Pearson Education, 2001).

Le Goff, Jacques, *Saint Francis of Assisi* (London/New York: Routledge, 2004).

—, *Saint Louis* (Paris: Editions Gallimard, 1996).

Lehmijoki-Gardner, Maiju, 'Denial as Action – Penance and its Place in the Life of Catherine of Siena', in *A Companion to Catherine of Siena*, ed. Carolyn Muessig, George Ferzoco, and Beverly Kienzle (Leiden: Brill, 2012), pp. 113-26.

—, 'Laywomen, Religious', in *Women and Gender in Medieval Europe: An Encyclopedia* (London/New York: Routledge, 2006) pp. 462-64.

—, *Worldly Saints: Social Interaction of Dominican Penitent Women in Italy, 1200-1500* (Helsinki: Finnish Literature Society, 1999).

Lett, Didier, '*Judicium Medicine* and *Judicium Sanctitatis*: Medical Doctors in the Canonization Process of Nicholas of Tolentino (1325); Experts Subject to the Inquisitorial Logic', in *Church and Belief in the Middle Ages: Popes, Saints, and Crusaders*, ed. Sari Katajala-Peltomaa and Kirsi Salonen (Amsterdam: Amsterdam University Press, 2016), pp. 153-70.

—, 'La parole des humbles comme resource: l'utilisation de la procedure inquisitoire par les postulateurs de la cause dans la procès de canonisation de Nicolas de Tolentino (1325)', in *Hagiography and Popular Cultures: in Ricordo di Pietro Boglioni*, ed by Paolo Golinelli (Bologna: Cooperativa Libraria Universitaria Editrice Bologna, 2012), pp. 233-40.

—, *L'Enfant des miracles: enfance et société au Moyen Âge (XIIe-XIIIe siècle)* (Paris: Aubier, 1997).

—, *Un procès de canonisation au Moyen Âge: essai d'histoire sociale; Nicolas de Tolentino, 1325* (Paris: Presses Universitaires de France, 2008).

Lewis, Katherine J., 'Gender and Sanctity in the Middle Ages', in *Gendering the Middle Ages*, ed. Pauline Stafford and Anneke Mulder-Bakker (Oxford: Blackwell, 2001), pp. 205-14.

—, '"Imitate, too, this king in virtue, who could have done ill, and did it not": Lay Sanctity and the Rewriting of Henry VI's Manliness', in *Religious Men and Masculine Identity in the Middle Ages*, ed. P. H. Cullum and Katherine J. Lewis (Woodbridge: Boydell Press, 2013), pp. 126-42.

—, 'Male Saints and Devotional Masculinity in Late Medieval England', *Gender & History*, 24 (2012): 112-33.

Loconte, Aislinn, 'Constructing Female Sanctity in Late Medieval Naples: The Funerary Monument of Queen Sancia of Majorca', in *Representing Medieval Genders and Sexualities in Europe: Construction, Transformation, and Subversion, 600-1530*, ed. Elizabeth L'Estrange and Alison More (Farnham: Ashgate, 2012), 107-26.

Lugano, Placido Tommaso, 'Introduzione', in *I processi inediti per Francesca Bussa dei Ponziani (Santa Francesca Romana) 1440-1453*, ed. Placido Tommaso Lugano, Studi e Testi 120 (Vatican City: Biblioteca Apostolica Vaticana, 1945), i-xl.

MacDougall, Simone C., 'The Surgeon and the Saints: Henri de Mondeville on Divine Healing', *Journal of Medieval History*, 26 (2000): 256-67.

McAvoy, Liz Herbert, 'Bathing in the Blood: The Medicinal Cures of Anchoritic Devotion', in *Medicine, Religion and Gender in Medieval Culture*, ed. Nao Yoshikawa (Cambridge: D. S. Brewer, 2015), pp. 85-102.

McCleery, Iona, 'Isabel of Aragon (d. 1336): Model Queen or Model Saint?', *Journal of Ecclesiastical History*, 57 (2006): 668-92.

McClure, George W., *Sorrow and Consolation in Italian Humanism* (Princeton: Princeton University Press, 2014).

McNamer, Sarah, *Affective Meditation and the Invention of Medieval Compassion* (Philadelphia: University of Pennsylvania Press, 2010).

McVaugh, Michael, *Medicine before the Plague: Practitioners and their Patients in the Crown of Aragon, 1285-1345* (Cambridge: Cambridge University Press, 1993).

Maniura, Robert, *Pilgrimage to the Images in the Fifteenth Century: The Origins of the Cult of Our Lady of Częstochowa* (Woodbridge: Boydell Press, 2004).

Marini, Alfonso, 'Introduzione', in *Il processo di canonizzazione di Celestino V*, ed. Alessandra Bartolomei Romagnoli and Alfonso Marini, 2 vols. (Florence: Sismel, 2015), I, pp. 3-72.

Mattei, Mario, 'Introduzione', in *Il processo di canonizzaione di Fra Giovanni Bono (1251-1253/54) fondatore dell'ordine degli eremiti*, ed. Mario Mattei (Rome: Institutum historicum Augustinianum, 2002), pp. 9-134.

Matter, E. Ann, 'The Undebated Debate. Gender and the Image of God in Medieval Theology', in *Gender in Debate From the Early Middle Ages to the Renaissance*, ed. Thelma S. Fenster and Clare E. Lees (New York: Palgrave, 2002), pp. 41-56.

Menestò, Enrico, 'The Apostolic Canonization Proceedings of Clare of Montefalco, 1318-1319', in *Women and Religion in Medieval and Renaissance Italy*, ed. Daniel Ethan Bronstein and Roberto Rusconi (Chicago: University of Chicago Press, 1996), pp. 104-29.

—, 'Introduzione', in *Il processo di canonizzazione di Clare of Montefalco*, ed. Enrico Menestò (Florence/Perugia: La Nuova Italia, 1984), pp. xxi-lxix.

—, 'La biografia di Chiara scritta da Bérangar de Saint-Affrique', in *Santa Chiara da Montefalco monaca agostiniana (1268-1308) nel contesto socio-religioso femminile dei secoli XIII-XIV*, ed. Enrico Menestò (Spoleto: Fondazione Centro italiano di studi sull'alto medioevo, 2009), pp. 163-80.

Metzler, Irina, *Disability in Medieval Europe: Thinking about Physical Impairment during the High Middle Ages, c.1100-1400* (London/New York: Routledge, 2006).

—, *Fools and Idiots? Intellectual Disability in the Middle Ages* (Manchester: Manchester University Press, 2016)

—, 'Indiscriminate Healing Miracles in Decline: How Social Realities Affect Religious Perception', in *Contextualizing Miracles in the Christian West, 1100-1500: New Historical Approaches*, ed. Matthew M. Mesley and Louise E. Wilson, Medium Aevum Monographs 32 (Oxford: Society for the Study of Medieval Languages and Literature, 2014), pp. 155-76.

—, *A Social History of Disability: Cultural Considerations of Physical Impairment*, Routledge Studies in Cultural History (London/New York: Routledge, 2013).

Miller, Sarah Alison, *Medieval Monstrosity and the Female Body* (London/New York: Routledge, 2010).

Miller, Tanya Stabler, *The Beguines of Medieval Paris: Gender, Patronage, and Spiritual Authority* (Philadelphia: University of Pennsylvania Press, 2014).

Mills, Robert, *Suspended Animation: Pain, Pleasure and Punishment in Medieval Culture* (London: Reaktion Books 2005).

Minnis, Alastair J. and Rosalynn Voaden, eds., *Medieval Holy Women in the Christian Tradition c. 1100-c. 1500* (Turnhout: Brepols, 2010)

Mitchell, Piers D., 'The Infirmaries of the Order of the Temple in the Medieval Kingdom of Jerusalem', in *The Medieval Hospital and Medical Practice*, ed. Barbara S. Bowers (Aldershot: Ashgate, 2007), pp. 225-34.

Mollat, Michel, *The Poor in the Middle Ages: An Essay in Social History*, trans. Arthur Goldhammer (New Haven/London: Yale University Press, 1990).

Mooney, Catherine M., ed., *Gendered Voices: Medieval Saints and their Interpreters* (Philadelphia: University of Pennsylvania Press, 1999).

—, '*Imitatio Christi* or *Imitatio Mariae*? Clare of Assisi and her Interpreters', in *Gendered Voices: Medieval Saints and their Interpreters*, ed. Catherine M. Mooney (Philadelphia: University of Pennsylvania Press, 1999), pp. 52-77.

—, 'Voice, Gender, and the Portrayal of Sanctity', in *Gendered Voices: Medieval Saints and their Interpreters*, ed. Catherine M. Mooney (Philadelphia: University of Pennsylvania Press, 1999), pp. 1-15.

Moore, R. I., 'Between Sanctity and Superstition: Saints and their Miracles in the Age of Revolution', in *The Work of Jacques le Goff and the Challenges of Medieval History*, ed. Miri Rubin (Woodbridge: Boydell Press, 1997), pp. 55-67.

—, *The War On Heresy: Faith and Power in Medieval Europe* (London: Profile Books, 2012).

More, Alison, 'Convergence, Conversion, and Transformation: Gender and Sanctity in Thirteenth-Century Liège', in *Representing Medieval Genders and Sexualities in Europe: Construction, Transformation, and Subversion, 600-1530*, ed. Elizabeth L'Estrange and Alison More (Farnham: Ashgate, 2011), pp. 33-48.

Morelli, Francesca, 'Malattie e medicina a Roma nel XV secolo. Un'analisi delle testimonianze di guarigione miracolosa nei processi di canonizzazione per Santa Francesca Romana (1440-1453)', *Archivio della Società Romana di Storia Patria*, 131 (2008): 87-116.

Mormando, Franco, *The Preacher's Demons: Bernardino of Siena and the Social Underworld of Early Renaissance Italy* (Chicago/London: University of Chicago Press, 1999).

Morris, Bridget, *St. Birgitta of Sweden* (Woodbridge: Boydell Press, 1999).

Morrison, Susan S., *Women Pilgrims in Late Medieval England: Private Piety as Public Performance*, Routledge Research in Medieval Studies 3 (London/New York: Routledge, 2004 [2000]).

Muessig, Carolyn, 'Learning and Mentoring in the Twelfth Century: Hildegard of Bingen and Herrad of Landsberg', in *Medieval Monastic Education*, ed. George

Ferzoco and Carolyn Muessig (London/New York: Leicester University Press, 2000), pp. 87-104.

Mulder-Bakker, Anneke B., 'The Invention of Saintliness: Texts and Contexts', in *The Invention of Saintliness*, ed. Anneke B. Mulder-Bakker (London/New York: Taylor & Francis, 2003 [2002]), pp. 3-24.

Muravyeva, Marianna G. and Raisa Maria Toivo, 'Introduction: Why and How Gender Matters?', in *Gender in Late Medieval and Early Modern Europe* (London/New York: Routledge, 2012), pp. 1-16.

Neal, Derek G., *The Masculine Self in Late Medieval England* (Chicago/London: University of Chicago Press, 2008).

Newman, Barbara, *From Virile Woman to WomanChrist: Studies in Medieval Religion and Literature* (Philadelphia: University of Pennsylvania Press, 1995).

Newman, Martha G., 'Crucified by the Virtues: Monks, Lay Brothers, and Women in Thirteenth-Century Cistercian Saints' Lives', in *Gender and Difference in the Middle Ages*, ed. Sharon Farmer and Carol Braun Pasternack (Minneapolis: University of Minnesota Press, 2003), pp. 182-209.

Nie, Giselle de, 'Fatherly and Motherly Curing in Sixth-Century Gaul: Saint Radegund's *Mysterium*', in *Women and Miracles Stories: A Multidisciplinary Exploration*, ed. Anne-Marie Korte (Leiden: Brill, 2004), pp. 53-86.

Nieuwland, Jeannette, 'Motherhood and Sanctity in the Life of Saint Birgitta of Sweden: An Insoluble Conflict?', in *Sanctity and Motherhood: Essays on Holy Mothers in the Middle Ages*, ed. Anneke Mulder-Bakker (New York: Garland Publishers, 1995), pp. 297-329.

Nissi, Jyrki, 'Quomodo Scit Quod Mortuus Erat? Signs of Death in 15th-Century Italy', *SVMMA*, 7 (2016).

Nocentini, Sylvia, 'The *Legenda maior* of Catherine of Siena', *in A Companion to Catherine of Siena*, ed. Carolyn Muessig, George Ferzoco, and Beverly Mayne Kienzle (Leiden: Brill, 2012), pp. 339-57.

Norri, Juhani, *Dictionary of Medical Vocabulary in English, 1375-1550: Body Parts, Sicknesses, Instruments, and Medicinal Preparations* (London/New York: Routledge, 2016).

Nyberg, Tore, 'The Canonization Process of St. Birgitta of Sweden', in *Procès de canonisation au Moyen Âge: aspects juridiques et religieux*, ed. Gábor Klaniczay, Collection de l'École française de Rome 340 (Rome: École française de Rome, 2004), pp. 67-85.

O'Tool, Mark, 'Caring for the Blind in Medieval Paris', PhD thesis, University of California, 2007.

Paciocco, Roberto, *Canonizzazioni e culto dei santi nella Christianitas (1198-1302)* (Assisi: Edizioni Porziuncola, 2006).

Paoli, Emore, 'Le visioni di Chiara da Montefalco', in *Santa Chiara da Montefalco monaca agostiniana (1268-1308) nel contesto socio-religioso femminile dei secoli XIII-XIV*, ed. Enrico Menestò (Spoleto: Fondazione Centro italiano di studi sull'alto medioevo, 2009), pp. 233-50.

Parigi, Paolo, *The Rationalization of Miracles* (Cambridge: Cambridge University Press, 2012).

Park, Katharine, 'The Criminal and the Saintly Body: Autopsy and Dissection in Renaissance Italy', *Renaissance Quarterly*, 47 (1994): 1-33.

—, 'Relics of a Fertile Heart: The "Autopsy" of Clare of Montefalco', in *The Material Culture of Sex, Procreation, and Marriage in Premodern Europe*, ed. Anne L. McClanan and Karen Rosoff Encarnación (New York: Palgrave Macmillan, 2002), pp. 115-33.

Pearman, Tory Vandeventer, *Women and Disability in Medieval Literature* (New York: Palgrave Macmillan, 2010).

Pellegrini, Letizia, 'Introduzione', in *Il processo di canonizzazione di Bernardino da Siena (1445-1450)*, ed. Letizia Pellegrini, Analecta Franciscana, XVI, n.s., Documenta et Studia 4 (Grottaferrata: Frati editori di Quaracchi, 2009), pp. 1-107.

—, 'La sainteté au XVe siècle entre procès et droit canonique: avant et après Bernardin de Sienne', in *Procès de canonisation au Moyen Âge: aspects juridiques et religieux*, ed. Gábor Klaniczay, Collection de l'École française de Rome 340 (Rome: École française de Rome, 2004), pp. 309-26.

—, 'Sui miracoli di Bernardino da Siena: pratiche notarili e stratificazione documentaria', in *Notai, miracoli e culto dei santi: pubblicità e autenticazione del sacro tra XII e XV secolo*, ed. R. Michetti (Milan: Giuffrè, 2004), pp. 369-96.

—, 'Testifying to Miracles: A Report on the Canonization Process of Bernardin of Siena', in *Miracles in Medieval Canonization Processes*, ed. Christian Krötzl and Sari Katajala-Peltomaa (Turnhout: Brepols, 2018), pp. 105-30.

Peyroux, Catherine, 'The Leper's Kiss', in Sharon Farmer and Barbara H. Rosenwein, eds., *Monks and Nuns, Saints and Outcasts. Religion in Medieval Society: Essays in Honor of Lester K. Little* (Ithaca/London: Cornell University Press, 2000), 172-88.

Pfau, Alexandra, 'Madness in the Realm: Narratives of Mental Illness in Late Medieval France', PhD thesis, University of Michigan, 2008.

Pincikowski, Scott E., *Bodies of Pain: Suffering in the Works of Hartmann von Aue*, Routledge Studies on Medieval History and Culture (London/New York: Routledge, 2002)

Pomata, Gianna, *Contracting a Cure. Patients, Healers, and the Law in Early Modern Bologna* (Baltimore: Johns Hopkins University Press, 1998).

Pratt, Karen, '*De vetula*: The Figure of Old Woman in Medieval French Literature', in *Old Age in the Middle Ages and Renaissance: Interdisciplinary Approaches to a Neglected Topic*, ed. Albrecht Classen, Fundamentals of Medieval and Early Modern Culture 2 (Berlin: De Gruyter, 2007), pp. 321-42.

Prudlo, Donald, *The Martyred Inquisitor: The Life and Cult of Peter of Verona (d. 1252)*, Church, Faith, and Culture in the Medieval West (Aldershot: Ashgate, 2008).

Räsänen, Marika, 'Making a Saint for the Monastery of Fossanova: The Dispute on the Ownership of the Corpse of Saint Thomas Aquinas at the Time of his Canonisation (1323)', in *Changing Minds. Communication and Influence in the High and Later Middle Ages*, ed. Christian Krötzl and Miikka Tamminen, Acta Instituti Romani Finlandiae 39 (Rome: Institutum Romanum Finlandiae, 2013), pp. 107-26.

—, *Thomas Aquinas's Relics as Focus for Conflict and Cult in the Late Middle Ages: The Restless Corpse* (Amsterdam: Amsterdam University Press, 2017).

Rawcliffe, Carole, 'Curing Bodies and Healing Souls: Pilgrimage and the Sick in Medieval East Anglia', in *Pilgrimage: The English Experience from Becket to Bunyan*, ed. Colin Morris and Peter Roberts (Cambridge: Cambridge University Press, 2002) pp. 108-40.

—, *Leprosy in Medieval England* (Woodbridge: Boydell & Brewer, 2006).

—, *Medicine and Society in Later Medieval England* (Stroud: Sutton Publishing, 1995)

Riches, Sam and Sarah Salih, 'Introduction: Gender and Holiness, Performance and Representation in the Later Middle Ages', in *Gender and Holiness: Men, Women and Saints in Late Medieval Europe*, ed. Sam Riches and Sarah Salih (London/New York: Routledge, 2011 [2002]), pp. 1-8.

—, eds., *Gender and Holiness: Men, Women and Saints in Late Medieval Europe* (London/New York: Routledge, 2011 [2002]).

Rider, Catherine, *Magic and Religion in Medieval England* (London: Reaktion Books, 2012).

Rittgers, Ronald K., *The Reformation of Suffering: Pastoral Theology and Lay Piety in Late Medieval and Early Modern Germany* (Oxford: Oxford University Press, 2012).

Rocke, Michael, *Forbidden Friendships: Homosexuality and Male Culture in Renaissance Florence* (Chicago/London: University of Chicago Press, 1996).

Rogers, Clifford J., 'Sir Thomas Dagworth in Brittany, 1346-7: Restellou and La Roche Derrien', in *The Journal of Medieval Military History*, III, ed. Kelly DeVries and Clifford J. Rogers (Rochester and Woodbridge: The Boydell Press, 2005), pp. 127-54.

Rosenwein, Barbara H., *Emotional Communities in the Early Middle Ages* (Ithaca/London: Cornell University Press, 2007).

Rubin, Miri, 'The Body, Whole and Vulnerable, in Fifteenth-Century England', in *Bodies and Disciplines: Intersections of Literature and History in Fifteenth-Century*

England, ed. David Wallace and Barbara Hanawalt (Minneapolis: University of Minnesota Press, 1996), pp. 19-28.
—, *Charity and Community in Medieval Cambridge* (Cambridge: Cambridge University Press, 1987).
—, *Corpus Christi: The Eucharist in Late Medieval Culture* (Cambridge: Cambridge University Press, 1991).
—, *Emotion and Devotion: The Meaning of Mary in Medieval Religious Cultures* (Budapest: Central European University Press, 2009).
Rusconi, Roberto, *L'Ordine dei peccati: la confessione tra Medioevo ed età moderna* (Bologna: Il Mulino, 2002).
—, 'St. Bernardino of Siena, the Wife, and Possessions', in *Women and Religion in Medieval and Renaissance Italy*, ed. Daniel Bornstein and Roberto Rusconi (Chicago: University of Chicago Press, 1996), pp. 183-84.

Sahlin, Claire Lynn, *Birgitta of Sweden and the Voice of Prophecy*, Studies in Medieval Mysticism (Woodbridge: The Boydell Press, 2001).
Salih, Sarah, *Versions of Virginity in Late Medieval England* (New York: Boydell & Brewer, 2001).
Salmesvuori, Päivi, *Power and Sainthood: The Case of Birgitta of Sweden* (New York: Palgrave Macmillan, 2014).
Salonen, Kirsi, 'What Happened to Aged Priests in the Late Middle Ages?', in *On Old Age: Approaching Death in Antiquity and the Middle Ages*, ed. Christian Krötzl and Katariina Mustakallio (Turnhout: Brepols, 2011), pp. 183-96.
— and Jussi Hanska, *Entering a Clerical Career at the Roman Curia 1458-1471*, Church, Faith and Culture in the Medieval West (Aldershot: Ashgate, 2013).
Scanlan, Suzanne M., *Divine and Demonic Imagery at Tor de'Specchi 1400-1500: Religious Women and Art in 15th-Century Rome* (Amsterdam: Amsterdam University Press, 2018).
Schäfer, Daniel, 'More than a Fading Flame: The Physiology of Old Age between Speculative Analogy and Experimental Method', in *Concepts of Physiology from Antiquity into Early Modern Europe*, ed. Manfred Horstmanshoff, Helen King, and Claus Zittel (Leiden: Brill, 2012), pp. 241-66.
Schulenburg, Jane Tibbetts, *Forgetful of their Sex: Female Sanctity and Society, ca. 500-1100* (Chicago/London: University of Chicago Press, 1998).
Scott, Karen, 'Mystical Death, Bodily Death: Catherine of Siena and Raymond of Capua on the Mystic's Encounter with God', in *Gendered Voices: Medieval Saints and their Interpreters*, ed. Catherine M. Mooney (Philadelphia: University of Pennsylvania Press, 1999), pp. 136-67.
Scott, Robert A., *Miracle Cures: Saints, Pilgrimage, and the Healing Powers of Belief* (Berkeley/Los Angeles: University of California Press, 2010).

Scheer, Monique, 'Are Emotions a Kind of Practice (and Is that What Makes Them Have a History)? A Bourdieuian Approach to Understanding Emotion', *History and Theory*, 51 (2012): 193-220.

Sears, Elizabeth, *The Ages of Man: Medieval Interpretations of the Life Cycle* (Princeton: Princeton University Press, 1986).

Shahar, Shulamith, *Growing Old in the Middle Ages: 'Winter Clothes Us in Shadow and Pain'* (London/New York: Routledge, 1997).

Sheehan, Michael M., '*Maritalis Affectio* Revisited', in *The Olde Daunce: Love, Friendship, Sex, and Marriage in the Medieval World*, ed. Robert Edwards (New York: State University of New York Press, 1991), pp. 32-43.

Sigal, Pierre-André, 'Les témoins et les témoignages au procès du canonisation de Dauphine de Puimichel (1363)', *Provence Historique*, 49 (1999): 461-71.

—, *L'Homme et le miracle dans la France médiévale (XIe-XIIe siècle)* (Paris: Les Éditions du Cerf, 1985).

Signori, Gabriela, 'Anchorites in German-Speaking Regions', in *Anchoritic Traditions of Medieval Europe*, ed. Liz Herbert McAvoy (Woodbridge: Boydell Press, 2010), pp. 43-61.

Simons, Walter, *Cities of Ladies: Beguine Communities in the Medieval Low Countries 1200-1565* (Philadelphia: University of Pennsylvania Press, 2001).

Singer, Julie, *Blindness and Therapy in Late Medieval French and Italian Poetry*, Gallica (Woodbridge: Boydell & Brewer, 2011).

Siraisi, Nancy, *Medieval and Early Renaissance Medicine: An Introduction to Knowledge and Practice* (Chicago: Chicago University Press, 2009).

Skinner, Patricia, *Living with Disfigurement in Early Medieval Europe* (New York: Palgrave Macmillan, 2016).

Smith, David M., 'The *Officialis* of the Bishop in Twelfth- and Thirteenth-Century England: Problems of Terminology', in *Medieval Ecclesiastical Studies: In Honour of Dorothy M. Owen*, ed. Dorothy Mary Owen, Michael J. Franklin, and Christopher Harper-Bill (Rochester: Boydell & Brewer, 1995), pp. 201-20.

Smoller, Laura Ackerman, 'Defining the Boundaries of the Natural in Fifteenth-Century Brittany: The Inquest into the Miracles of Saint Vincent Ferrer (d. 1419)', *Viator*, 28 (1997): 333-60.

—, 'Miracle, Memory, and Meaning in the Canonization of Vincent Ferrer, 1453-54', *Speculum*, 73 (1998): 429-54.

—, 'Northern and Southern Sanctity in the Canonization of Vincent Ferrer: The Effects of Procedural Differences on the Image of the Saint', in *Procès de canonisation au Moyen Âge: aspects juridiques et religieux*, ed. Gábor Klaniczay, Collection de l'École française de Rome 340 (Rome: Ecole française de Rome, 2004), pp. 289-309.

—, *The Saint and the Chopped-Up Baby: The Cult of Vincent Ferrer in Medieval and Early Modern Europe* (Ithaca/London: Cornell University Press, 2014).

Sorrell, Roger D., *St. Francis of Assisi and Nature: Tradition and Innovation in Western Christian Attitudes toward the Environment* (Oxford: Oxford University Press, 1988).

Stargardt, Ute, 'Dorothy of Montau', in *Medieval Holy Women in the Christian Tradition c. 1100-c. 1500*, ed. Alastair J. Minnis and Rosalynn Voaden (Turnhout: Brepols, 2010), pp. 475-96.

Suerbaum, Almut, 'An Urban Housewife as a Saint: Dorothea of Montau and Johannes Marienwerder', in *A Companion to Mysticism and Devotion in Northern Germany in the Late Middle Ages*, ed. Elizabeth Andersen, Henrike Lähnemann, and Anne Simon (Leiden: Brill, 2014), pp. 179-204.

Tamminen, Miikka, 'The Crusaders' *Stigmata*: True Crusading and the Wounds of Christ in the Crusade Ideology of the Thirteenth Century', in *Infirmity in Antiquity and the Middle Ages: Social and Cultural Approaches to Health, Weakness and Care*, ed. Christian Krötzl, Katariina Mustakallio, and Jenni Kuuliala (Aldershot: Ashgate, 2015), pp. 103-17.

Taylor, Chloe, *The Culture of Confession from Augustine to Foucault: A Genealogy of the 'Confessing Animal'* (London/New York: Routledge, 2010).

Toivo, Raisa Maria, 'Gender Performance in Early Modern Religious Life', in *Revisiting Gender in European History, 1400-1800*, ed. Elise M. Dermineur, Åsa Karlsson Sjögren, and Virginia Langum (London/New York: Routledge 2018), pp. 169-86.

Touati, François-Olivier, *Maladie et société au Moyen Âge: la lèpre, les lépreux et les léproseries dans la province ecclésiastique de Sens jusqu'au milieu du XIVe siècle* (Paris: De Boeck & Larcier, 1998).

Toynbee, Margaret R., *S. Louis of Toulouse and the Process of Canonisation in the Fourteenth Century* (Manchester: Manchester University Press, 1929).

Trembinski, Donna, *Illness and Authority: Disability in the Life and Lives of St. Francis of Assisi* (Toronto: University of Toronto Press, forthcoming).

—, 'Illness and Authority: The Case of Francis of Assisi', in *Disability and Medieval Law: History, Literature, Society*, ed. Cory James Rushton (Newcastle: Cambridge Scholar's Press, 2013), pp. 112-33.

—, 'An Infirm Man: Reading Francis of Assisi's Retirement in the Context of Canon Law', in *Medicine and the Law*, ed. Wendy Turner and Sara Butler (Leiden: Brill, 2014), pp. 269-87.

Turner, Wendy J., *Care and Custody of the Mentally Ill, Incompetent, and Disabled in Medieval England*, Cursor Mundi 16 (Turnhout: Brepols, 2012).

Van Dam, Raymond, *Saints and their Miracles in Late Antique Gaul* (Princeton: Princeton University Press, 1993).

Van Mulder, Jonas, 'Miracles and the Body Social. *Infirmi* in the Middle Dutch Miracle Collection of Our Lady of Amersfoort', in *Infirmity in Antiquity and the Middle Ages: Social and Cultural Approaches to Health, Weakness and Care*, ed. Christian Krötzl, Katariina Mustakallio, and Jenni Kuuliala (Aldershot: Ashgate, 2015), pp. 241-53.

Vauchez, André, 'Canonisation et politique au XIVe siècle: documents inédits des Archives du Vatican relatifs au procès de canonisation de Charles de Blois, duc de Bretagne (d. 1364)', in *Miscellanea in onore di Monsignor Martino Giusti, Prefetto dell'Archivio Segreto Vaticano II*, Collectanea Archivi Vaticani 6 (Vatican City: Archivio Vaticano, 1978), pp. 381-404.

—, *Francis of Assisi: The Life and Afterlife of a Medieval Saint*, trans. Michael F. Cusato (New Haven/London: Yale University Press, 2012).

—, *The Laity in the Middle Ages: Religious Beliefs and Devotional Practices*, trans. Margery J. Scheider (Notre Dame, IN: University of Notre Dame Press, 1993).

—, 'Lay People's Sanctity in Western Europe: Evolution of a Pattern (Twelfth and Thirteenth Centuries)', in *Images of Sainthood in Medieval Europe*, ed. Renate Blumenfeld-Kosinski and Timea Szell (Ithaca/London: Cornell University Press, 1991), pp. 21-32.

—, *Sainthood in the Later Middle Ages*, trans. Jean Birrell (Cambridge: Cambridge University Press, 2005).

—, *Santi, profeti e visionari: il soprannaturale nel medioevo* (Bologna: Il Mulino, 2000).

Vogüé, Adalbert de, *La règle de Saint Benoît*, VI: *Commentaire historique et critique*, Sources Chrétiennes 186 (Paris: Cerf, 1971).

Vuille, Juliette, '"Maybe I'm Crazy?" Diagnosis and Contextualisation of Female Medieval Mystics', in *Medicine, Religion and Gender in Medieval Culture*, ed. Nao Yoshikawa (Cambridge: D. S. Brewer, 2015), pp. 103-21.

Waugh, Robin, *The Genre of Medieval Patience Literature: Development, Duplication, and Gender* (New York: Palgrave Macmillan, 2012).

Webb, Diana, *Pilgrimage in Medieval England* (London/New York: Continuum, 2000).

—, *Pilgrims and Pilgrimage in the Medieval West* (London: Bloomsbury Academic, 2001).

Weinstein, Donald and Rudolph M. Bell, *Saints and Society: The Two Worlds of Western Christendom, 1000-1700* (Chicago: University of Chicago Press, 1987).

Weissenberg, Marita von, 'Generations of Men and Masculinity in Two Late-Medieval Biographies of Saints', in *Men at Home: Domesticities, Authority, Emotions, Work*, ed. Raffaella Sarti, special issue of *Gender & History*, 27 (2015): 669-83.

—, 'Men, Marriage, and Masculinity in Late Medieval Hagiography, 1100-1500', PhD thesis, Yale University, 2013.

—, '"What man are you?" Piety and Masculinity in the *vitae* of a Sienese Craftsman and a Provençal Nobleman', in *Religious Men and Masculine Identity in the Middle Ages*, ed. P. H. Cullum and Katherine J. Lewis (Woodbridge: Boydell Press, 2013), pp. 112-25.

Wells, Scott, 'The Exemplary Blindness of Francis of Assisi', in *Disability in the Middle Ages: Reconsiderations and Reverberations*, ed. Joshua R. Eyler (Aldershot: Ashgate, 2010), pp. 67-80.

Wetzstein, Thomas, *Heilige vor Gericht: das Kanonisationserfahren im europäischen Spätmittelaltern* (Cologne/Vienna: Böhlau, 2004).

Wheatley, Edward, 'Blindness, Discipline, and Reward: Louis IX and the Foundation of the Hospice des Quinze-Vingts', *Disability Studies Quarterly*, 22 (2002): 194-212.

—, *Stumbling Blocks before the Blind: Medieval Constructions of a Disability, Corporealities; Discourses of Disability* (Ann Arbor: University of Michigan Press, 2010).

Wilson, Louise E., 'Conceptions of the Miraculous: Natural Philosophy and Medical Knowledge in the Thirteenth-Century *Miracula* of St. Edmund of Abingdon', in *Contextualizing Miracles in the Christian West, 1100-1500: New Historical Approaches*, ed. Matthew M. Mesley and Louise E. Wilson, Medium Aevum Monographs 32 (Oxford: Society for the Study of Medieval Languages and Literature, 2014), pp. 99-125.

—, 'Hagiographical Interpretations of Disability in the Twelfth-Century *Miracula* of St. Frideswide of Oxford', in *The Treatment of Disabled Persons in Medieval Europe: Examining Disability in the Historical, Legal, Literary, Medical, and Religious Discourses of the Middle Ages*, ed. Wendy J. Turner and Tory Vandeventer Pearman (Lewiston: Edwin Mellen Press, 2010), pp. 135-65.

Wittmer-Butsch, Maria and Constanze Rendtel, *Miracula: Wunderheilungen im Mittelalter; eine historisch-psychologische Annäherung* (Cologne: Böhlau, 2003).

Wogan-Browne, Jocelyn, 'How to Marry Your Wife with Chastity, Honour, and Fin' Amour', in *Thirteenth Century England IX: Proceedings of the Durham Conference 2001*, ed. Michael Prestwich, R. H. Britnell, and Robin Frame (Rochester/Woodbridge: Boydell Press, 2001), pp. 131-50.

Wolf, Kenneth Baxter, ed. and trans., *The Life and Afterlife of St. Elizabeth of Hungary: Testimony from her Canonization Hearings* (Oxford: Oxford University Press, 2010).

Woolgar, C. F., *The Senses in Late Medieval England* (New Haven/London: Yale University Press, 2006).

Yarrow, Simon, *Saints and their Communities: Miracle Stories in Twelfth-Century England*, Oxford Historical Monographs (Oxford: Oxford University Press, 2006).

Yearl, Mary K. K., 'Medieval Monastic Customaries on *Minuti* and *Infirmi*', in *The Medieval Hospital and Medical Practice*, ed. Barbara S. Bowers (Aldershot: Ashgate, 2007), pp. 175-94.

Ziegler, Joseph, 'Practitioners and Saints: Medical Men in Canonization Processes in the Thirteenth to Fifteenth Centuries', *Social History of Medicine*, 12 (1999): 191-225.

Index

For Product Safety Concerns and Information please contact our EU
representative GPSR@taylorandfrancis.com
Taylor & Francis Verlag GmbH, Kaufingerstraße 24, 80331 München, Germany

www.ingramcontent.com/pod-product-compliance
Ingram Content Group UK Ltd.
Pitfield, Milton Keynes, MK11 3LW, UK
UKHW021721240926
475702UK00029BA/1745
9781041185710